Endorsements

"This book offers the most authoritative, up-to-date and easy-to-understand advice for the treatment of diabetes. Dr. Seymour L. Alterman, a respected endocrinologist for 35 years, provides guidance on every issue of concern for todays d̶...

...kin, Director
...a, California

"If you're ...oved one, the first thing ...s the layman can easily ...s and medical jargon in ...e can imple- ment. In a ...book is your appointme ...in the field."

...land, Oregon

"Dr. Alter ...tes and meta- bolic disc ..., concise and informati ...he significant issues and ...aily basis."

...ng Physician
...each, Florida

"The best ...m the patients themsel... ...g their knowl- edge co ...ormation on all the l ...nat."

...es Educator
...trol Center,
...ach, Florida

"The pa ...e cornerstone of trea... ...rman has of- fered, i ...or blood glu- cose co ...e in reducing the risl ...ecommend it highly. ...M.D., Chief,
...nd Diabetes,
...ach, Florida

"In a practical and easy-to-understand manner, Dr. Alterman addresses every significant issue facing diabetic patients of all ages. He offers information regarding travel, sports activity, and excellent advice to teenagers and young adults in the management of their disease. The importance of life-long glucose monitoring is emphasized along with special precautions regarding "tight control" in the very young. This book should be kept handy by all diabetic patients and those responsible for their care. I highly recommend this book."

—**C. Sanchez, M.D.**
Assistant Professor Pediatric Endocrinology
University of Miami School of Medicine

"Dr. Seymour Alterman, a well known diabetologist, has written a most helpful book for those afflicted with diabetes (Type 1 or Type 2) and their families. Not only is this book informative but it is also a pleasure to read, easy to understand and simple to follow. He covers both the cause and management of the disease and how to deal with the psychological problems that living with diabetes creates. I recommend the book to anyone who has been recently diagnosed as having diabetes as well as those who have been living with it for years. They will find much new information that will make their life pleasanter, healthier and more hopeful."

—**Dr. Alice Ginott, Ph.D. Psychology**
New York, New York

"A valuable contribution to the needs of patients with diabetes and their physicians. *How to Prevent, Control and Cure Diabetes* gives encouraging data that shows when proper relationships with physicians and health providers is maintained, along with reliable sources of information, the diabetic can have a much improved outlook in terms of the quality of life."

—**Yank D. Coble, Jr., M.D. F.A.C.P.**
Past President, Florida Medcal Association

HOW TO PREVENT, CONTROL &
CURE DIABETES

MINIMIZE THE IMPACT DIABETES HAS ON YOUR LIFE

- Straightforward Answers to Everyday Questions
- Eliminate or Lessen the Need for Anti-Diabetic Medication
- Reduce the Risk of Long-Term Complications
- Gain the Many Hidden Benefits of Good Blood Sugar Control

Seymour L. Alterman, M.D., F.A.C.P.
Donald A. Kullman, M.D.

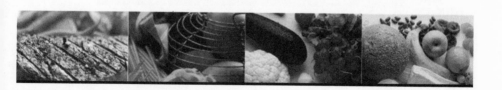

Published by Frederick Fell Publishers, Inc.
www.fellpub.com

CAUTION: Please Read Carefully

Diabetes is a life-threatening disease. It is mandatory that a diabetic be under the care of a physician to whom he/she should look for advice and guidance. This book should be considered only as a general overview of diabetes. It is not intended to replace the services of a trained physician, nor is it intended to encourage self-treatment of illness or other medical condition by the layman. Only one's own personal physician can advise him/her about information described in this book and its application to any individual patient. Everyone's circumstances vary; only your doctor can prescribe treatment appropriate for you.

Library of Congress Cataloging-in-Publication Data

Alterman, Seymour L., 1930-
   How to Prevent, Control & Cure Diabetes / by Seymour Alterman, Donald Kullman.— 2004 ed.
      p. cm.
   ISBN 0-88391-125-6 (Paperback : alk. paper)
   1. Diabetes—Popular works. I. Kullman, Donald A., 1928- II. Title.
RC660.4.A483 2004
616.4'62—dc22
                                        2003025131

Cover/Interior Design by Chris Hetzer
Printed in USA
10 9 8 7 6 5 4 3 2 1

*To Joanne and Janine for their
encouragement and patience, this
book is affectionately dedicated.*

Physicians Statement

The 2004 Update of *How to Prevent, Control and Cure Diabetes* contains the most recent advances and beneficial management of diabetes to minimize the impact this metabolic disorder has on your life and prevent long-term complications. The following are some of the more significant advances that have occurred since the last edition.

* A twenty year search by a leading research group has at last succeeded in regrowing the burned out or destroyed insulin-producing pancreatic tissue. Only a short time ago, this safe non-surgical cure for diabetes would have seemed impossible. However, this experimental cure is now in the final phase of human trials before being awarded FDA approval. This amazing diabetes cure holds the promise of revolutionizing the treatment of diabetes for many Type 1 and Type 2 patients.

* Great strides have been made in preventing Type 2 diabetes in those with a strong family history of the disorder and therefore a high likelihood of developing diabetes as they grow older.

* Newly developed insulins have made it possible to offer patients treatment regimens which can closely simulate the pancreas' normal release of insulin in response to dietary intake thus significantly improving blood sugar control.

* In the past year, medical thinking about hormone replacement therapy (HRT) has made a complete about face. What we thought was cardio-protective turns out to cause an increased risk for coronary artery disease as well as breast cancer. Much confusion remains regarding the safe use of HRT. The current status and safe use is fully explained.

* C-reactive protein (CRP), a substance in the blood which can be measured, is now known to be a better risk indicator for coronary artery disease than cholesterol levels. How to treat elevated CRP levels is explained.

The publisher plans yearly revisions and updates of *How to Prevent, Control and Cure Diabetes* which will make this book the most current and authoritative diabetes guide available.

Seymour L. Alterman, M.D., F.A.C.P.

Donald A. Kullman M.D

Table of Contents

Foreword

DIABETES IN AMERICA TODAY:
THE SILENT EPIDEMIC

Diabetes can now be prevented, controlled and even cured. Nevertheless, despite the progress scientists have made in recent years in our understanding and treatment of diabetes, it remains an increasingly serious health problem in the United States that is rising at an alarming rate.

This complex metabolic disorder affects more than eighteen million Americans, many of whom are unaware of their disease. Like high blood pressure, their diabetes has a gradual, insidious and silent onset and may remain "silent" for many years because in the early stages the elevation of the blood sugar is often not sufficiently elevated to produce the classic symptoms of the disease. However, the long-term complications of diabetes can progress asymptomatically in anyone with even relatively minor degrees of chronic elevation of the blood sugar. During the initial seven to twelve year symptom-free phase, diabetes can be diagnosed only by routine testing of the blood sugar level. For many undiagnosed diabetics, medical care is not sought until one of the long-term complications of diabetes, such as kidney failure, loss of vision or nerve damage, becomes symptomatic and motivates the patient to seek treatment. Furthermore, of those who know they have diabetes, some are not getting adequate, aggressive treatment. The derangement in sugar metabolism that frequently gets all of the attention is but the "tip of the iceberg." The associated dyslipidemia, high blood pressure, and silently progressive kidney and cardiovascular disease are co-morbidities that are often not addressed with the aggressive vigorous treatment necessary to significantly alter the course of these disorders. This is not meant to minimize the importance of strict control of the blood sugar. The landmark Diabetes Control and Complications Trial (DCCT) laid to rest any doubt about the benefits derived from tight blood sugar control.

The purpose of this book is not to encourage self-treatment—that can be hazardous; nor is it intended to replace the clinical judgment and guidance of a trained physician. However, the more knowledge you have about diabetes, the better prepared you will be to play an active role with your physician in selecting treatment alternatives that minimize the impact diabetes has on your life. Many physicians render adequate routine medical care, but all too often Type 2 diabetic patients "out eat" their treatment. Ultimately, only you—the diabetic patient—are responsible for the management of your diabetes. Your health care team can point the way, but only you can take the necessary steps to control or reverse your diabetes.

For over twenty years Drs. Aaron Vinik and Lawrence Rosenberg have collaborated in their search for a safe effective diabetes cure. Their joint effort has at last successfully stimulated the worn out pancreases of diabetic animals to neogenesis —to regrow functioning pancreatic islet tissue. This cure in laboratory animal was accomplished without the use of any toxic drugs. Stage II human trials for safety have already been successfully completed. Currently stage III (the last stage before FDA approval) human trials are underway. Not long ago the idea of regrowing functioning pancreatic tissue would have seemed like a science fiction, hope of the future.....too good to be true, but the future is now here. The outlook for a safe effective cure for diabetes has never been brighter.

WHERE TO FIND HELP

To find a diabetes educator (nurse, registered dietitian, pharmacist, or other professional with experience in diabetes education), call the American Association of Diabetes Educators, toll-free, at 1-800-TEAM-UP-4 (1-800-832-6874). The operator can give you the names of diabetes educators in your zip code.

To find a diabetes education program that has received recognition from the American Diabetes Association, call 1-800-DIABETES (1-800-342-2383). This toll-free call reaches the American Diabetes Association office in your state. Ask for the names and telephone numbers of recognized diabetes education programs near you.

To find a registered dietitian, call toll-free to the Consumer Nutrition Hotline at 1-800-366-1655. This is The National Center for Nutrition and Dietetics of The American Dietetic Association. Ask for the names of registered dietitians in your area that provide diabetes and nutrition counseling. Many insurance companies pay for the services of a registered dietician.

To protect your job, the Disability Rights Education Defense Fund, Inc., 2212 6th Street, Berkeley, CA, 94710, provides technical assistance and information to employers and individuals with disabilities on disability rights legislation and policies, as well as assistance with legal representation. Call (510) 644-2555 or fax (510) 841-8645 for additional information.

The Family and Medical Leave Act allows up to 12 weeks of unpaid leave for illness. The sick leave can be taken for a single 12-week period or at intervals. The law applies only to companies with 50 or more local employees. Eligibility requires that you have worked for the company for more than one year.

Acknowledgments

This book covers many aspects of the complex metabolic disorder called Diabetes Mellitus. It is designed for diabetics to be used under the guidance and approval of their physician. The many clinicians and researchers throughout the world whose published works have contributed to our present understanding of diabetes have made this book possible.

So many direct and indirect sources have been utilized in writing this book, it would be impossible to acknowledge all of them. However, special thanks are in order for the Eli Lilly Company, Indianapolis, Indiana, who have graciously contributed the material on *Insulin* in Chapter 8 as well as *Guidelines to Healthier Eating with Diabetes*, in Chapter 7.

Appreciation is also due the Bayer Company, Diagnostic Division for material utilized in Chapter 13, *Patterns of Control and Sick Day Care* and Chapter 25, *Straight Talk to Teenagers and Young Adults With Diabetes.*

Acknowledgment is also in order for Becton Dickinson and Co., the U.S. Department of Health and Human Services, the National Institute of Health, and the Veterans Administration for their assistance.

—**Seymour Alterman, M.D., FACP**

—**Donald A. Kulman, M.D.**

C H A P T E R
•1•

Diabetes Mellitus: An Overview

What is Diabetes Mellitus?
Type 1 & Type 2 Diabetes
Historical Perspective

Diabetes mellitus, or "diabetes" as it is commonly known, is a disorder of metabolism—the way our bodies use food to obtain energy. The most apparent disturbance in diabetes is with carbohydrate metabolism and is classically characterized by an elevated blood sugar and often the excretion of sugar in the urine. To understand diabetes, it is necessary to know how the body functions normally to convert food substances into energy. The human body may be thought of as a machine that requires "fuel" to function.

As we walk down the street, hit a baseball, or just take a breath, we expend energy. The body's fuel is obtained from the food we eat—carbohydrates (sugars and starches), proteins, and fats. Food must be digested —broken down in the gastrointestinal tract—before it can be absorbed. Complex carbohydrates such as those in vegetables and whole grains are composed of long-chain molecules that are broken down by the digestive enzymes into their simple sugar components. All the simple sugars are eventually converted into glucose, the body's main fuel which is the form of sugar required by the body's cells for energy. Proteins are broken down by the digestive enzymes into their constituent amino acids. Fats are digested to fatty acids.

Your body is composed of billions of cells, the smallest units of living matter. Each cell is surrounded by a cell membrane that protects the inside of the cell from its environment. For glucose to get into the cells, where it can be used, it must cross this protective barrier. The hormone insulin, manufactured by specialized cells in the pancreas,* called *beta* cells, is secreted directly into the bloodstream and transported throughout the body, where it plays a vital role in the conversion of glucose into usable energy by escorting it across cell membranes. It is the key that opens the cell door to allow glucose in.

Once taken up by the tissues, glucose is either metabolized (burned) to supply the energy for all body functions, or is stored away for future use, to be drawn upon later when needed.

The pancreas secretes a steady, constant basal amount of insulin

In a healthy person, rising blood sugar levels after eating serve as a signal for the pancreatic beta cells to secrete insulin. The beta cells act like a tiny thermostat, constantly measuring the blood sugar and releasing precisely the right amount of insulin to ensure the correct balance between the blood glucose level and the quantity of insulin needed to metabolize the glucose and keep the blood sugar within a fairly narrow range. When blood glucose levels are high, insulin helps muscle and liver cells respond to the body's need to lower the blood sugar by removing glucose molecules from the blood and stringing them together to form long, complex molecules, called *glycogen*—an efficient form for glucose storage in the muscles and liver. Glucose that is not used by the body or exceeds its capacity for glycogen storage is converted into triglycerides- a storage form of fat.

The liver may be thought of as a food processing center. Insulin enables the liver to not only convert glucose into glycogen, but also to synthesize, from amino acids, proteins that the body needs for cell growth and repair. Any surplus amino acids are converted by the liver into glucose or glycogen, depending on bodily needs. This process of manufacturing glucose from non-carbohydrate food sources, known as *gluconeogenesis*, helps the body function efficiently as it prevents any excess fuel from being wasted. Any carbohydrate or protein intake that exceeds the body's immediate energy needs and glycogen storage capacity is rapidly converted by

---

The pancreas is a flat abdominal organ situated in the posterior abdomen below and behind the stomach. It functions as though it were two organs. As a digestive organ, it secretes enzymes into the intestinal tract that help to break down food into constituents that the body can use. As an endocrine organ, it secretes insulin and other hormones into the bloodstream that regulate the metabolism of glucose, proteins and fats. Normally, in non-diabetic persons, the pancreas can store approximately 200 units of insulin and it secretes about twenty-five to forty units daily to meet metabolic needs.

the body—with an efficiency greater than any machine—into fat and stored away. Thus, any of the body's three sources of fuel—carbohydrates, protein or fat—can end up as body fat. This explains why one gains weight, regardless of the type of food consumed, when the caloric content of the diet exceeds the caloric expenditure by the body.

After a full meal, the insulin-producing beta cells of the pancreas secrete adequate amounts of insulin to transport the glucose from the bloodstream into the cells, thereby keeping the blood sugar level from rising too high. Between meals—during the fasting state—blood sugar levels gradually decline, as do blood insulin levels. However, should the blood glucose level fall too low, the alpha cells, another group of specialized pancreatic cells, secrete a hormone, *glucagon*, which acts in an opposite or antagonistic manner to insulin. Glucagon raises the blood sugar by signaling the liver to break down its glycogen stores and release glucose into the bloodstream. Glucagon can also mobilize stored fat and muscle protein which are then transformed by the liver into glucose.

The brain, our body's most important organ, relies primarily on glucose for fuel. It has evolved its own glucose regulatory mechanisms to ensure an adequate, continuous fuel supply. A special glucose-monitoring sensor within the brain responds to rapid falls in the blood sugar level by stimulating the adrenal glands to secrete epinephrine, another insulin antagonist hormone. Epinephrine is responsible for causing many of the symptoms associated with mild episodes of hypoglycemia (low blood sugar).

There are two main types of diabetes mellitus. Type 1 diabetes arises from the destruction of the insulin-producing beta cells of the pancreas, which causes an absolute deficiency of insulin. Without daily injections of insulin to replace what their bodies cannot produce, Type 1's are unable to survive. In Type 2 diabetes, the pancreas produces insulin, but the body's cells become resistant to its glucose lowering action—an inability to use it efficiently. Before future Type 2's develop diabetes, their bodies require extra insulin to keep their blood sugar within the normal range. This compensatory mechanism of increased insulin output by the pancreas may suceed in controlling the blood sugar for years. However, over time, as insulin resistance gradually increases and the tired, overworked pancreas' output of insulin decreases, the blood sugar rises—initially to levels beyond normal but below those needed to make a diagnosis of diabetes, the so-called impaired glucose tolerance phase. Eventually the blood sugar rises to diabetic levels and the patient becomes symptomatic.

In Type 2 diabetes, the body manufactures the insulin keys, but many of the cell door locks (insulin receptors) are blocked or defective, which prevents the insulin keys from doing their job.

HISTORICAL PERSPECTIVE

Diabetes is an ancient disorder, recognized by its symptoms as early as 1500 B.C. in an Egyptian medical text called the *Ebers Papyrus*. In the second century A.D., Aretaeus, a Greek physician, gave the disease its present name from a Greek word meaning "to run through a siphon" (originally referring to the large volume of urine excreted in uncontrolled diabetes). The Latin word for honey, "mellitus," appeared much later, and was employed to describe the honey-like odor and sweet taste of the urine. In 1775, Matthew Dobson, an Englishman, proved that the sweet taste of the urine of diabetics was actually due to sugar. In the 1860s, a medical student, Paul Langerhans identified the patches of unique cells, scattered as small islands throughout the pancreas, which now bear his name. In 1889, two German physiologists, Drs. Von Mering and Minkowski, were the first to note that removal of the pancreas caused the syndrome known as diabetes mellitus. It was later demonstrated that the Islets of Langerhans actually manufactured, stored and released the hormone insulin into the bloodstream.

For centuries, the symptoms of diabetes—marked thirst, frequency of urination and weight loss—were well known. As the disease progressed, patients would try the various nostrums of the day: special diets, fasting, opium, barley water and even blood-letting. Of course, these therapeutic efforts were to no avail because the real culprit was an absolute or a relative absence of the hormone insulin. As recently as the first two decades of the 1900s, there was no unanimity of medical opinion about the type of diet and medications that should be prescribed for diabetics. Most physicians speculated that a low carbohydrate diet would be beneficial. However, some believed that the sugar lost in the urine should be replaced, and accordingly recommended a high carbohydrate diet. The guesswork treatment of diabetes came to an abrupt end in 1921 when a young surgeon, Frederick Banting, with the assistance of Charles H. Best, a medical student working in the physiology department at the University of Toronto, made an extract of the tiny pancreatic islet cells. When injected into laboratory animals, the extract caused a dramatic fall in blood sugar levels. Soon, human patients with diabetes were given this "new insulin treatment," and the modern era of what had been a long and dismal history of diabetes treatment was to begin. Dr. Banting received the Nobel Prize for this important discovery.

Purification and standardization of insulin was undertaken, and prolongation of its action was finally achieved by adding proteins and zinc to the insulin extracted from animals, primarily cows and pigs. Today we use "human" insulin made semi-synthetically from pork insulin, or biologically engineered, utilizing complicated recombinant-DNA technology. This has been of great value in reducing the allergic reactions that were sometimes seen with animal insulins.

In later chapters, we shall take an in-depth look at the different types of insulin and their use, as well as oral anti-diabetic medications.

C H A P T E R
• 2 •

Type 1 & Type 2 Diabetes: Two Different Disorders

Type 1 Diabetes
Type 2 Diabetes
Atypical Variations

Type 1 diabetes was formerly known as Insulin-Dependent Diabetes Mellitus (IDDM), Juvenile Diabetes or Ketosis Prone Diabetes. Type 2 diabetes was formerly called Non-Insulin Dependent Diabetes Mellitus (NIDDM), Maturity-Onset Diabetes, or Non-Ketosis Prone Diabetes. The designations Juvenile Diabetes or IDDM for Type 1, and Maturity-Onset or NIDDM for Type 2 diabetes are outmoded, misleading and inaccurate. Age of onset does not necessarily determine the type of diabetes nor does dependence on insulin occur exclusively with Type 1 diabetes.

The underlying causes of Type 1 and Type 2 diabetes differ fundamentally, but both are ultimately caused by a lack of insulin, or its effectiveness. The end results therefore are similar—glucose builds up in the blood and is not available to the body's cells for fuel. The differences are those of degree. Persistent elevated blood sugar is the hallmark feature of both forms of diabetes. This explains why there are many similarities in the symptoms and complications they produce.

Type 1 Diabetes

Type 1 diabetes is a chronic autoimmune disease. An autoimmune disease occurs when the body's immune defense system for fighting infections turns against itself and mistakenly attacks a part of its own body. In Type 1 diabetes, the immune system produces antibodies that attack the

7

insulin producing beta cells of the pancreas and destroy them. The pancreas then produces little or no insulin. To correct the insulin deficit, people with this form of diabetes must take insulin by injection.*

Normally insulin serves to suppress glucose production by the liver and its release from storage depots into the bloodstream. In the absence of insulin, glucose pours out of the liver, and is one of the main factors that contribute to the elevated blood sugar in uncontrolled diabetes.

Without insulin, the glucose in the blood remains virtually useless and body cells are starved for fuel despite an elevated blood sugar level. Fats are mobilized from storage reserves as an alternative fuel and burned for energy. This results in the production of toxic by-products called ketones and fatty acids. This abnormal metabolic state is known as diabetic ketoacidosis (DKA). If untreated, DKA can lead to coma and even death.

Type 1 diabetes is far more common in whites than in non-caucasian ethnic/racial populations such as African Americans, Native Americans and Pacific Islanders. It affects about 5 percent to 10 percent of the diabetic population. In Type 1, the onset of elevated blood sugar levels usually begins abruptly in a fairly dramatic way, before age 30. About half of all cases of Type 1 diabetes appear during childhood, with a peak incidence between 12-14 years of age. Increased thirst, hunger, frequency of urination, fatigue, and apathy associated with unexplained weight loss, in spite of increased appetite, herald the onset of Type 1 diabetes in its classical form.

In the early stage of Type 1 diabetes patients may experience periods of remission for varying lengths of time, the so-called "honeymoon period," that result from a temporary, partial recovery of islet cell function. Eventually, however, the disorder returns and becomes constant. It is clear that although genetic factors—diabetic genes—play an important role in Type 1 diabetes, they are only a predisposing component which must interact with environmental influences such as damage to the beta cells from common viral infections (influenza, mumps, measles, etc.) or other forms of physiologic stress to produce diabetes.

Since Type 1 patients are unable to produce insulin, the foundations of treatment are the administration of two or more divided doses of insulin daily, checking blood sugars, proper diet and exercise, and working with a health team (physician, dietician, diabetic educator, and physical trainer).

---

* Since insulin is a protein, it must be taken by injection because it would be destroyed by the digestive enzymes if taken by mouth. However, bio-engineered forms of human insulin which is stable and capable of intestinal absorption is currently the subject of clinical study. Insulin can be absorbed through the nasal mucosa or the lungs. Delivery systems for these routes have been developed.

With modern knowledge and treatment, there is no longer a need for fear, anger, and confusion to weigh heavily on the young diabetic. Type 1 diabetes can be controlled and the risk of complications markedly reduced.

Experimental cures have already been accomplished in laboratory animals including primates, our closest mamalian relatives with whom we share more than 90 percent of our DNA (genes). See Chapter 27, **Diabetes: The Cure.** *These promising results point to the potential for successful human application. A practical permanent cure for Type 1 diabetes cannot be far behind.*

Type 2 Diabetes

Type 2 diabetes differs sharply from Type 1 in many important respects. The onset is usually gradual rather than sudden. Incidence increases with age, and is far more common after age 40, reaching a peak between 60-65 years of age. Type 2 patients make up about 90 percent of the total diabetic population in the United States. Approximately 85 percent of Type 2 patients are obese. Those who are not obese often have an increased percentage of body fat distributed to the abdominal area—so-called central obesity—which poses a special risk for glucose intolerance. (Obesity is not believed to be a risk factor for Type 1 diabetes.) During the early years of their disease, Type 2 patients often have no noticeable symptoms or only mild ones. They may remain asymptomatic for many years because their blood sugar elevation develops gradually and is often not sufficiently high during the early years of the disease to cause the classic symptoms of diabetes. It is not unusual for Type 2s to go unrecognized for ten to twelve years, during which time damage to body organs may silently progress. Fifteen to twenty percent of those with Type 2 diabetes already have diabetic retinopathy—eye damage—and five to ten percent already have micro-proteinuria, indicative of kidney disease, before the disease is detected during a medical exam that includes laboratory testing of blood and urine.

It is estimated that more than seventeen million people in the United States have Type 2 diabetes, half of whom are unaware of their disorder. Blood glucose levels in Type 2 diabetes do not usually rise or fall rapidly as in Type 1, and ketoacidosis is quite rare. In Type 2 diabetes, the beta cells still manufacture and release insulin in response to dietary needs, but not enough is produced to keep the blood sugar within the normal range. Generally though, there is sufficient insulin to move enough glucose into the cells to prevent the development of ketoacidosis.

The presenting symptoms of Type 2 diabetes may include, in varying degrees, those seen with Type 1 diabetes: blurring of vision, increased thirst,

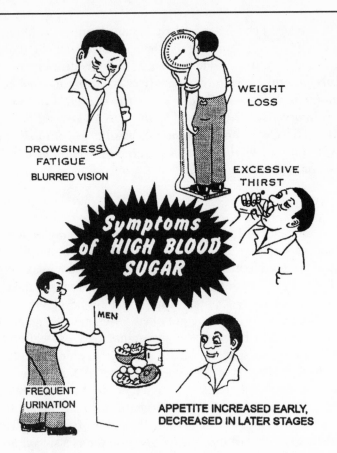

DROWSINESS
FATIGUE
BLURRED VISION

WEIGHT
LOSS

EXCESSIVE
THIRST

Symptoms of HIGH BLOOD SUGAR

MEN

FREQUENT
URINATION

APPETITE INCREASED EARLY,
DECREASED IN LATER STAGES

fatigue, excessive urination and weight loss despite increased appetite. In addition, Type 2's may present with a loss of feeling in the hands or feet as a consequence of nerve damage. A decreased resistance to infections manifested by frequent boils or carbuncles is sometimes seen. Female patients often experience vaginal and urinary tract infections as initial symptoms. Genital itching may be the first symptom noted.

As we have seen, Type 2 diabetes is associated with metabolic defects in both the action of insulin and insulin secretion. The beta cells of the pancreas are able to produce insulin, but for various reasons, the body's cells are resistant to its physiologic action. Although the pancreas manufactures and secretes insulin, it cannot churn it out fast enough and in sufficient quantity to overcome the resistance. In most cases, the amount of insulin produced is even greater than normal, but still inadequate to overcome the body's resistance to insulin's action. This deficiency is therefore a relative deficiency of insulin, unlike the absolute insulin deficiency—the inability to produce insulin—seen with Type 1 diabetes. Ultimately, however, the basis of the abnormalities of the carbohydrate, fat and protein metabolism that characterize both types of diabetes stem from deficient insulin action at the cellular level.

Most Type 2's have inherited a predisposition to develop diabetes. A high percentage have a close relative with Type 2 diabetes. Fortunately, despite an inherited vulnerability for developing this metabolic disorder, it is not necessarily a destiny. Lifestyle patterns—chiefly lack of exercise and obesity—are often prerequisites for the disease to manifest itself. In later chapters, the measures that can prevent or reverse the course of Type 2 diabetes will be explored.

Strong genetic determinants for obesity and insulin resistance are responsible for the definite racial and ethnic differences in the incidence of Type 2 diabetes. There is a very high rate, for example, among Pima American Indians in Arizona, Hispanics, and black Americans. Environmental factors as well as genetic factors undoubtedly contribute to the increased incidence in these ethnic groups. Some studies have indicated that when excessive obesity is factored out, the incidence of diabetes may not be much greater for black Americans than for Caucasians. As people around the world gradually adopt a Western lifestyle and diet, abandoning simple native foods in favor of high fat, low fiber, highly processed foods, the incidence of obesity and diabetes has risen.

People with Type 2 diabetes may be treated with oral medications that stimulate pancreatic insulin production or sensitize the body's cells to insulin's action. Usually, they do not require insulin to control their disease—at least in the early years, and for many not throughout their lifetime. Most will respond to weight loss, exercise, diet, and if necessary oral medications. However, for some, over time, as their insulin resistance increases and the insulin output of their worn-out pancreas declines, injections of insulin are required for glycemic (blood sugar) control.

The chronically elevated blood sugar in Type 2 diabetes impairs insulin production. This adverse effect is called *glucose toxicity*. Paradoxically, glucose toxicity contributes to and perpetuates elevation of the blood sugar. In other words, the elevated blood sugar in Type 2 diabetes is both a cause and the result of impaired insulin secretion by the pancreatic beta cells. However, glucose toxicity is responsive to blood sugar control. *Glycemic control enhances pancreatic insulin production and helps to overcome glucose toxicity.* During periods of poor blood sugar control in Type 2 diabetes, temporary insulin therapy can play an important role in breaking the glucose toxicity cycle and restoring the effectiveness of oral hypoglycemic agents. This temporary need for more aggressive treatment to achieve glycemic control is in accord with the old clinical aphorism, "It is easier to maintain glucose control than to attain glucose control."

NORMAL CARBOHYDRATE METABOLISM

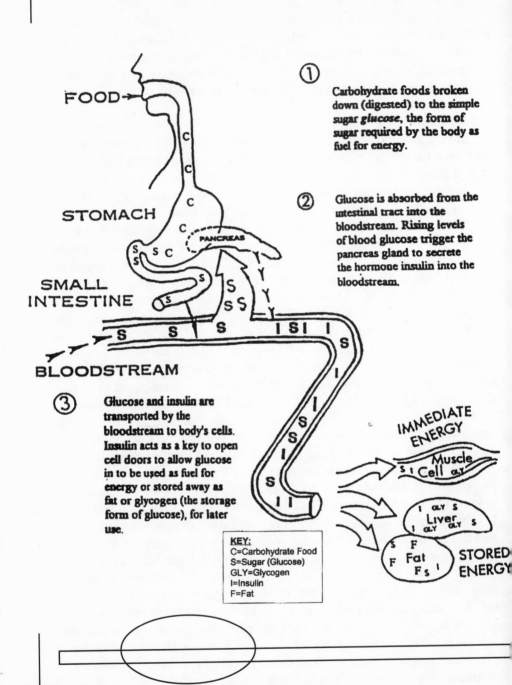

① Carbohydrate foods broken down (digested) to the simple sugar *glucose*, the form of sugar required by the body as fuel for energy.

② Glucose is absorbed from the intestinal tract into the bloodstream. Rising levels of blood glucose trigger the pancreas gland to secrete the hormone insulin into the bloodstream.

③ Glucose and insulin are transported by the bloodstream to body's cells. Insulin acts as a key to open cell doors to allow glucose in to be used as fuel for energy or stored away as fat or glycogen (the storage form of glucose), for later use.

FOOD→

STOMACH

PANCREAS

SMALL INTESTINE

BLOODSTREAM

IMMEDIATE ENERGY

Muscle Cell

Liver

Fat

STORED ENERGY

KEY:
C=Carbohydrate Food
S=Sugar (Glucose)
GLY=Glycogen
I=Insulin
F=Fat

CARBOHYDRATE METABOLISM: DIABETES

①

Type 1 diabetes: Little or no insulin produced.

Type 2 diabetes: Body tissues are resistant to insulin's action. Insulin is unable to work efficiently because cell door locks (insulin receptors) are blocked or defective.

Without (or a deficiency of) insulin, glucose builds up in the bloodstream because it cannot gain entry into the cells.

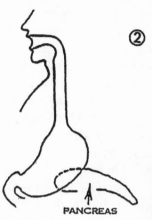

PANCREAS

②

Without available glucose symptoms of diabetes develop: fatigue, weakness, blurring of vision, excessive thirst, frequent urination, weight loss despite increased appetite.

③

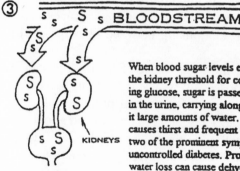

S S S S BLOODSTREAM

S S

KIDNEYS

URINE

When blood sugar levels exceed the kidney threshold for conserving glucose, sugar is passed out in the urine, carrying along with it large amounts of water. This causes thirst and frequent urination, two of the prominent symptoms of uncontrolled diabetes. Progressive water loss can cause dehydration.

④

In untreated Type 1 diabetes fats are burned as an alternative fuel for glucose. This abnormal fat metabolism produces toxic by-products called ketones, which build up in the blood causing a serious metabolic disorder called diabetic keto-acidosis (DKA). DKA rarely occurs in Type 2 diabetes because unlike Type 1 diabetes, where very little or no insulin is produced, Type 2's generally manufacture at least enough insulin to prevent DKA.

⑤

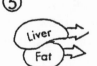

Liver

Fat

$$\frac{SS + SS}{Ketones} + DEHYDRATION = \text{Diabetic Ketoacidosis} \xrightarrow[\text{Untreated}]{\text{If}} \text{Diabetic Coma}$$

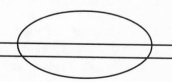

There are multiple factors cited as possible causes of Type 2 diabetes. Although diabetes does not result from an overindulgence in sweets, eating large amounts of sugar and other rich, fatty foods can cause weight gain. Most people who develop Type 2 diabetes are overweight. Even in non-diabetic persons, obesity is associated with insulin resistance. The progressive development of insulin resistance that accompanies weight gain is a key factor contributing to the association of diabetes and obesity. Also, a large body mass requires more insulin for its metabolism.

The more a person eats, the greater the amount of insulin required to process the glucose derived from the ingested food. Caloric intake beyond body needs is stored away as fat. As fat cells enlarge and become engorged they become insulin resistant. This leads to a demand for more insulin to process a given quantity of glucose. The pancreas attempts to compensate for the insulin resistance by increasing insulin output. This compensatory mechanism may succeed in keeping the blood sugar within a normal range. However, for those predisposed to developing diabetes—future Type 2 patients—the pancreas gradually loses its ability to manufacture sufficient quantities of insulin to control the blood sugar. The blood sugar levels rise progressively and eventually diabetes manifests itself. Although this explanation is an over simplification of the many physiologic processes involved, it does help to explain the relationship between obesity, insulin resistance and Type 2 diabetes.

Scientists are still investigating the exact cause of insulin resistance. Current research is focused on two possibilities. The first points to a defect in the insulin cell receptors. The receptors are special protein molecules that are present on the surface of cells. These bind to insulin and allow it to gain entry into the cell. Like an appliance that must be plugged into an electrical outlet, insulin needs to bind to a cell receptor to function. Several things can go wrong with the receptor mechanism. There may be too few receptors for insulin to bind to, or there may be a defect in the receptors that prevents the insulin from binding. Another possible factor may be a defect in the process that occurs after insulin plugs into the receptor. Insulin may successfully bind to the receptors, but the signal to transport glucose across the cell membrane is blocked, thus preventing glucose from gaining entry into the cell where it can be metabolized.

ATYPICAL VARIATIONS OF TYPE 1 AND TYPE 2

The vast majority of diabetic patients can be readily diagnosed and their type of diabetes categorized when they are first seen by a physician. However, although Type 1 and Type 2 diabetes generally represent two distinctly different disease complexes in their classic form, at times the distinction between them may be blurred. Impairment of insulin secretion and defects in insulin's physiologic action—insulin resistance—can be present in the same patient, and the main type of deficiency in an individual case may be unclear before a complete medical evaluation is completed. The predominant features in any one isolated case can cover a wide spectrum, ranging from predominantly insulin resistant, with relative insulin deficiency, to predominantly deficient in insulin secretion accompanied by some insulin resistance.

Type 2 patients, whose disease initially shows primarily insulin resistance, may experience decreased insulin output with age that may require injections of insulin to keep their blood sugar within a satisfactory range. Although they require insulin and may resemble Type 1 patients, they should not be so classified based solely on their insulin regimen. These patients take insulin for blood sugar control rather than as a life-sustaining therapy to prevent fatal ketoacidosis. If they omit their insulin, they usually do not develop DKA. A test of their blood for auto-antibodies would most likely be negative.

Some older patients who develop diabetes have a gradual onset to their disease and may resemble Type 2 diabetics. This sub-group of adult-onset diabetes is associated with slow destruction of the beta cells of the pancreas. Their immune attack is less aggresive and does not wreak as much havoc as is usually seen with Type 1 diabetes. These patients are positive for auto-immune antibodies in their blood. This sub-group, known as Latent Autoimmune Diabetes in Adults (LADA), accounts for approximately 10 percent of the entire diabetic population, thereby making it as common as the usual rapidly progressing typical Type 1 diabetes. They are more sensitive to insulin than their Type 2 counterparts and require smaller amounts of insulin to control their blood sugar.

DO YOU HAVE TYPE 1 OR TYPE 2 DIABETES?

If blood tests reveal that you have diabetes, your doctor will determine whether you have Type 1 or Type 2 diabetes. Although the symptoms and laboratory tests of the two main types of diabetes may resemble each other, the causes and treatment are quite different. A physician can differentiate them by taking a detailed medical history, evaluating the patient's signs and symptoms, and by reviewing the results of laboratory examinations of urine and blood.

TABLE 1
Characteristic Features of the Two Major Types of Primary Diabetes Mellitus

	Type 1 Diabetes Mellitus Formerly called insulin dependent; Juvenile-onset diabetes mellitus; Ketosis-prone diabetes mellitus; Insulin-deficient diabetes mellitus	Type 2 Diabetes Mellitus Formerly called non-insulin dependent; Maturity-onset diabetes mellitus; Ketosis-resistant diabetes mellitus; insulin-resistant diabetes mellitus
CLINICAL FEATURES		
Age of Onset	Usually before age 30; peak incidence at age 12-14	Usually after age 40; peak incidence at age 60-65
Clinical Onset	Usually abrupt, may be gradual	Usually very gradual excessive thirst, urination
Symptoms	Excessive thirst and urination, excessive hunger, weight loss, fatigue	May have symptoms of Type 1, vaginal or urinary tract infections, loss of feeling in an extremity, impotence, blurred vision delayed wound healing
Nutritional Status	Usually normal	Obesity in 80-90%
Underweight When Diagnosed	Sometimes	Not Likely
Overweight When Diagnosed	Not Likely	Probably, obesity in 80-90%
Ketosis-Proneness	Frequent, especially if treatment not sufficient; large amount of ketones in urine when diabetes not controlled	Uncommon, but may occur during infection or unusual stress
Carbohydrate-Intolerance	Marked	Mild, moderate, or marked

	Type 1	Type 2
Remission Phase	Often occurs temporarily in early stage	Following weight reduction and exercise
Stability	Labile—wide fluctuations in blood glucose common	Relatively stable - blood glucose fluctuations less marked
Insulin Responsiveness	Sensitive	Usually resistant
Control of Diabetes	Often difficult	Usually less difficult

EPIDEMIOLOGY

	Type 1	Type 2
Proportion of Total Diabetes Cases	@10%; Common in caucasians, rare in non-caucasian ethnic, racial populations	@90%; Most common in non-caucasian ethnic/racial groups, black Americans, Pacific Islanders, Hispanics, American Indians
Sex Predilection	About equal distribution	Female preponderance
Family History	Maybe	Often
Concordance in Identical Twins	Less than 50%	Greater than 90%

AUTO-(SELF) ANTIBODIES

	Type 1	Type 2
Islet Cell Antibodies	Present in 80-90% at onset	Less than 3%
Insulin Antibodies	30-50%	Less than 1%
GAD Antibodies	80-95%	Less than 3%

ENDOGENOUS INSULIN (Pancreatic Insulin)

	Type 1	Type 2
(Pancreatic Insulin)	"Low-output"	"High-output"
Fasting Plasma Insulin	Absent or very low	Normal or elevated early, late diminished

	Type 1	Type 2
Response to Glucose	None to negligible	(1) Early: adequate but delayed (2) Later Stages: diminished but not absent
C-Peptide Secretion*	Absent or very low	Present

PATHOLOGY

	Type 1	Type 2
Islet Cell Mass	Markedly diminshed	Minimally altered
Beta Cell Mass	Markedly diminished	Variable - may be slightly decreased or hypertropic (enlarged)
Insulitis	Present at onset in 60-90%	Not present

THERAPEUTIC REQUIREMENTS

	Type 1	Type 2
Diet	Mandatory to balance food intake and energy expenditure with insulin dosage	Diet alone may be adequate for therapy; clinical remission may follow weight reduction
Insulin	Necessary for all patients; patients require at least two doses daily	Usually not necessary early; % of patients requiring insulin depends on severity and duration; most eventually require insulin; single, daily dose often adequate
Oral Agents Sulfonylureas, Prandin, Avandia, Metformin, Actos, etc.)	Not efficacious	Usually efficacious
Physical Activity	Must be balanced with food intake and insulin	May improve insulin action, improve glucose control and decrease need for oral antidiabetic medications

*For each insulin molecule released by the pancreas a C-Peptide molecule is also released. C-Peptide levels in the blood can be measured and serve as an indicator of pancreatic insulin production

LONG-TERM COMPLICATIONS OF DIABETES

Many people are under the mistaken impression that Type 2 diabetes is not as serious a disorder as Type 1 diabetes. This is incorrect. If ignored and untreated, Type 2 can be associated with many of the same complications as Type 1.

The long-term complications of diabetes are usually divided into two main categories—those that primarily affect the large blood vessels (macrovascular disease) and those that primarily affect the small blood vessels (microvascular disease). Small vessel disease of the kidneys affects renal function and may lead to progressive kidney failure requiring dialysis. Nervous system damage—neuropathy—may cause loss of feeling and numbness in various parts of the body. Neuropathy of the autonomic nervous system can cause diverse symptoms of the gastro-intestinal tract and genito-urinary abnormalities, including sexual dysfunction. Although large vessel disease may predominate in Type 2 diabetes and small vessel disease may be the dominant feature in Type 1 diabetes, long-term tissue damage attributable to both portions of the vascular system usually co-exist, in varying degrees, in both Type 1 and Type 2 diabetes. Generally, the complications that arise from small vessel disease—retinopathy (eye disease), nephropathy (kidney disease), and neuropathy (nerve disease) appear at an earlier stage of Type 2 diabetes than those caused by large vessel disease. In other words, cardio-vascular disease, the main large vessel abnormality, takes a longer time to develop. Cardiovascular disease includes such varied disorders as heart attacks, strokes, peripheral vascular disease, aneurysms, and impotence—all manifestations of atherosclerosis (hardening of the arteries). The long-term microvascular complications of diabetes are examined in detail in Chapter 19, *Long-term Complications of Diabetes*. Atherosclerosis, its cause, consequences and prevention, is discussed in Chapter 18, *Cardiovascular Disease and Diabetes*.

OTHER SPECIFIC TYPES OF DIABETES

Genetic Defects of the Beta Cells—Several different genes are believed to be responsible for variations of the syndrome known as Maturity Onset Diabetes of the Young (MODY). This form of diabetes is responsible for approximately 1 to 2 percent of the cases of diabetes encountered in young persons. The failure of these patients to exhibit ketosis, even under periods of stress, can serve to differentiate MODY from Type 1 diabetes. Furthermore, the disease usually exhibits a strong family genetic link with cases apparent over several generations. The commonly encountered type of MODY is transmitted as a single dominant chromosomal pattern. The clinical picture is one of mild hyperglycemia (elevated blood sugar) in childhood, which does not progress. Even in old age, this group of MODY patients is usually asymptomatic. It is important to make the diagnosis of MODY because unrecognized elevated blood sugars—even only moderate elevations—over time, can cause organ damage. Another type of MODY is associated with normal glucose metabolism until adolescence or early adulthood, when blood sugars rise. Many in this category can be controlled with diet alone, but about one third require oral agents or insulin.

Idiopathic Diabetes—Some forms of diabetes which would seem to belong in the Type 1 category have no known cause. These patients have low insulin levels, are prone to ketoacidosis, but have no evidence of autoimmune antibodies. Only an extremely small percentage of diabetic patients fall into this category.

Secondary Diabetes—These forms of diabetes occur when there is damage to the pancreas from trauma, tumors, deposits of iron, inflammation of the pancreas (particularly chronic pancreatitis associated with alcoholism), liver disease, medications, certain endocrinopathies and other hormonal abnormalities including those that result from the administration of steroids. These causes of diabetes are relatively rare. Diabetes associated with pregnancy requires special monitoring. Non-diabetics who develop glucose intolerance during pregnancy have what is called gestational diabetes. The relationship between pregnancy and diabetes is dealt with separately in Chapter 6, *Diabetes and Pregnancy.*

Drug or Chemical-Induced Diabetes—Many drugs can impair the production and secretion of insulin and precipitate diabetes, particularly in those with pre-existing insulin resistance. Pentamidine, a medication used to treat pneumonia, and L-Asparaginase, an anti-cancer drug, can cause diabetes. A list of all of your medications should be given to your physician.

CHAPTER
• 3 •

Criteria for Establishing the Diagnosis of Diabetes

New Criteria
Impaired Category
Screening Guidelines
Treatment Goals

I n the nineteenth century, the diagnosis of diabetes was established by some physicians actually tasting and taking note of the sweetness of the urine. Today diabetes is suspected in persons with the classic signs and symptoms of the disorder, as well as those without symptoms, who have abnormally elevated levels of glucose in the blood and urine. In asymptomatic individuals, high blood sugar levels alone are usually sufficient to establish the diagnosis. However, it is possible to have some minor elevation of the blood sugar and sugar in the urine from other, non-diabetic causes.

New evidence that the long-term complications of diabetes begin and progress asymptomatically at blood sugar levels lower than previously thought has recently prompted the American Diabetes Association (ADA) Expert Committee on the Diagnosis and Classification of Diabetes Mellitus, to modify the accepted blood sugar cut-off point for making a diagnosis of diabetes. Blood glucose titers below the previously accepted diabetic levels are now recognized to be sufficient to cause end organ damage to the eyes, kidneys, nerves and the cardiovascular system. During this asymptomatic (symptom-free) period it is possible to predict these changes from measurements of the blood glucose in the fasting state or after an oral glucose load. Screening of high risk populations should be conducted to detect the disorder when it is most amenable to treatment. When detected early, prompt measures can be undertaken to sometimes forestall the development of classical diabetes and/or prevent the long-term complications of the disorder.

BLOOD SUGAR MEASUREMENT

In the United States, the level of glucose in the blood is reported in metric units — milligrams per deciliter (mg/dl) of blood plasma. Plasma is the fluid portion of the blood that remains after the red blood cells have been centrifuged to the bottom of a test tube. The United Kingdom and many other countries employ the Système International D'Unites, which is based on a unit of substance called a mol. The prefix milli means one thousandth. A milli mol (mMol) is 1/1000th of a mol. Those using the Système International report blood glucose levels in milli mols per liter (mMol/L). To convert from one system to the other :

mMol/dl x 18 = mg/dl

$$\frac{mg/dl}{18} = mMol/dl$$

Recommendations for Screening, Diagnosing and Classifying Diabetes Mellitus by the Expert Committee of the American Diabetes Association: The New Criteria for Making a Diagnosis of Diabetes

The committee stated that diabetes can be diagnosed by any one of the following three methods:

1. The presence of classic clinical symptoms of diabetes (excessive thirst, urination, unexplained weight loss, etc.) AND a plasma glucose level in excess of 200mg/dl (11.1mMol/dl) done at any time without regard to meals.

2. Fasting plasma glucose greater than 126mg/dl (7.0mMol/dl) (no food intake for at least eight hours prior to the test).

3. A 2 hour plasma glucose level of 200mg/dl (11.1mMol/dl) or greater during an oral glucose tolerance test with a 75 gram oral glucose load. This test consists of drinking a solution containing 75 grams of glucose (after an overnight fast) and measuring the blood glucose at prescribed intervals (1/2 hour, 1 hour, 2 hour, 3 hour). Normally the blood sugar level rises after drinking the glucose but does not exceed 140mg/dl (7.8 Mmol/dl)and then returns rather quickly to normal.

NOTE: Unless there is a blood sugar elevation in association with metabolic changes characteristic of diabetes, such as ketoacidosis, a positive test should be confirmed by a repeat examination on a subsequent day. The oral glucose tolerance test is no longer routinely recommended. A single sugar examination as outlined is preferred because of patient convenience and cost containment.

Intermediate Group:

The committee recognized an intermediate group whose glucose levels were too low to qualify for a diagnosis of diabetes, but whose levels were too high to be considered altogether normal. Those in this category are believed to be at greater risk for developing diabetes and cardiovascular disease in the future. The intermediate group has two categories:

1. Impaired fasting glucose (IFG). This newly created category includes those with a fasting blood plasma glucose greater than 110mg/dl (6.1mMol/dl), but less than 126mg/dl (7.0mMol/dl).

2. The committee left essentially unchanged the impaired glucose tolerance category (IGT)—plasma glucose levels following an oral glucose tolerance test, greater than 140mg/dl (7.8 Mmol/dl), but less than 200mg/dl (11.1mMol/dl)

Many diabetiologists believe that the intermediate group may represent an early stage in the development of diabetes. This group is associated with a greater risk for developing macrovascular disease (coronary artery, peripheral vascular and cerebrovascular). *Weight reduction, improved diet and increased physical activity may prevent those with IGT from progressing to Type 2 diabetes.*

The term "borderline diabetes" is no longer used to describe those with IGT. The current classification has also eliminated the poorly understood terms "latent diabetes," subclinical and chemical diabetes, and placed them in the IGT category.

Summary of the Currently Accepted Categories For Screening, Diagnosing and Classifying Diabetes

> = Greater than
< = Less than
FPG = Fasting Plasma Glucose
IFT = Impaired Fasting Glucose
FPG <110mg/dl (6.1mMol/dl) = normal fasting plasma glucose
FPG >110mg/dl (6.1mMol/dl) and <126mg/dl (7.0mMol/dl) = IFG
FPG >126mg/dl (7.0mMol/dl) = provisional diagnosis of diabetes (diag-
        nosis must be confirmed with a repeat test on a subsequent day)

Corresponding Categories When the Oral Glucose Tolerance Test (OGTT) is used are:

2 hour post 7dl) = normal glucose tolerance
2hPG >140mg/dl (7.8mMol/dl) and <200mg/dl
        (11.1mMol/dl) = IGT
2hPG >200mg/dl (11.1mMol/dl0 = provisional diagnosis
    of diabetes (the diagnosis must be confirmed)

NOTE: The HbA₁c* level is not currently recommended for diagnosing diabetes. Although the HbA₁c, FPG and OGTT are all reflections of plasma glucose levels—long-term for the former and immediate for the latter—the lack of laboratory standardization nationwide has prevented the HbA₁c test from being utilized for screening purposes. However, the HbA₁c and the FPG are the measurements of choice for monitoring diabetes and making treatment decisions.

* A laboratory blood test that correlates with the average blood sugar level during the two to three month period prior to the test

SCREENING FOR DIABETES

Guidelines for Testing for Diabetes in Undiagnosed Asymptomatic Individuals:

1. Routine test for everyone 45 years of age or older, if normal repeat at three year intervals.

2. Consider testing younger individuals who:
    • are obese
    • have a close relative with diabetes
    • are members of high-risk ethnic population (black American,

Hispanic, Asian or American Indian)
- have had gestational diabetes or delivered a baby weighing more than 9 pounds
- have an HDL-cholesterol level 35mg/dl or less or a triglyceride level greater than 250mg/dl
- have blood pressure 140/90 or greater
- have previously had tests that revealed impaired glucose tolerance or impaired fasting blood sugar

TREATMENT GOALS

Treatment goals were not altered by the committee. The ADA's target goal of a fasting plasma glucose level less than 120mg/dl (6.7mMol/L) and HbA1c less than 7% remain unchanged.

Other Therapeutic Goals in Type 2 Diabetes

- Eliminate symptoms
- Prevent long-term complications
- Control obesity (attain normal body weight)
- Normalize plasma total cholesterol
- Normalize plasma LDL-cholesterol
- Normalize plasma triglycerides
- Normalize blood pressure
- Stop smoking

C H A P T E R
• 4 •

The Genetics of Diabetes

Risk of Inheriting Type 1 Diabetes
Risk of Inheriting Type 2 Diabetes
Gestational Diabetes Risk

W hy does a person get diabetes? The question is simple, but the answers are not. They are part of a very complex genetic puzzle that researchers are trying to decode through genetic research. Diabetes may have multiple etiological factors, including a gene code that causes it to function abnormally under some circumstances. For instance, if a person has a gene that predisposes him or her to become diabetic, eating a high-fat diet over time may cause obesity and increase his or her chance of getting the disease. On the other hand, eating low-fat food and exercising each day may help to prevent the disease from manifesting itself. You can't choose your genes, but you can choose what to eat and whether or not to exercise. Genes undoubtedly influence some people's bodies to burn energy at a slow rate, and/or to want to eat more, making it more likely that they will become overweight, which puts them at a higher risk for Type 2 diabetes.

Scientists have already identified some of the genes that may increase the risk for getting diabetes. This enables them to study how these genes work, and how the changes they cause contribute to the disease. This knowledge provides clues to design new treatments.

Diabetes has long been considered a geneticist's nightmare. Genetic factors are clearly important in both Type 1 and Type 2 diabetes, but the genetic predisposition must interact with environmental factors to produce the disease. Some of the genes involved in making a person susceptible to diabetes have been identified, but the story is far from complete. We do know, for example, that susceptibility to Type 1 diabetes is associated with definite characteristics on chromosome 6, involving a portion known as the Human Leukocyte Antigen (HLA) Complex. The HLA's are coded to assemble antigens (protein substances) that instruct the immune system to recognize "self." The defective HLA's are believed to incorrectly identify one's own beta cells as foreign "non-self" tissue. This genetic defect explains the worldwide differences in prevalence and incidence of diabetes in different ethnic groups.

We can now routinely test for auto-antibodies that serve as markers for beta cell destruction in Type 1 diabetes, which makes it possible to tell if high risk individuals have inherited the relevant genes and to predict their chance of developing diabetes. Auto-antibodies may be present in the blood for 10 to 12 years before the disease becomes symptomatic. Type 2 diabetes has an even stronger genetic predisposition than Type 1 diabetes and also requires interaction with environmental factors.

What are the odds of a child getting diabetes if one or both parents are diabetic? A woman with Type 1 diabetes, who gives birth after the age of twenty-five, has approximately a 1 in 25 chance of having a diabetic child. If the child is born to a mother younger than 25 years, the risk drops to roughly one in a hundred, a risk that is similar to that of a child born to a non-diabetic mother.

A man with Type 1 diabetes has about a 1 in 17 chance of producing a diabetic child. However, if either parent had Type 1 diabetes before age 11, the risk to the child is doubled. If both parents have Type 1 diabetes, the risk for the child ranges from one in four to one in ten.

Approximately 90 percent of Type 2 diabetics have a positive family history of the disorder. As noted, Type 2 diabetes seems to run in families to a greater degree than Type 1. Aside from the genetic predisposition, family lifestyle, eating patterns, obesity and lack of exercise, play a significant role in the development of Type 2 diabetes. A parent with Type 2 diabetes, whose diagnosis was made before age 50, has a 1 in 7 chance of producing a diabetic child. If the diagnosis was made after age 50, the odds increase to 1 in 2 for the child to develop Type 2 diabetes later in life. Some studies suggest that the child's risk is greater if the parent with diabetes is the mother.

If you have an identical twin who develops Type 1 diabetes as a young person, you have only a 30-50 percent chance of developing the disease. If your identical twin develops Type 2 diabetes that does not require insulin, there is a 60-90 percent chance that you, too, will get the disease unless you slim down and adopt a healthy lifestyle with a regular exercise regime and balanced diet.

THE GENETICS OF GESTATIONAL DIABETES

The genetics of gestational diabetes (diabetes which develops during pregnancy) is still not fully understood. We do know, however, that women with a family history of diabetes—especially on the mother's side—are more likely to get gestational diabetes. We also know that older women, minorities and those who are overweight are more prone to gestational diabetes.

C H A P T E R
• 5 •

Diabetic Ketoacidosis (DKA)

Causes
Symptoms
Treatment
Non-Ketotic Syndrome

T he lack of insulin in Type 1 diabetes results in an inability of the body's cells to "take in" glucose and convert it into energy for vital life processes or store it away for future use. Even though the blood sugar is high, the cells are unable to get their fuel. Another important function of insulin is to suppress glucose production and its release into the bloodstream by the liver. Without this inhibiting action, glucose pours out of the liver unchecked and is one of the main factors that contribute to very high blood sugar levels in uncontrolled diabetes. When the concentration of glucose in the blood exceeds the kidney's threshold to conserve this nutrient, glucose begins to "spill over" into the urine. As the glucose is excreted by the kidneys, it exerts an osmotic effect, carrying large amounts of water and electrolytes along with it. The electrolytes are charged minerals that play important roles in physiologic functions. Electrolytes are lost whenever there is excessive fluid loss from the body. This loss of body fluids and electrolytes results in dehydration which causes extreme thirst accompanied by frequent urination—two of the prominent symptoms of uncontrolled diabetes.

Physiologically, the untreated Type 1 patient responds to his disorder as though he were starving—which indeed he is. Despite the high blood sugar level, his body is starved for fuel. To sustain itself the body makes a desperate effort to find an alternative fuel source. Stored fat is metabolized and burned to provide the energy the body needs. This abnormal fat metabolism causes the serious metabolic derangement called Diabetic Ketoacidosis (DKA). As the fats are burned, they produce toxic by-products called ketones and fatty acids. Ketones "spill" into the urine and are easily detected by a simple paper dip-stick home laboratory test.

KETOSTIX®

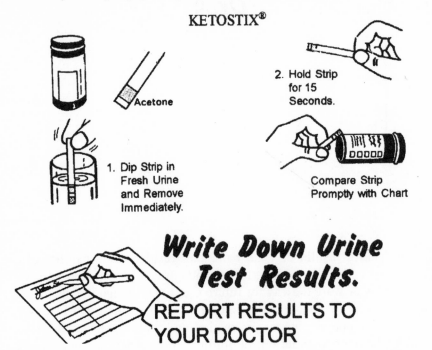

Acetone

2. Hold Strip
for 15
Seconds.

1. Dip Strip in
Fresh Urine
and Remove
Immediately.

Compare Strip
Promptly with Chart

Write Down Urine Test Results.
REPORT RESULTS TO
YOUR DOCTOR

Some ketones are also excreted by the lungs, giving rise to the unique, fruity acetone (nail polish-like) breath associated with this condition. Because ketone acids are formed faster than the body can get rid of them, the blood level of these poisonous substances rises and life-threatening ketoacidosis develops.

The persistent loss of water from DKA dehydrates the brain cells, which can lead to coma. This scenario of diabetic ketoacidosis is seen primarily in untreated Type 1 diabetes, and only rarely is it encountered with Type 2 patients. Although Type 2 diabetics are not ketosis prone, they, too, can develop ketoacidosis when subjected to stress from trauma, infections or other illness, and should check their urine for ketones at such times.

DKA generally gives plenty of warning before it happens. It is the end result of uncontrolled diabetes. DKA is an important, and at times a life threatening, acute complication of diabetes that must be promptly recognized and appropriately treated.

> *Caution: Diabetics who are sick and can't eat may believe they don't need their insulin. However, their body is still synthesizing glucose and insulin is required to prevent DKA. Keep in close contact with your physician during any acute illness.*

Test for Ketones
- When blood sugar levels exceed 250mg/dl.
- During any illness, especially when associated with high fever, nausea, vomiting or diarrhea.
- When you feel chronically fatigued.
- Routinely during pregnancy (daily prior to breakfast).
- When you have difficulty concentrating, disturbances in breathing, or your breath has a fruity "acetone" (nail polish) odor.

It is not necessary to understand the biochemical changes of ketoacidosis in order to recognize the signs and symptoms that will alert you to seek prompt treatment for this condition.

Symptoms of Ketoacidosis
- Increased thirst and urination
- Fatigue
- Lack of appetite
- Nausea, vomiting, abdominal pain
- Shortness of breath
- Headaches, muscle aches

Signs of Ketoacidosis
- Ketones in the urine.
- High blood sugar (most range between 200mg/dl - 800mg/dl).
- Acetone breath (fruity nail-polish odor).
- Abdominal tenderness—muscle tightness over abdomen, decreased bowel sounds.
- Dehydration with poor skin tone.
- Rapid pulse, rapid labored breathing.

- Decreased reflexes.
- Fever with warm, dry or flushed skin.
- Decreased body temperature.
- Uncoordinated eye movements and fixed, dilated pupils.
- Mental confusion which may progress to coma.

TREATMENT OF KETOACIDOSIS

When symptoms suggestive of ketoacidosis appear, it is important to check the blood sugar and urine at frequent intervals. Exercise should be avoided because the lack of insulin causes more fat to be burned. If a high blood sugar level is found and ketones are present in the urine in a significantly dehydrated Type 1 patient, there is no significant first-aid treatment of value. The patient should be transported to the nearest hospital with trained emergency physicians, where life-saving measures can be instituted. Treatment must be vigorous. The basic therapy consists of providing adequate insulin, intravenous fluids and electrolytes to reverse the metabolic changes and correct the deficit of body fluids and electrolytes.

The exact amount of insulin, fluid and electrolytes required to restore physiologic harmony must be carefully monitored by the physician. Fluid loss with ketoacidosis depends on the severity and duration of the condition. Typically, it averages about 10 percent of the body weight. Deaths from DKA have been dramatically reduced by improved therapy for young diabetics, but DKA remains a significant death risk in the elderly and patients who are in deep coma as a result of delayed treatment.

Aggressive treatment and hospitalization are not usually necessary for Type 2 patients with DKA. Often, an extra dose of regular fast-acting insulin and increased fluid intake—drinking plenty of water to correct dehydration—can keep ketoacidosis from progressing to the stage where hospitalization becomes necessary. With careful clinical monitoring and treatment, DKA patients generally respond favorably and return to their pre-acidotic state within a relatively short time, feeling much better.

HYPEROSMOLAR NON-KETOTIC SYNDROME (HNKS)

The Hyperosmolar Non-Ketotic Syndrome (HNKS) is the second most common form of coma associated with extremely high elevations of the blood sugar, dehydration and concentration of the blood elements (hyperosmolality). HNKS is often seen in patients with mild or undiagnosed diabetes. Most patients with HNKS are at least middle age or elderly and many have tolerated excessive thirst and high urine output for a prolonged period and consequently may have very significant fluid loss and electrolyte abnormalities when first seen by the physician. Elderly patients may be unaware of slowly developing dehydration that results from a decreased fluid intake because they lack normal thirst perception.

Underlying congestive heart failure or kidney disease is often present and the presence of these conditions worsen the prognosis. Precipitating factors include heart attacks, strokes, kidney failure, infections or recent surgery. Aside from correcting fluid loss and electrolyte abnormalities, additional treatment should be directed at the precipitating cause of the HNKS.

The clinical picture of HNKS shows mental aberrations ranging from disorientation and confusion to coma, in the absence of ketones in the urine, generally occurring in uncontrolled Type 2 diabetes. If the treating personnel are not aware that the patient is diabetic, these symptoms may appear to be those of a stroke, and valuable time may be lost. This is an important reason for patients to wear or carry on their person diabetes identification. The blood sugar elevation and dehydration are usually more severe than with DKA. HNKS resembles DKA in many ways, but since insulin is available in Type 2 diabetes, the derangement in fat metabolism that causes the incomplete burning of the fats with the formation of ketone bodies and free fatty acids does not occur.

As in DKA, in HNKS there is water loss and dehydration. Although the blood does not become acidotic in HNKS, as in DKA, it does become more concentrated as the blood volume decreases with the dehydration resulting from the loss of body fluids. The term "hyperosmolar" means, literally, "increased concentration" (of the blood).

The symptoms of HNKS are similar to those of diabetic ketoacidosis: thirst, frequent urination, nausea, labored breathing, dry skin, mental confusion, and drowsiness progressing to coma. Once significant dehydration has occurred, hospitalization is mandatory to correct the fluid and electrolyte balance. Fluid replacement is similar to that for ketoacidosis.

Prevention of HNKS is another reason why home monitoring of blood glucose plays such an important role in diabetes management.

C H A P T E R
• 6 •

Diabetes & Pregnancy

Gestational Diabetes
Diagnosis
Management & Prognosis

WARNING: ————————————————————————
Women with gestational diabetes whose disease is not controlled with diet and exercise alone, and women with Type 2 diabetes who become pregnant should be treated with insulin therapy alone because all oral agents are contraindicated during pregnancy.

In the past, pregnancy for women with diabetes posed a major threat to both the mother and the fetus. Today, the prognosis has changed due to more intensive control of diabetes before conception and meticulous management throughout the pregnancy.

Diabetic mothers-to-be should plan their pregnancies. Many studies have shown that achieving excellent control of blood sugar before and during pregnancy reduces maternal complications to about the same rate as the general population. It also substantially reduces infant mortality and complications as well as the risk for birth defects.

Tight control before getting pregnant and during the first three months of pregnancy is especially important because the first trimester is the period of formation of the major fetal organs and, therefore, the time when the developing fetus is most vulnerable to damage from elevated blood sugar levels. Poorly controlled diabetes may lead not only to fetal malformations, but also intrauterine death and a higher rate of miscarriage. Pregnancy has an affect on insulin dosage during the gestational period. Often, less insulin is needed in the first trimester. Insulin requirements then rise until term and delivery.

Women who have had no previous signs of diabetes prior to the pregnancy, but who develop any degree of glucose intolerance during pregnancy, have Gestational Diabetes Mellitus (GDM). In other words, the designation GDM is restricted to those whose glucose intolerance is first recognized during pregnancy, including diabetics whose disease went undiagnosed prior to the pregnancy. Many of these patients, as well as many of those who have mild Type 2 diabetes, probably do not require as "tight" or intensive management as do the pregnant Type 1 diabetics, unless their diabetic status deteriorates during the pregnancy. Frequent monitoring of glucose and evaluation of fructosamine or glycohemoglobin levels (blood tests that serve as barometers of long-term glucose control) is important throughout pregnancy.

The fasting blood glucose level is lower during pregnancy because of the constant transfer of glucose to the fetus as the mother supplies nourishment through the placenta — the organ that nourishes the baby. Additionally, many metabolic and hormonal changes occur in pregnancy that act physiologically to antagonize the action of insulin, creating a form of insulin resistance. This has the effect of raising blood sugar levels and making rigorous control more difficult.

GDM is more like Type 2 diabetes than Type 1 because, like the former, insulin resistance is the major metabolic defect with this form of diabetes.

Risks to the developing fetus are directly related to the mother's blood glucose level. The most desirable way to manage GDM is with diet, physical activity and, when necessary, insulin. Blood sugar control should be tight without being so overly intensive as to increase the risk for hypoglycemia. Goals must be individualized by the physician for each patient.

Typical Target Blood Sugar Schedule for GDM Patients:
Note: Must be individualized for each patient

Before meals 80 to 120mg/dl (4.4 mMol/L - 6.7 mMol/dl)
Before bedtime 100 to 140mg/dl (5.5mMol/L - 778 mMol/dl)

GDM patients taking insulin must monitor their blood glucose levels regularly. Many experience a decreased perception of low blood sugar levels—hypoglycemia unawareness—which makes them more prone to bouts of mild or moderate hypoglycemia. In addition to routine testing, it is especially important for GDM patients to monitor their blood when hypoglycemia is most likely, between meals and in the middle of the night. Any mother-to-be whose blood sugar is 60mg/DL or lower requires treatment.

BASIC MANAGEMENT RULES OF GDM

1. Oral hypoglycemic agents are contraindicated because they may cause fetal abnormalities.
2. Weight reduction is to be avoided because of possible adverse effects on the developing fetus.
3. Intensive insulin therapy when necessary with frequent, self-monitoring of blood glucose.
4. Daily monitoring for ketones.

> *Pregnant diabetic patients with high blood pressure should not take drugs of the class called Angiotensin-Converting Enzymes, better known as ACE inhibitors. These drugs can cause serious fetal abnormalities. They should be stopped PRIOR to getting pregnant.*

GDM occurs in about 3 percent to 5 percent of all pregnancies and is more apt to occur in women who are over thirty, overweight and/or have a family history of diabetes. Previous delivery of a large baby (nine pounds or more), increases the need for close surveillance of the blood sugar level by the obstetrician. GDM is more common in Hispanics, Asians, black Americans, and American Indians. GDM develops most frequently between the 24th and 28th weeks of pregnancy, but usually improves markedly or is undetectable after delivery of the baby.

Women who have elevated blood sugar levels prior to the 24th week of pregnancy probably had diabetes that was unrecognized prior to pregnancy. GDM is more common in obese women, and may be precipitated by obesity.

Because diabetes can have serious consequences for the fetus as well as the mother, it is now routine for obstetricians to test for GDM as soon as the diagnosis of pregnancy is made.

All pregnant women should be screened for GDM because selective screening based on special characteristics or past obstetrical history has been shown to be inadequate. * Mothers-to-be who have not been identified as having glucose intolerance before the 24th week of their pregnancy should have a screening blood sugar done between the 24th and 28th week.

---

* Women under twenty-five years of age who do not belong to a high risk ethnic group, are of normal weight, and have no family history of Type 2 diabetes, have such a low incidence of GDM that some obstetricians believe that routine screening for this group may not be necessary. Admittedly, the incidence in this sub-group is very low, but it is not non-existent.

This test consists of having a blood sugar done one hour after drinking a 50 gram glucose drink (without regard to the time of the last meal or the time of day). A blood sugar of 140mg/dl (7.8mMol/L) or greater is considered the threshold, which indicates the need for a 100 gram oral glucose tolerance test.

A definitive diagnosis of GDM can be made by performing an oral glucose tolerance test. A 100 gram glucose load is administered in the morning following an overnight fast of at least eight hours. The preceding three days should include an unrestricted diet that contains at least 150 grams of carbohydrate per day.

The normal upper limit of fasting plasma glucose in pregnancy is 105mg/dl, although some authorities feel this cutoff level is set too high. To diagnose GDM, two or more of the blood sugar levels after a 100 gram oral glucose load must meet or exceed the following values:

Sample 1 -	Fasting	95mg/dl	(5.3 mMol/dl)
Sample 2 -	1 Hour	180mg/dl	(10.0 mMol/dl)
Sample 3 -	2 Hour	155mg/dl	(8.6 mMol/dl)
Sample 4 -	3 Hour	140mg/dl	(7.8 mMol/dl)

Women who do not meet the criteria for gestational diabetes, but in whom there is increasing glucose intolerance during pregnancy, are at a higher risk for having large babies with jaundice, requiring phototherapy, caesarian section, and prolonged hospital stays.

Risks to the developing fetus are directly related to the mother's blood glucose level. The most desirable way to manage gestational diabetes is with diet, and when necessary, insulin, without an overly intensive intervention.

A serious complication of poorly controlled blood sugars during pregnancy is the possible development of ketoacidosis. Ketones are particularly hazardous to the fetus and ketoacidosis is associated with a marked increase in fetal mortality. Therefore, mothers-to-be must check their urines for ketones throughout pregnancy. It is best to check the urine for ketones in the morning before eating. Ketones in the urine may be due to simply missing a meal or snack and the body relying on the breakdown of stored fat for nutrition, at least on a temporary basis. Increasing the caloric intake of meals or taking more frequent snacks will correct this "ketonuria." Eating a snack before bedtime to protect against ketone formation during the night is recommended by some obstetricians.

When maternal blood glucose rises, it passes through the placenta into the baby's blood stream. Because insulin cannot penetrate the placenta, the fetus' blood sugar levels are abnormally high when the mother's diabetes is out of control. The chronically elevated fetal blood sugar supplies extra calories that cause excessive fetal weight gain in the last half of pregnancy, which can lead to a baby who is too large to be delivered safely by the vaginal route. The large size of the fetus often leads to premature birth, or in some cases, necessitates a caesarian section to facilitate delivery. A premature baby is at high risk for serious respiratory disorders because the lungs mature very late in pregnancy. Additionally, the baby's own pancreas may have become accustomed to making extra insulin to handle the increased sugar load. After birth, the baby's pancreas may continue to manufacture extra insulin when it is no longer needed, causing hypoglycemia. This is most likely to happen when the blood sugars were high during the last few days of pregnancy.

For reasons already noted, if a person has been diagnosed with diabetes before the onset of pregnancy, intensification of diabetic control and careful attention to diet, exercise, and insulin requirements become essential and urgent. Therefore, frequent glucose monitoring with finger-stick blood sugar must be done on a regimen advised by the patient's physician or diabetic educator. This usually requires determination of blood sugars before and sometimes after meals, before and sometimes after exercise, and whenever symptoms of excessive fatigue or illness occur.

Women who strive for tight blood sugar control increase their risk for hypoglycemia—a drop in blood glucose levels, which may cause a loss of consciousness. Obstetrical patients should be trained not to overtreat hypoglycemic reactions, in order to minimize rebound hypoglycemia. Frequent blood sugar testing is the best way to avoid hypoglycemia.

The keystone of tight control of diabetes during pregnancy is diet. Caloric intake must be adjusted to prevent weight loss or excessive weight gain (greater than 4 lbs. during the first trimester and 4 lbs. per month during the remainder of the pregnancy. Total weight gain should not exceed 25 to 35 pounds. Total caloric needs will vary with activity. Typically 13-14 cal/lb of ideal body weight meet daily caloric needs. However, a dietician should customize a meal plan to meet your individual needs. Throughout pregnancy it is particularly important to eat complex carbohydrates that are high in fiber—whole grains, breads, cereals, legumes, fruits and vegetables. Include all of the basic food groups in your meal plan. Caffeine, alcohol, concentrated sweets, and artificial sweeteners are to be avoided. Your doctor will prescribe a schedule for checking your blood sugars to suit your individual needs. A typical plan might require testing before breakfast, one hour after lunch, and one hour after dinner.

Although exercise is one of the mainstays of diabetic control, in the past, fear that it might harm the developing fetus, prompted some obstetricians to limit physical activities during pregnancy. New evidence now supports the belief that in the absence of any obstetrical or medical contraindications, most women can maintain a regular exercise program during pregnancy. However, all exercise regimens should be done under medical supervision.

Physical activity has been shown to reduce or eliminate entirely the need for insulin in many GDM patients. The American College of Obstetricians and Gynecologists now recommends exercise for 15-30 minutes, three or four times per week. Maximum heart rate should not exceed 130-140 beats per minute while exercising. Avoid dehydration by drinking plenty of fluids before, during and after exercising. Avoid strength exercises. Walking, swimming or stationary bike pedaling are excellent forms of exercise for pregnant women. Twenty to thirty minute walks after meals can help utilize excess blood sugar. It is best for you to let your doctor determine the correct amount of exercise for you during your pregnancy.

Always begin any exercise period slowly with a gradual warm up. After exercise cool down by decreasing activity gradually rather than stopping suddenly. During exercise don't let your body temperature go over 100 degrees F.

Have your obstetrician show you how to feel your uterus for contractions when exercising. Uterine contractions can be an indication that you are overdoing it. Should any signs of fetal distress or changes in your pregnancy status, such as uterine contractions or vaginal bleeding occur or if you feel light-headed, weak or short of breath, stop immediately and notify your obstetrician. Guard against over exertion and dehydration. Avoid exercises that involve risk of abdominal trauma or falls, such as contact sports, as well as vigorous racket sports that could cause excessive joint stress. Do not include activities that involve holding your breath, sudden jerky movements or lying on your back, after 3 months of pregnancy.

Some studies have shown that women who are well-conditioned experience fewer complications during delivery.

> *Caution: Only your physician can determine your special exercise needs or restrictions. BEFORE STARTING ANY EXERCISE PROGRAM SEEK MEDICAL ADVICE AND GUIDANCE.*

The complications of diabetes encountered in women who were diabetic prior to pregnancy usually are greater than for those who develop GDM. The former are at higher risk for cardiovascular, kidney, eye and nerve damage. They are also at greater risk for miscarriage, stillbirth, and birth defects, as well as an increased incidence of Type 1 diabetes in childhood for their offspring. However, with careful dietary control, home-glucose monitoring, physician-recommended exercise, and intensive diabetic control, the vast majority of diabetic pregnancies result in normal, healthy new-born babies.

The blood sugar ofthe vast majority of patients with GDM will return to normal after delivery. However, a small percentage have impaired glucose tolerance (IGT), blood sugars that are higher than normal, but not high enough to be called diabetes. All women who have had GDM are at a greater risk of developing Type 2 diabetes later in life. Obese women, particularly those who don't exercise, have the greatest risk of developing lifelong diabetes. Patients who maintain normal weight after pregnancy markedly reduce their chance of eventually developing diabetes.

All patients who have had elevated blood sugars during their pregnancy should have a blood sugar test six weeks after delivery and be re-evaluated. The majority of women return to normal glucose tolerance after delivery.

Jaundice, a slightly yellow skin color, frequently occurs in newborns. It is caused by a pigmented blood breakdown product called bilirubin. Usually, this is transient and resolves spontaneously without treatment. Jaundice is more likely to be severe in babies whose mothers develop gestational diabetes. A simple light treatment is usually all that is required to help absorb the extra build-up of bilirubin that causes the changes in skin color.

The management of the pregnant woman with diabetes before her pregnancy, and the pregnant woman who develops diabetes during pregnancy—GDM—is similar. Adherence to a well balanced meal plan (adjusted for insulin requirements), maintenance of prescribed target blood glucose levels, and regular exercise is essential.

The optimal time for delivery depends on fetal status and maturity. The goal is to allow pregnancy to go at least 35 weeks and then check the patient carefully until the 37th or the 38th week.

With modern management, pregnant women who have had either a previous diagnosis of diabetes or GDM, can now, with appropriate education, proper meal planning, careful control of blood sugar throughout pregnancy, adequate exercise, and proper motivation, look forward to a happy and healthy life for themselves as well as their newborn babies.

Children whose mothers had gestational diabetes require special monitoring because they are at greater risk for obesity and glucose intolerance later in life. Signs of obesity are often apparent as early as six or seven years of age. The child's risk of developing diabetes is reduced when mothers-to-be keep their blood sugars close to normal throughout pregnancy.

CHAPTER
•7•

Guidelines for Healthier Eating with Diabetes

Material in this chapter courtesy Eli Lily and Company, Indianapolis, Indiana.

Importance for Diabetes Control
Exchange Lists
Meal Planning

E ating healthy foods is one of the most basic and important tools of diabetes management. The right foods can help to control blood sugar and protect long-term health. Every person with diabetes should have a personal meal plan developed by a registered dietitian (RD) or other qualified professional. The meal plan must balance the amount of food eaten against the amount of anti-diabetic medication taken, and physical activity. The preplanned menu guide sheets in this section are a good start. Use the one that is closest to your caloric needs to begin to learn about diabetes meal planning and to guide your choices until you can get a personalized plan prepared by a dietician to meet your individual long-term needs.

What you need to do —

- Realize that the best food choices to control diabetes are healthy choices for the whole family.
- Reach and stay at a desirable body weight. Extra body fat makes it harder to control blood sugar.
- Eat a variety of foods—"well-balanced meals"—at regular times each day to balance diabetes medicines and control hunger.

- Be physically active. Do an activity or exercise you enjoy at least three or four times a week and look for ways to put more activity in your daily routine.
- See your health care team regularly to check your diabetes. Your doctor, dietitian, diabetes educator, and pharmacist can make the job of staying healthy much easier.

RECOMMENDED NUTRIENT INTAKE FOR AMERICANS

NUTRIENT	CONTENT
Carbohydrate	40-60% of calories
Protein	10-20% of calories
Fat	≤ 30% of calories
Saturated Fat	≤ 10% of calories <7% with elevated LDL
Cholesterol	< 300 mg/day
Fiber	20-35 g/day
Sodium	<3000 mg/day
Alcohol	<2 alcoholic beverages daily

EASY STEPS TO HEALTHIER EATING

Eat less fat, especially animal fat —
- Eat fewer high-fat foods like cold cuts, sausage, and nuts. Cut down on add-ons such as butter, margarine, lard, oil, shortening, salad dressing, and gravy.
- Eat less fried food. Try baking, broiling, steaming, grilling, and poaching instead.
- Reduce your use of high-fat cuts of red meat. Instead, have chicken and turkey (without skin), fish, lean meats, and vegetarian dishes.
- Choose low-fat and skim dairy products. Avoid whole milk, cream, high-fat cheeses, and eggs.
- Season food with low-fat flavorings. Try lemon or lime juice, flavored vinegars, low-calorie salad dressings, low-fat yogurt, or small amounts of wine instead of butter, margarine, sour cream, and other high-fat choices.

Eat more starches and foods high in fiber —

- Eat starches — like potatoes, pasta, grains, and vegetables — and fresh fruit every day. Choose whole-grain breads, cereals, and crackers.
- Regularly include peas, beans, rice, bran, and oats in your food choices.

Eat more vegetable protein —

- Animal protein may aggravate kidney disease (nephropathy). Many studies suggest that vegetable proteins are much less toxic to the kidneys. There are many palatable soy substitutes for animal products.

Eat less sugar —

- Drink low-calorie, sugar-free soda instead of the regularly sweetened type, (unless you are pregnant).
- Eat less table sugar, honey, jelly, candy, cookies, cake, pie, and other sweets.
- Find a sugar substitute you like and use it instead of table sugar. Look for prepared foods made with sugar substitutes instead of real sugar.
- Current ADA recommendations do not restrict the use of rapidly absorbed sugars, provided they are substituted for other carbohydrates in the meal plan. The fact that the ban on simple sugars has been relaxed by the ADA does not give you a license to eat large amounts of them. Although there certainly are differences and variations in the speed with which different carbohydrates are broken down and enter the bloodstream, it may not be nearly as much as was once believed. Sugars such as sucrose may not be digested significantly faster than starches. Although sucrose may not produce a significantly greater rise in blood sugar, it provides only empty calories, devoid of fiber and vitamins or minerals, which by itself is an adequate reason to limit your intake of simple sugars.

Use less salt —

- Keep the salt shaker off the table. Keep pepper, onion and garlic powders, and other low-salt seasonings handy instead.
- Cook without adding salt. Flavor foods with spices and herbs instead.
- Eat less salty food. Canned soups, pickles, hot dogs, bacon, sausage, snack chips, and convenience and fast foods often contain large amounts of salt and fat.

Space meals at 4-5 hour intervals —

- In Type 2 diabetes, insulin secretion by the pancreas is delayed. This delay in insulin response generally requires four to five hours to restore the elevated blood sugar following a meal to pre-meal levels. Therefore, spacing meals at four to five hour intervals is an important nutritional principle in the management of Type 2 diabetes.

HOW TO PLAN MEALS FOR BETTER DIABETES CONTROL

The 1,200-2,000 calorie charts in the next section show a method of planning meals that work well for people who have diabetes. In it, similar foods are divided into groups called "exchange lists."* For example, when your meal plan calls for 1 starch/bread exchange at a meal, you can select any food from List 1 in the amount shown: 1 slice of bread, half of an English muffin, or 1 corn tortilla, for example. If your plan calls for 2 or more servings from a group at 1 meal, you can either increase the serving size of 1 food (2 slices of bread or a whole English muffin, for example) or choose 2 items from the list (1 dinner roll AND 1/2 cup of mashed potatoes).

The foods in the exchange lists are marked to help you eat more fiber, and less salt and cholesterol, for better health, and to:

- *show the foods that are good sources of fiber.*
- *show foods that are high in salt.*
- *show foods that are high in cholesterol.*

The daily meal plan that follows is an example of how you can plan your meals using the exchange lists. When you plan your own meals, pick foods from the exchange lists that you enjoy and eat regularly. Eating the right number of servings from each exchange list will help you balance the right amounts of the foods you prefer. This is a big step toward good diabetes control.

Measuring foods —

Serving size is important. Notice that the sample menu includes the right serving sizes for the meal plan. To get the serving size right, measure all foods using standard measuring cups and spoons, or a food scale.

---

*These exchange lists are based on a meal planning system designed by a committee of the American Diabetes and the American Dietetic Association. Eli Lilly and Company gratefully acknowledge the assistance of Diabetes Cure and Education, a group of the American Dietetic Association, in developing this revised meal planning tool.

All measures are level (not rounded or heaping). Four ounces of raw meat with bone will shrink to three ounces after cooking. Use this general rule to estimate your serving of meat from its size before cooking. Other cooked foods should be measured after cooking.

Food preparation and selection —

Try preparing old favorites in new ways to meet your healthier eating goals. Stir-frying and steaming are two low-fat cooking methods you can try. Meats can be baked, broiled, roasted, or grilled. Pan broiling is a low-fat method when a nonstick pan or vegetable oil spray is used instead of butter, margarine, or shortening. NOTE: Everyone with diabetes should have his own individually designed meal plan!

FOOD EXCHANGE LISTS
List 1-Starches/Breads

(15 grams carbohydrate, 3 grams protein, a trace of fat, and 80 calories per serving)

Breads, starchy vegetables, and other starchy foods are the cornerstone of every healthy eating plan. Most of their calories come from carbohydrates, which are good sources of energy. Many choices from this group also provide needed fiber, vitamins, and minerals. For better health, prepare and eat these foods with as little added fat as possible, using less butter, margarine, shortening, and oil.

Use the following guide to estimate servings of any plain starch or bread not listed.

- Starchy vegetables, grains, pasta .... 1/2 cup
- Breads and cereals .... 1 oz

Cereals/Grains/Pasta/ Starchy Vegetables   **Serving Size**

Cereal, cooked
    (oatmeal, ☒ oat bran,
    cream of wheat, rice, etc) .... 1/2 cup
Dry cereal,
    any type containing less than
    100 calories per 1-oz serving .... 1 oz
    (Serving sizes may vary; check box.)

Macaroni, noodles, spaghetti,
and other pasta, cooked ....1/2 cup

Rice, brown, white, cooked ....1/3 cup

Bulgur, barley, other grains ....1/2 cup

⬛ Dried beans, peas,
lentils, cooked...1/3 cup

⬛ Lima beans, cooked ....1/2 cup

⬛ Corn..1/2 cup

⬛ Corn on the cob (6" piece) 1

⬛ Peas, green, cooked ....1/2 cup

Potato, baked, boiled, steamed ....1 small (3 oz)

Potato, mashed with
nothing added ....1/2 cup

Squash, winter, acorn, hubbard ....3/4 cup

Yam, sweet potato ....1/3 cup

Breads

Breads, whole wheat, ⬛ rye, white,
pumpernickel, raisin, other...................1 slice (1 oz)

Bagel, plain, small.......................................1/2 (1 oz)

Bun, hamburger, hot dog ....1/2 (1 oz)

Dinner roll ....1 small

Sandwich roll, kaiser ....1/2 small

English muffin..1/2

Pita pocket (6"-8"across)...............................1/2

Pita pocket (4"across) 1

Tortilla, flour, corn...1

Crackers/Snacks

Animal crackers..8

Graham crackers (2 1/2" square) 3

Melba toast, oblongs...5

Melba toast, rounds 7

Whole wheat or rye crackers
(80 calories/serving)................................4-6

Saltines, unsalted tops..6

Pretzels...3/4 oz

Popcorn, plain, popped ....3 cups
Sherbet, any flavor...1/4 cup
Yogurt, frozen, fruit flavor................................1/3 cup

Starches/Breads With Fat

(15 grams carbohydrate, 3 grams protein,
5 or more grams fat, and 125-150 calories per serving)
Count as 1 Starch/Bread serving AND 1 Fat serving.
Biscuit (2 1/2") 1
Cornbread (2" cube) 1
Crackers, butter type..6
French fries (2"- 3 1/2" long)................................10
◩ Potato chips 10
Muffin, small, plain (2"-3")...............................1/2
Taco shell (6")...2

List 2-Meat and Meat Substitutes

Small servings of meat and meat substitutes provide ample protein for daily needs. For better health, choose lean meats, fish, and poultry more often than medium- and high-fat meats and cheeses.

Lean Meats

(7 grams protein, 3 grams fat, and 55 calories per serving)
Serving Size
Chicken or turkey, skin removed ....1 oz
Lean cuts of beef
   (round, extra lean
   ground round, flank steak, etc)..............................1 oz
Lean cuts of pork
   (◩ Canadian bacon, ◩ ham, etc).......................1 oz
Veal (lean chops and roasts) ....1 oz
Fish, fresh or frozen ....1 oz
Shellfish (clams, crab, lobster,
   scallops, ◒ shrimp)...2 oz
◩ Tuna, canned in water ....1/4 cup

Cottage cheese, lowfat .... 1/4 cup
Egg substitute .... 1/4 cup

Medium-fat Meats

(7 grams protein, 5 grams fat, and 75 calories per serving)

Beef, pork, lamb (most cuts) .... 1 oz
Veal cutlet, ground or cubed,
    unbreaded .... 1 oz
⬛ Liver .... 1 oz
⬛ Egg 1
Cheese, low-fat, part skim .... 1 oz

High-fat Meats

(7 grams protein, 8 grams fat, and 100 calories per serving)

⬛ Prime beef, ⬛ corned beef .... 1 oz
⬛ Spareribs .... 1 oz
⬛ ⬛ Sausage, ⬛ ⬛ luncheon meat .... 1 oz
⬛ ⬛ Hot dog .... 1 oz
⬛ ⬛ Regular cheese .... 1 oz
Peanut butter .... 1 Tbsp

List 3-Vegetables

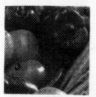

(5 grams carbohydrate, 2 grams protein, and 25 calories per serving)

Vegetables are a very good source of vitamins and minerals. Many choices from this group also provide some fiber.

A serving is 1/2 cup of cooked vegetables, 1/2 cup of vegetable juice, or 1 cup of raw vegetables. (Starchy vegetables like potatoes, corn, and peas appear on List 1-Starches/Breads. Vegetables that have fewer than 20 calories per serving appear on List 7-Free Foods.)

Asparagus
Beans, green, wax,
    Italian
Bean sprouts

Mushrooms
Okra
Onion
Pea pods (snow peas)

Beets
Broccoli
Brussels sprouts
Cabbage
Carrots
Cauliflower
Eggplant
Green onion
Greens, collard,
   mustard, etc

Peppers, red, green,
   yellow
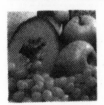Sauerkraut
Spinach
Squash, summer,
   crookneck, zucchini
Tomato
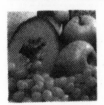Tomato or vegetable
   juice
Turnip
Water chestnuts

List 4-Fruits

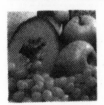

(15 grams carbohydrate and 60 calories per serving)

Fruits provide important vitamins and minerals and are a good source of fiber.

To obtain the most fiber from fruits, eat the edible peelings too, such as those of apples, apricots, and pears.

Use the following guide to estimate servings of any fruit not listed.

■ Fresh, canned, or frozen
   fruit, no sugar added ....1/2 cup
■ Dried fruit..1/4 cup

Serving Size

Apple, raw (2") 1
Applesauce, no sugar added...................................1/2 cup
Apricot, raw (medium) 4
Banana (9" long)...1/2
Blackberries or blueberries, raw ....3/4 cup
Cantaloupe or honeydew melon ....1 cup
Cherries, raw (large)...12

Fig, raw (2" across)..2
Grapefruit (medium)..1/2
Grapes (small)..15
Kiwi (large)...1
Mandarin oranges...3/4 cup
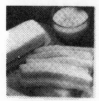 Nectarine (2 1/2" across)..................................1
Orange (2 1/2" across) 1
Papaya...1 cup
Peach (2 3/4" across)..........................1 whole or 3/4 cup
Pear...1/2 large or 1 small
Pineapple, fresh...3/4 cup
Plum, raw (2" across) 2
Strawberries, raw (whole).............................1 1/4 cup
Tangerine (2 1/2" across) 2
Watermelon...1 1/4 cup

Dried Fruit
Apricots ....7 halves
Prunes (medium)...3
Raisins...2 Tbsp

Fruit Juices
Apple, orange, grapefruit......................................1/2 cup
Cranberry, grape, prune..1/3 cup

List 5-Milk and Milk Products

Milk and milk products are needed throughout life. Choose 2 or more servings a day. Milk products supply calcium and other minerals, vitamins, protein, and carbohydrate. Choose low-fat and skim varieties for better health since these choices have less fat, calories, and cholesterol than whole milk products.

Skim Milk and Skim Milk Products

(12 grams carbohydrate, 8 grams protein, 1 gram fat, and 90-110 calories per serving)

Serving Size

Skim, 1/2%, 1% milk...8 oz
Buttermilk, low-fat ....8 oz
Evaporated skim milk..4 oz
Nonfat dry milk powder ....2 2/3 oz (1/3 cup)
Yogurt, nonfat, plain..8 oz
Yogurt, nonfat, fruited,
    artificially sweetened ....8 oz
Hot cocoa, artificially sweetened.....................1 envelope

Low-fat Milk and Low-fat Milk Products

(12 grams carbohydrate, 8 grams protein, 3 or more grams fat, and 120-150 calories per serving)
2% milk..8 oz
Yogurt, low-fat, plain ....8 oz

Whole Milk and Whole Milk Products

(12 grams carbohydrate, 8 grams protein, 5 or more grams fat, and 150-170 calories per serving)
To reduce your intake of cholesterol and saturated fat, limit or avoid foods in this group.
Whole milk...8 oz
Evaporated whole milk...4 oz
Yogurt, regular, plain...8 oz

List 6-Fats

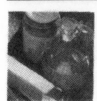

(5 grams fat and 45 calories per serving) Fats add flavor and moisture to foods but provide few additional nutrients, such as vitamins and minerals. Note that serving sizes of fats are small. Choose unsaturated fats instead of saturated fats to help lower blood cholesterol levels.

Unsaturated Fats   Serving Size

Margarine, stick ....1 tsp
Margarine, tub ....1 tsp
Margarine, diet..1 Tbsp
Mayonnaise, regular ....1 tsp
Mayonnaise, reduced-calorie ....1 Tbsp
Salad dressing, regular ....1 Tbsp
▚ Salad dressing, reduced-calorie....................2 Tbsp
Oil, corn, cottonseed, soybean,
    olive, sunflower, safflower, peanut..................1 tsp
Nuts and seeds...1 Tbsp

Saturated Fats

Bacon ....1 slice
Butter ....1 tsp
Nondairy creamer, liquid....................................2 Tbsp
Nondairy creamer, powdered.................................4 tsp
Cream, light, table, coffee, sour........................2 Tbsp
Cream, heavy, whipping ....1 Tbsp
Cream cheese ....1 Tbsp

List 7-Free Foods

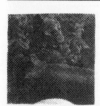

Each free food or drink contains fewer than 20 calories per serving. You may eat as much as you want of free foods that have no serving size listed; you may eat 2 or 3 servings per day of free foods that have serving sizes listed. For better blood sugar control, spread your servings of these extra foods throughout the day.

Drinks

🔖 Bouillon or broth, no fat

Cocoa powder, unsweetened baking type (1 Tbsp)

Coffee or tea

Soft drinks, calorie-free, including carbonated drinks

Fruits

Cranberries or rhubarb, no sugar added (1/2 cup)

Vegetables

Celery
Cucumber
Peppers, hot
Radishes
Salad greens, all types

Sweet Substitutes

Gelatin, sugar-free

Jam or jelly, sugar-free (2 tsp)

Whipped topping (2 Tbsp)

Spreadable fruit, no sugar added (1 tsp)

Condiments

Catsup (l Tbsp)

🔖 Dill pickles, unsweetened

Horseradish

Hot sauce

Mustard

Salad dressing, nonfat, low-calorie, including mayonnaise-type (2 Tbsp)

Taco sauce (2 Tbsp)

Vinegar

Seasonings can be used as desired. If you are following a low-sodium diet, be sure to read the labels and choose seasonings that do not contain sodium or salt.

Flavoring extracts (vanilla, almond, butter, etc)
Garlic or garlic powder
Herbs, fresh or dried
Lemon or lemon juice
Lime or lime juice

Onion powder
Paprika
Pepper
Pimento
Spices
🔖 Soy sauce
Worcestershire sauce

🔖 High in fiber.
🔖 High in sodium.
🔖 High in cholesterol.

	Sample Menu 1	Sample Menu 2
Breakfast		
1 Starch/Bread (List 1)	1/2 cup bran flakes cereal	1/2 bagel (whole wheat or pumpernickel)
1 Fruit (List 4)	1/2 banana	3/4 cup mandarin oranges, drained and mixed with
1 Milk (List 5)	8 oz skim or 1% milk	1 cup lemon nonfat yogurt
Lunch		
1 Starch/Bread (List 1)	1 slice whole wheat bread	1 slice rye bread
2 Meat (List 2)	2 oz sliced lean ham	2 oz sliced turkey
0-1 Vegetable (List 3)	Carrot sticks, radishes*	Sliced tomato, lettuce on sandwich*
1 Fruit (List 4)	1 apple	1 1/4 cups watermelon
1 Fat (List 6)	1 Tbsp reduced-calorie mayonnaise OR 1 tsp margarine	1 Tbsp reduced-calorie mayonnaise
Dinner		
2 Starch/Bread (List 1)	1 small dinner roll 1/3 cup brown rice	1 small dinner roll or tortilla 1/2 cup corn or malanga
2 Meat (List 2)	2 oz baked chicken	2 oz flank steak, broiled or grilled
1 Vegetable (List 3)	1/2 cup cooked broccoli	1/2 cup green beans
1 Fruit (List 4)	1 1/4 cup strawberries	1 cup cantaloupe/honeydew melon salad
2 Fat (List 6)	1 tsp margarine 1 Tbsp regular salad dressing Green salad*	1 tsp margarine for corn 1 Tbsp slivered almonds for green beans
Evening Snack		
1 Starch/Bread (List 1)	3 cups hot air popcorn	1 oz (1 1/2 cups) puffed wheat or rice cereal
1 Milk (List 5)	8 oz sugar-free hot cocoa	8 oz skim or 1% milk

*From List 7 - Free Foods

Key: oz = ounce
Tbsp = tablespoon
tsp = teaspoon

Carbohydrate: 149 g. 49% of total calories
Protein: 61 g. 20% of total calories
Fat: 42 g. 31% of total calories

These two menus show some of the ways the exchange lists can be used to add variety to your meals. Use the exchange lists to plan your own menus.

1200 Calories

Sample Menu 1

Breakfast

Starch/Bread (List 1) — 2
- 1/2 cup bran flakes cereal
- 1 slice whole wheat toast

Fruit (List 4) — 1
- 1/2 banana

Milk (List 5) — 1
- 8 oz skim or 1% milk

Fat (List 6) — 1
- 1 tsp margarine

Lunch

Starch/Bread (List 1) — 2
- 2 slices whole wheat bread

Meat (List 2) — 2
- 2 oz sliced lean ham

Vegetable (List 3) — 0-1
- Carrot sticks, radishes*

Fruit (List 4) — 1
- 1 apple

Fat (List 6) — 1
- 1 Tbsp reduced-calorie mayonnaise
  OR 1 tsp margarine

Dinner

Starch/Bread (List 1) — 2
- 1 small dinner roll
- 1/3 cup brown rice

Meat (List 2) — 3
- 3 oz baked chicken

Vegetable (List 3) — 1
- 1/2 cup cooked broccoli

Fruit (List 4) — 1
- 1 cup raspberries

Fat (List 6) — 2
- 1 tsp margarine
- 1 Tbsp regular salad dressing
- Green salad*

Evening Snack

Starch/Bread (List 1) — 1
- 3 cups hot air popcorn

Milk (List 5) — 1
- 8 oz sugar-free hot cocoa

From List 7 - Free Foods

Sample Menu 2

Breakfast
- 1 bagel (whole wheat or pumpernickel)
- 3/4 cup mandarin oranges, drained and mixed with
- 1 cup lemon nonfat yogurt
- 1 Tbsp cream cheese

Lunch
- 2 slices rye bread
- 2 oz sliced turkey
- Sliced tomato, lettuce on sandwich*
- 1 1/4 cups watermelon
- 1 Tbsp reduced-calorie mayonnaise

Dinner
- 1 small dinner roll or tortilla
- 1/2 cup corn or malanga
- 3 oz flank steak, broiled or grilled
- 1/2 cup green beans
- 1 cup cantaloupe/honeydew melon salad
- 1 tsp margarine for corn
- 1 Tbsp slivered almonds for green beans

Evening Snack
- 1 oz (1 1/2 cups) puffed wheat or rice cereal
- 8 oz skim or 1% milk

Key: *oz = ounce*
Tbsp = tablespoon
tsp = teaspoon

Carbohydrate:	179 g.	48% of total calories
Protein:	74 g.	20% of total calories
Fat:	54 g.	32% of total calories

These two menus show some of the ways the exchange lists can be used to add variety to your meals. Use the exchange lists to plan your own menus.

1500 Calories

	Sample Menu 1	Sample Menu 2
Breakfast		
2 Starch/Bread (List 1)	1/2 cup bran flakes cereal 1 slice whole wheat toast	1 bagel (whole wheat or pumpernickel)
1 Fruit (List 4)	1/2 banana	3/4 cup mandarin oranges, drained and mixed with
1 Milk (List 5)	8 oz skim or 1% milk	1 cup lemon nonfat yogurt
1 Fat (List 6)	1 tsp margarine	1 Tbsp cream cheese
Lunch		
2 Starch/Bread (List 1)	2 slices whole wheat bread	2 slices rye bread
3 Meat (List 2)	3 oz sliced lean ham	3 oz sliced turkey
0-2 Vegetable (List 3)	Carrot sticks, radishes*	Sliced tomato, lettuce on sandwich*
1 Fruit (List 4)	1 apple	1 1/4 cups watermelon
1 Fat (List 6)	1 Tbsp reduced-calorie mayonnaise OR 1 tsp margarine	1 Tbsp reduced-calorie mayonnaise
Dinner		
3 Starch/Bread (List 1)	1 small dinner roll 2/3 cup brown rice	1 small dinner roll or tortilla 1 cup corn or malanga
3 Meat (List 2)	3 oz baked chicken	3 oz flank steak, broiled or grilled
2 Vegetable (List 3)	1 cup cooked broccoli	1 cup green beans
1 Fruit (List 4)	1 cup raspberries	1 cup cantaloupe/honeydew melon salad
2 Fat (List 6)	1 tsp margarine 1 Tbsp regular salad dressing Green salad*	2 tsp margarine for corn
Evening Snack		
1 Starch/Bread (List 1)	3 graham cracker squares	1 oz (1 1/2 cups) puffed wheat or rice cereal
1 Fruit (List 4)	1 small peach or pear	1/2 banana
1 Milk (List 5)	8 oz sugar-free hot cocoa	8 oz skim or 1% milk

*From List 7 - Free Foods

Key: *oz = ounce*
Tbsp = tablespoon
tsp = teaspoon

Carbohydrate:	224 g.	50% of total calories
Protein:	90 g.	20% of total calories
Fat:	60 g.	30% of total calories

These two menus show some of the ways the exchange lists can be used to add variety to your meals. Use the exchange lists to plan your own menus.

1800 Calories

	Sample Menu 1	Sample Menu 2
Breakfast		
2 Starch/Bread (List 1)	1/2 cup bran flakes cereal 1 slice whole wheat toast	1 bagel (whole wheat or pumpernickel)
1 Fruit (List 4)	1/2 banana	3/4 cup mandarin oranges, drained and mixed with
1 Milk (List 5)	8 oz skim or 1% milk	1 cup lemon nonfat yogurt
1 Fat (List 6)	1 tsp margarine	1 Tbsp cream cheese
Lunch		
3 Starch/Bread (List 1)	2 slices whole wheat bread 1/2 cup noodles in broth*	2 slices rye bread 1 oz pack tortilla or potato chips
2 Meat (List 2)	2 oz sliced lean ham	2 oz sliced turkey
0-1 Vegetable (List 3)	Carrot sticks, radishes*	Sliced tomato, lettuce on sandwich*
1 Fruit (List 4)	1 apple	1 1/4 cups watermelon
1 Milk (List 5)	8 oz skim or 1% milk	8 oz skim or 1% milk
2 Fat (List 6)	2 Tbsp reduced-calorie mayonnaise OR 2 tsp margarine	Mustard on sandwich (Fats in chips — see above)
Afternoon Snack		
1 Starch/Bread (List 1)	3/4 oz pretzels	8 animal crackers
Dinner		
2 Starch/Bread (List 1)	1 small dinner roll 1/3 cup brown rice	1 small dinner roll or tortilla 1/2 cup corn or malanga
4 Meat (List 2)	4 oz baked chicken	4 oz flank steak, broiled or grilled
2 Vegetable (List 3)	1 cup cooked carrots	1/2 cup green beans 1/2 cup mushrooms, sauteed in 1 tsp margarine
1 Fruit (List 4)	1 cup raspberries	1 cup cantaloupe/honeydew melon salad
2 Fat (List 6)	1 tsp margarine 1 Tbsp regular salad dressing Green salad*	1 tsp margarine for corn (1 tsp margarine for mushrooms — see above)
Evening Snack		
1 Starch/Bread (List 1)	3 cups hot air popcorn	1 oz (1 1/2 cups) puffed wheat or rice cereal
1 Fruit (List 4)	1 small peach or pear	1/2 banana
1 Milk (List 5)	8 oz sugar-free hot cocoa	8 oz skim or 1% milk

*From List 7 - Free Foods

Key: oz = ounce Tbsp = tablespoon tsp = teaspoon

Carbohydrate:	246 g.	48% of total calories
Protein:	99 g.	20% of total calories
Fat:	72 g.	32% of total calories

These two menus show some of the ways the exchange lists can be used to add variety to your meals. Use the exchange lists to plan your own menus.

2000 Calories

	Sample Menu 1	Sample Menu 2
Breakfast		
3 Starch/Bread (List 1)	1/2 cup bran flakes cereal 2 slices whole wheat toast	1 1/2 bagel (whole wheat or pumpernickel)
1 Fruit (List 4)	1/2 banana	3/4 cup mandarin oranges, drained and mixed with
1 Milk (List 5)	8 oz skim or 1% milk	1 cup lemon nonfat yogurt
2 Fat (List 6)	2 tsp margarine	2 Tbsp cream cheese
Lunch		
4 Starch/Bread (List 1)	2 slices whole wheat bread 1/2 cup noodles in broth* 6 saltine crackers	4 slices rye bread (for 2 sandwiches)
3 Meat (List 2)	3 oz sliced lean ham	3 oz sliced turkey
0-1 Vegetable (List 3)	Carrot sticks, radishes*	Sliced tomato, lettuce on sandwich*
2 Fruit (List 4)	1 apple 2 Tbsp raisins	2 1/2 cups watermelon
1 Milk (List 5)	8 oz skim or 1% milk	8 oz skim or 1% milk
2 Fat (List 6)	2 Tbsp reduced-calorie mayonnaise OR 2 tsp margarine	2 Tbsp reduced-calorie mayonnaise
Afternoon Snack		
1 Starch/Bread (List 1)	1 pita pocket (4")	8 Melba toast rounds
1 Meat (List 2)	1/4 cup tuna	1 oz mozzarella string cheese
Dinner		
3 Starch/Bread (List 1)	1 small dinner roll 2/3 cup brown rice	1 small dinner roll or tortilla 1 cup corn or malanga
4 Meat (List 2)	4 oz baked chicken	4 oz flank steak, broiled or grilled
2 Vegetable (List 3)	1 cup cooked broccoli	1/2 cup green beans 1/2 cup mushrooms, sauteed in 1 tsp margarine
1 Fruit (List 4)	1 cup raspberries	1 cup cantaloupe/honeydew melon salad
3 Fat (List 6)	2 tsp margarine 1 Tbsp regular salad dressing Green salad*	1 tsp margarine for corn 1 Tbsp slivered almonds for green beans (1 tsp margarine for mushrooms — see above)
Evening Snack		
1 Starch/Bread (List 1)	3 cups hot air popcorn	1 oz (1 1/2 cups) puffed wheat or rice cereal
1 Fruit (List 4)	1 small peach or pear	1/2 banana
1 Milk (List 5)	8 oz sugar-free hot cocoa	8 oz skim or 1% milk

*From List 7 - Free Foods

Key: oz = ounce   Tbsp = tablespoon   tsp = teaspoon

Carbohydrate:	306 g.	49% of total calories
Protein:	122 g.	19% of total calories
Fat:	90 g.	32% of total calories

These two menus show some of the ways the exchange lists can be used to add variety to your meals. Use the exchange lists to plan your own menus.

2500 Calories

CHAPTER
• 8 •

Insulin

Insulin Needs
Sources of Insulin
Different Types and Mode of Action
Cautions Regarding Use

P eople with Type 1 diabetes can't make their own insulin. They must take insulin injections every day to live. People with Type 2 diabetes may make insulin but can't use it efficiently. They can survive without insulin injections, but taking insulin often helps them keep their blood sugar closer to normal. About 40 percent of people with Type 2 diabetes eventually require insulin injections to achieve satisfactory blood sugar control.

Insulin cannot be taken in a pill or tablet form. It must be injected under the skin, using a syringe.

HOW MUCH INSULIN DO YOU NEED?

Each person is different. The amount of insulin you need depends on your:
- body weight
- body build (how much fat and muscle you have)
- level of physical activity
- daily food intake

- other medicines
- emotions
- general health
- amount of stress

HOW MANY TIMES EACH DAY?

Because people can be different in all of the ways listed above, their needs for insulin will also be different. People also differ in when they need to take insulin.
- Some people can control their diabetes with only one shot of insulin a day.
- Most people need two or more shots every day to keep their blood sugar in control.
- Some people need more than one TYPE of insulin.

THE GOAL IS CONTROL

Taking more shots does not mean your diabetes is worse. Control, not treatment, is the best way to judge how much of a problem your diabetes is. A person with Type 2 diabetes who takes three shots a day and has near-normal blood sugar is much better off than someone who takes diabetes pills or one shot a day and has high blood sugar.

CHANGING YOUR DOSE(S) AND SCHEDULE

When you first start taking insulin, your doctor will probably change the dose or schedule several times. These changes will be made when your blood sugar tests show that a change is needed. Ask questions. It's important that you understand when and how your particular schedule of insulin works. Follow the doctor's instructions carefully. Together, you and your doctor can find the insulin routine that is best for your needs and lifestyle.

WHERE DOES BOTTLED INSULIN COME FROM?

"Human insulin" does not come from human beings, but is made to be the same as the insulin made by the human body. Human insulin is made in one of two ways:

1. Recombinant DNA technology—a chemical process that makes it possible to make unlimited amounts of human insulin from cultures of rapidly multiplying bacteria that have had the human gene, which

directs the cell to sequence amino acids to form insulin, incorporated into their chromosomal chain.

2. Through a process that chemically changes pork insulin to make human insulin.

Note: Beef insulin from cows and pork insulin from pigs is no longer manufactured in the United States.

RECENT ADVANCES IN INSULIN THERAPY

Tight blood sugar control has clearly been shown to be the key to preventing the dreaded long-term complications of diabetes. Accomplishing strict blood sugar control without causing significant hypoglycemia (precipitous drop in the blood sugar) is the main goal of insulin therapy. Regular insulin, the short-acting insulin commonly employed in the past, has a slow rate of absorption which coincided poorly with meals. Background basal insulin was supplied with long-acting Lente or Ultralente insulin. The traditional regimens employed multiple injections of intermediate-acting insulin such as NPH and mixed-regular insulin. This therapeutic approach, the best available for many years, fell short of controlling the blood sugar in a manner that simulates the pancreas' normal beta cells physiologic activity. A major challenge with the older insulins was a day-to-day variation, which at times could be as high as 30% in the absorption of the insulin as well as a variation between individual patients that could reach 50%. Another disadvantage of the older traditional insulins was their peaking at unwanted and unpredictable times of the day or night, causing hypoglycemia. In recent years novel forms of insulin analogs have been developed which offer advantages over the traditional insulins. These new fast-acting insulin analogs are rapidly absorbed and show less variation in absorption time thus closely mimicking the body's normal insulin secretion as required to keep the blood sugar within a narrow safe range. The fast-acting insulin analogs are given within fifteen minutes of ingesting a meal. Their rapid action coincides with dietary intake and prevents post-prandial blood sugar elevations closely imitating the body's natural insulin response to food. Background basal insulin is supplied by Glargine, a new long-acting insulin analog that is peakless with a 24 hour duration of action similar to the body's normal basal insulin release. Regimens utilizing the new insulin analogs are not only more physiological but offer the patient greater flexibility in his daily life enabling meals to be skipped without serious consequences and fast-acting insulin to be taken only at actual mealtimes. The new insulin analogs also avoid the disadvantage of the traditional insulins which sometimes peak at unpredictable times of the day or night causing hypoglycemia. In short, regiments that combine basal bolus insulin with Glargine, mealtime bolus insulin as needed with fast-acting insulin Lispro or Aspart can physiologically maintain satisfactory blood sugar control. The insulin analogs are also available in premixed combination for patient convenience and accuracy, and better post-prandial sugar control. For example, 75NPL/25 Lispro is a premixed combination of insulin Lispro Protamine suspension (similar to NPH) and insulin Lispro. This fixed combination offers the benefit of the separate response of each component which is preserved with a single injection.

CHARACTERISTICS OF HUMAN INSULIN PREPARATION

Category	Proprietary or Other Name	Onset Hours	Peak Concentration	Duration of Action (h) Effective	Maximum	Description
Rapid acting	Lispro® (Humalog)	<0.25	0.5 - 1.5	3 - 4	4 - 6	Insulin analog
Rapid acting	Aspart ® (Novolog)	0.17 - 0.33	0.67 - 0.83	1 - 3	3 - 5	Insulinanalog
Long acting	Glargine® (Lantus®)	2	none	24	24	Insulin analog
Short acting	Regular	0.5 - 1.0	2 - 3	3 - 6	6 - 8	Insulin
Intermediate acting	NPH	2 - 4	6 - 10	10 - 16	14 - 18	Insulin
Intermediate acting	Lente	3 - 4	6 - 12	12 - 18	16 - 20	Insulin zinc (suspension)
Long acting	Ultralente	6 - 10	10 - 16	18 - 20	20 - 24	Insulin zinc (suspension) extended

Characteristics of Human Insulin Preparations

* Lispro (Humalog®) and Aspart (Novolog ®) have a very rapid onset of action and short duration.

* Glargine (Lantus ®) is long-acting insulin that is peakless and thus able to simulate the body's normal release of basal insulin.

* NPH and Lente are intermediate-acting insulins.

* 70/30 insulin combines the action of regular insulin and NPH. The 30 percent Regular in the premixed insulin begins to work quickly. The 70 percent NPH begins to work as the Regular is finishing.

* 75NPL/25 Lispro combines insulin Lispro protamine suspensions (similar to NPH) with insulin Lispro. As with 70/30 insulin, each component preserves its individual action in a single injection.

* Ultralente insulin is a long-acting insulin with a minimal peak.

INSULIN IN TYPE 2 DIABETES

The basic defect of Type 2 diabetes, insulin resistance, requires the pancreas to secrete ever increasing amounts of insulin to maintain the blood sugar. Over time, the tired over-worked pancreas can no longer keep up its compensatory activity and symptoms of diabetes develop as the blood sugar rises and diabetes becomes symptomatic. Oral agents are capable of maintaining blood sugar control initially, and sometimes for many years. However, for the majority of Type 2 patients the progressive decline in beta cell function through the years makes the addition of insulin necessary in order to achieve satisfactory control. **Type 2 patients must realize the progressive nature of their disease and the frequent need of insulin to delay or prevent long-term complications.** In the light of the recent development of the more physiological insulin analogs, many Type 2 diabetes patients are being introduced to insulin early in their treatment rather than waiting for its use as a last resort when the disease is advanced. In fact, rapid acting insulin is often now used preferentially by patients because of its use to coincide with meals. Combination therapy reduces the number of injections. For convenience, pump therapy has also gained popularity in recent years (see Chapter 15, *The Insulin Pump*). As more new insulins and therapeutic treatments become available, patients are able to gain the ability to control their Type 2 diabetes more effectively. Many patients have an unreasonable fear of "the needle". Newer methods of insulin delivery and smaller needles make any pain involved minimal.

The false belief that insulin is the "end of the road" is frequently encountered, particularly in certain minority groups. In brief, patients must be made to understand that diabetes is a progressive disease with gradual failure of the insulin producing beta cells of the pancreas.Tight controls are the therapuetic goal to be accomplished by whatever combination of oral agents and/or insulin required to achieve satisfactory control

INSULIN STORAGE AND DISPOSAL

Insulin is quite stable and may be kept at room temperature, above 36 degrees and below 86 F° if it is to be utilized within one month and not exposed to sunlight. If it will not be used within thirty days, it should be kept in the refrigerator, but not allowed to freeze.*

Always allow the insulin filled syringe to reach room temperature prior to use, to avoid discomfort. Storage at high temperatures (such as inside a locked car during the summer) can damage insulin. Discard any unused insulin after the expiration date printed on the bottle. Opened bottles of insulin should be discarded after three months of storage in the refrigerator. As noted, opened bottles of insulin that have been kept at room temperature should be discarded after one month.

HOW MUCH INSULIN IS IN THE BOTTLE

Just as height is measured in inches, insulin is measured in "units." A unit is a small amount of pure insulin. All bottles of insulin sold in the U.S. have 100 units of insulin in each milliliter of fluid. Such bottles have "U-100" on the label. The amount of insulin in a milliliter (U100), is called the insulin's concentration.

Since each insulin bottle holds 10 milliliters of fluid, a bottle of U-100 insulin contains 1,000 units. Bottles of U-100 insulin have orange caps. (Bottles of U-40 insulin are available in some countries outside the U.S. These bottles have red caps.)

Check the expiration date printed on the insulin box before you buy it. The date must allow enough time for you to use the whole bottle. To find out how long the bottle will need to last, divide the number of units in the bottle by the number of units you take each day.

---

*Certain insulins, such as Novo Nordisk's 70/30 prefilled, should not be kept at room temperature for more than seven days. Follow the manufacturer's directions for insulin storage as described in the package insert with each new vial of insulin.

CHAPTER
• 9 •

Preparing and Injecting Insulin

Preparing & Injecting a Single Dose of Insulin
Selection of Injection Sites
How to Use an Insulin Pen Injector
How to Dispose of Syringes & Needles

These instructions explain how to draw insulin into a syringe and give yourself an injection. The pictures will help remind you of the steps to follow.

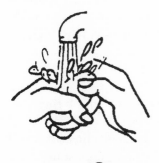

1. Wash your hands.

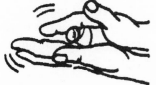

2. Gently mix the insulin. You can mix it by rolling the bottle between the palms of your hands, turning the bottle over from end to end a few times, or by shaking the bottle gently.

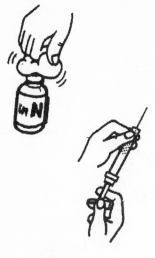

3. If this is a new bottle of insulin, remove the flat, colored cap. Do not remove the rubber stopper or the metal band under the cap. Clean the rubber stopper with an alcohol swab.

4. Remove the cover from the needle. Pull the plunger back until the tip of the plunger is at the line for _____ (X) units. This will pull air into the syringe.

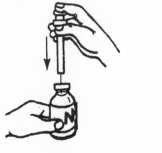

5. Push the needle through the rubber stopper. Press in the plunger to push the air into the bottle of insulin.

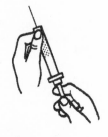

6. Turn the bottle and syringe upside down. Hold the bottle with one hand. The tip of the needle should be in the insulin. Use the other hand to pull back on the plunger until its tip is at the line for _____(X) units. This will pull insulin in to the syringe.

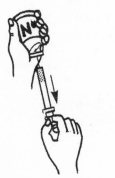

7. Look at the insulin in the syringe. Are there any air bubbles? If so, use the plunger to push the insulin back into the bottle. Then slowly pull insulin into the syringe again. Pull the plunger back to the line for your dose of insulin. Repeat this until there are no large air bubbles in the syringe.

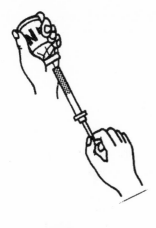

8. Make *sure* the tip of the plunger is at the line for the number of units to be injected. Double-check your dose. Magnifiers that connect to your syringe are available if needed. They can help you see the lines on the syringe more clearly.

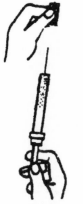

9. Pull the needle out of the rubber stopper. (If you need to lay the syringe down before taking the injection, put the cover back on the needle to protect it.)

10. Now you are ready to give yourself an injection. (See the *Injecting Your Insulin* section that follows.)

INJECTING YOUR INSULIN

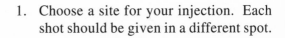

These instructions explain how to inject your insulin dose (single or mixed dose).

1. Choose a site for your injection. Each shot should be given in a different spot.

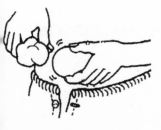

2. Clean the skin at the place for injection with an alcohol swab.

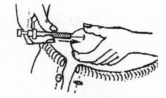

3. Pinch up a large area of skin. Push the needle into the skin, going straight in at a 90 degree angle. Be sure the needle is "way in."

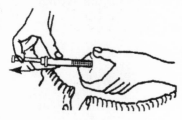

4. Pull back slightly on the syringe. If blood comes into the syringe, the needle has entered a blood vessel. Remove the needle and put it in another location.

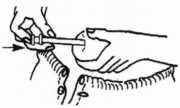

5. Push the plunger all the way down. This will push the insulin into your body. Release pinched skin.

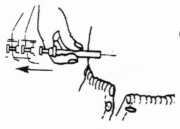

6. Pull the needle straight out. Don't rub the place where you gave the injection.

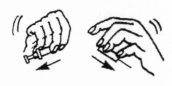

7. Safely dispose of used needles and syringes. Your doctor, pharmacist, or diabetes educator can show you how.

CHOOSING THE SITE FOR AN INSULIN INJECTION

Choosing exactly where on your body you will give the injection each day is very important.

Front

Back

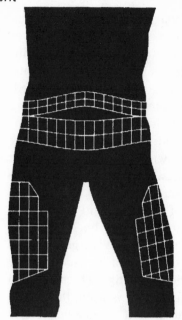

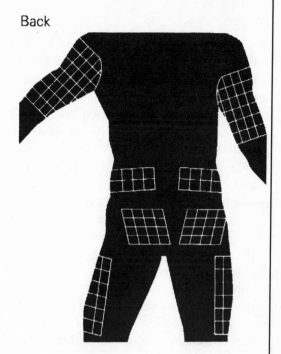

The boxed areas or drawings show suitable sites for your insulin shots. You may need a family member to give you the injection in some of the areas. Each square is an injection site, an exact place to give the shot. To keep skin, fat and muscle healthy, use a different site for each injection.

Note: Do not inject insulin into an area where the muscles will be exercised vigorously shortly thereafter. For example, avoid the legs prior to jogging.

INSERTION AIDS

Automatic injectors are an excellent aid for patients who are afraid of needles or who have difficulty reaching some injection sites. Automatic injectors hold an insulin filled syringe and insert the needle into the skin at the touch of a button. The B-D automatic injector, called the inject-ease, is a popular model that fits all single use insulin syringes.

Insulin Pen Injectors

The case for tight blood glucose control has never been stronger. As more people with diabetes have begun to use multiple daily injections of insulin, pen use has grown in popularity. The insulin pen injector looks like a fountain pen case. Instead of an ink cartridge and writing tip, the pen holds an insulin containing cartridge with a disposable needle and a dial that permits the user to preset the desired insulin dose. Some pens deliver insulin in half-unit increments, some in one-unit and some in two-unit increments. A disposable needle quickly penetrates the skin and automatically injects the pre-selected insulin dose when a release clip is pressed. The injections are virtually painless and eliminate the need for carrying bottles of insulin and syringes wherever you go. Insulin pen injectors provide an insulin delivery system that makes insulin therapy discreet, easy and convenient. Some units come pre-loaded with 150 units of insulin; others employ replaceable disposable cartridges. Each pen holds a single cartridge of insulin that has a pen needle attached to it.

Before dialing the dose, one or two units of insulin should be shot into the air to ensure that the mechanism is functioning properly. The disposable needle should be kept covered prior to use, to prevent germs from contaminating the insulin reservoir. Alcohol should not be used to wipe the needle because this could dissolve the silicone coating which helps to make the injection painless. Each time a pen injector is used, the needle must be changed to avoid problems that could arise if the needle were to become clogged.

Cartridges are available for the commonly employed insulins including Eli Lilly's NPH, regular 70/30 and Humulog, as well as, Novolin and Penfil insulins.

The convenience of having insulin, needle and syringe in one device, and the simplicity of the dial-in method for drawing up the dose, leaves less room for error, making them a good choice for children and adolescents.

The main drawback of insulin pens is that you cannot give combinations of insulin, making them unsuitable for those who require mixed dose therapy.

The same general precautions apply to the insulin pens as bottled insulin: avoid freezing or exposure to high temperatures. When used to administer regular insulin they may be kept unrefrigerated for up to one month; the longer-acting insulins should not remain unrefrigerated for more than one week.

How to Use an Insulin Pen Injector

An insulin pen and pen needle can be used instead of a syringe to inject insulin, but they are not suitable for everyone. Check with your doctor first, and be sure to read the directions that come with your pen. If it is OK for you to use an insulin pen, there are three important things you should know: Always prime your insulin pen before injecting. Always attach a new pen needle right before each injections. Never leave the pen needle attached between injections. When you inject, keep the needle in your skin at least until you count to five.

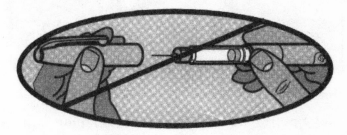

1. Always prime your insulin pen before injecting.

Shoot some insulin into the air—2 drops or more—to make sure it is working. (This is called an "air shot" or "priming" the pen.) The directions that come with your pen will tell you how to do this. If you do not see at least 2 drops of insulin after repeated priming, do not use the pen. The cartridge could be empty or the pen may not be set up right. You might not get the insulin you need.

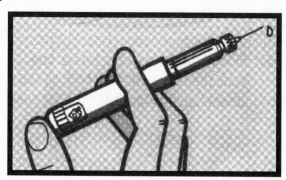

Sometimes, when you put a needle on a pen, one drop of insulin will come out. This does not mean the pen has been primed. You still need to do an "air shot" before you use the pen.

2. Always attach a new pen needled before each injection. Never leave the pen needle attached between injections. If you leave a needle on the insulin pen:

- you may get air in the insulin cartridge

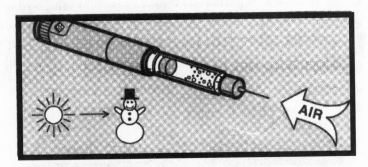

- or the fluid may run out and the insulin strength will change

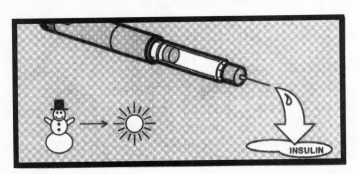

Either way, you will not get the correct dose of insulin with your next injection. Put the needle on the pen just before you use it. Take the needle off right after you use it.

3. When you inject, keep the needle in your skin at least until you count to five.

Don't take the needle out of your skin too fast. The insulin pen is not like a syringe. It takes longer for the insulin to come out. If there is insulin dripping from the needle after you take it out of your skin, you did not hold it in long enough. Next time, leave the needle in your skin longer.

If you take larger (25+ units) doses, you may have to hold the needle until you count to 10.

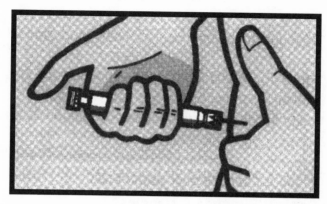

Learn how to use a syringe, too, in case you lose your pen. Most pharmacies have syringes if you need them. Not all pharmacies have insulin pens and pen needles.

Note : Becton-Dickinson and Company manufactures insulin pens and pen needles that are suitable for use with cartridges of the Eli Lilly Company insulins, NPH, regular, 70/30 and Humalog. Additional information about B-D insulin pens, syringes and other products can be obtained by calling B-D consumer services at 1-800-237-4554. They maintain a web site at www.BD.com/diabetes.

Insulin Jet Injectors

Jet injectors are needleless, high pressure injectors that can deliver insulin through the skin so fast that the insulin acts like a liquid needle. Insulin dose adjustments can be made in half-unit increments, from one-half unit to fifty units. The pressure under which the insulin penetrates the skin can be adjusted to accommodate variations in individual discomfort. A single type of insulin can be given or the insulin can be mixed.

When transferring from standard injections to a jet injector, special monitoring is required during the transition period because it can take time to ascertain the correct depth of injection.

Jet injectors are more accurate than any other delivery system when dealing with small amounts of insulin, but they are heavy, expensive and not as portable as insulin pens. Jet injectors must be taken apart and sterilized every two weeks.

To help patients decide if a jet injector would be suitable for them, most manufacturers permit those who are contemplating the purchase of a jet injector device a ten day trial period before deciding if it meets their needs.

HOW TO DISPOSE OF YOUR USED
SYRINGES AND NEEDLES PROPERLY

Check with your town for local rules for disposing of used syringes and lancets. If there are no rules, the following guidelines may be helpful:

How to Destroy Your Own Syringes—Preferred Method
- Never throw loose syringes or lancets into the trash.
- Clip the syringe needle with a clipping device such as the B-D safe-clip, which stores a years supply.
- Never use scissors to cut off a syringe needle. This could cause the needle to become a dangerous projectile.

How to Contain Syringes & Needles
- Put your syringe and used lancet into a sharps collector or hard plastic or metal container with a screw-on or tightly secured lid.
- Keep this container away from children.
- Seal the container when it is full.
- Mark the container "Used Syringes and Lancets."
- Place the container into the trash or other appropriate disposal receptacle. Do not put the filled container into the recycling bin.

Alternative Method for Disposing of
Your Own Syringes & Needles
Using a device such as the B-D safe-clip is the preferable method of destroying syringes and needles. When necessary, you may also remove the syringe plunger and push the needle into the rubber end — taking special care not to stick yourself while performing this procedure. The plunger with the embedded needle can then safely be bent back and forth until the needled breaks off. The syringe and needle can then be placed in an empty hard plastic (bleach or similar) bottle with a re-sealable cap. Do not use a breakable container, or one that could allow the needles to puncture its walls.

How to Dispose of Someone Else's Syringes & Needles
- Don't try to recap or clip a needle that has been used by or on another person. This can lead to accidental needlesticks which may cause serious infections. Follow the "contain" guidelines above.

Remember, syringes are not recyclable.

C H A P T E R
• 10 •

Hypoglycemia (Low Blood Sugar)

Causes of Low Blood Sugar Reactions
How To Recognize Hypoglycemia
Importance of Early Treatment
Comparison of Diabetic Coma & Insulin Reactions

Review of Diabetes Physiology: To understand the dynamics of hypoglycemia and its prevention or correction, it is necessary to understand the body's normal physiologic mechanisms for avoiding wide swings of the blood sugar level. Mother Nature designed a finely tuned regulatory and counter-regulatory system to keep the blood sugar within a relatively narrow safe range. The brain, our body's most important organ, relies primarily on glucose for fuel. It has evolved its own glucose regulatory mechanisms to ensure an adequate, continuous blood supply. A special glucose-monitoring sensor within the brain responds to rapid falls in the blood sugar level by stimulating the autonomic nervous system to activate the adrenal glands to secrete epinephrine, an insulin antagonist. Epinephrine is responsible for causing many of the symptoms associated with mild episodes of hypoglycemia. Another important counter-regulatory mechanism to raise the blood sugar when it falls too low is the secretion of the hormone glucagon by specialized cells within the pancreas. Glucagon exerts a strong anti-insulin effect and raises the blood sugar by mobilizing—breaking down and releasing—glucose stored as glycogen in the liver and muscles. Glucagon also plays a key role in gluconeogenesis—the process of converting non-carbohydrate food substances into glucose when needed.

The multi-syllable word *hypoglycemia* is derived from the Greek "hypo," meaning "too little," "gly," meaning "sugar" and the suffix "emia," meaning "in the blood." The word hypoglycemia, therefore, means "low blood sugar"—too little sugar in the blood to meet the body's needs. When the blood sugar falls, the cells cannot get their glucose, the body's equivalent of an automobile's fuel. Like a car running out of gas, hypoglycemia—low body fuel—gives rise to multiple symptoms (to be described later), as disrupted physiologic functions sputter and fail.

As we will see in Chapter 14, *Intensive Management of Diabetes*, the Diabetes Control and Complications Trial (DCCT) study clearly demonstrated that the long-term complications of diabetes are related to the level of blood sugar elevation. In this study, meticulous control of the blood sugar decreased the frequency and the severity of damage to the kidneys (nephropathy), to the nervous system (neuropathy) and to the eyes (retinopathy) by 50-70%. The study showed a continuous linear relationship between the blood sugar level and the risk of long-term diabetic complications, including heart disease.

The DCCT put to rest any doubt about the benefits that could be derived from tight blood sugar control. *Accordingly, the main goal of diabetes therapy today, is to keep the blood sugar within a satisfactory range—as close to normal as possible—without causing hypoglycemia.* Unfortunately, the tighter the blood sugar control regimen, the greater the risk of hypoglycemia. The most common causes of hypoglycemia are an overdose of insulin and/or oral agents, too little food or too much physical activity.

The backbone of drug therapy for Type 1 diabetics is the administration of insulin to replace the insulin their body can no longer produce. Type 2's generally retain the ability to produce insulin, but their output is insufficient to meet physiologic needs. The pancreatic insulin output of Type 2's can be increased by drugs called insulin secretogogues, such as the sulfonylureas, which stimulate the pancreas to produce more insulin.

Significant hypoglycemia occurs most often in patients taking insulin by injection or insulin secretogogues. The dosage of these medications is determined by an estimation of the amount needed to achieve a balance between the anticipated dietary intake (the amount of food to be consumed), the level of physical activity and such other contributory factors as shown in Table 1. When this balance is disrupted, the blood sugar can fall precipitously, causing hypoglycemia.

TABLE 1
Factors That May Play a Role in
Precipitating Hypoglycemia

1. Too much medication (insulin or oral agents such as sulfonylureas).
2. Errors of insulin administration. The injection of too much medicine by mistake or the administration of the wrong type of insulin erroneously (For example: taking regular insulin instead of a long-acting insulin).
3. Too little food for the amount of insulin or oral agent taken. This is most likely to happen when meals are skipped or delayed, or a between-meal snack is omitted.
4. Nausea or vomiting without replacement of food and/or body fluids lost. (Ginger ale or Coca Cola can serve as a well tolerated temporary source of glucose and fluid replenishment.)
5. The excessive utilization of glucose from unscheduled or excessively vigorous physical activity.
6. Drug interactions. Certain medications may boost the blood lowering effects of insulin or oral agents. The most notable examples are drugs belonging to a class known as beta blockers.
7. Taking a sauna bath. Injected insulin may be absorbed much more rapidly in the hot, steamy sauna environment. Eat before going to the sauna, or keep a snack on hand to treat any drop in the blood sugar.
8. Ingesting alcohol, particularly on an empty stomach.
9. Intercurrent illness that adversely affects blood sugar control.

ALCOHOL AND HYPOGLYCEMIA

The consumption of alcohol, particularly on an empty stomach (when glycogen stores and the blood glucose level may already be partially depleted), can induce significant hypoglycemia, even at blood alcohol levels well below the common legal limits. Alcohol, by itself, can lower blood sugar levels in non-diabetics as well as in diabetics, although its affect on the latter is often particularly severe. Accordingly, when it is not known that someone has diabetes, the symptoms of hypoglycemia can be mistaken for drunkenness. Thus, a slightly "tipsy" diabetic may develop hypoglycemia requiring urgent treatment, but be neglected because his symptoms are dismissed as purely those of inebriation. This danger makes it advisable to wear a diabetic medic-alert bracelet or pendant. In addition, a wallet-sized diabetic identification and information card should be kept on your person at all times.

EXERCISE AND HYPOGLYCEMIA

Diabetics are prone to hypoglycemia when they exercise, particularly following strenuous or prolonged physical activities. They are also especially vulnerable to hypoglycemic episodes when physical activity is undertaken during late evening or early a.m. hours, when blood sugar levels normally decline. As noted, alcohol poses an additional risk factor for hypoglycemia and is to be avoided, especially when consumed in conjunction with unusual physical activities—including sexual intimacy.

SYMPTOMS OF HYPOGLYCEMIA

Mild episodes of hypoglycemia typically cause the brain to signal the adrenal glands to secrete epinephrine (adrenaline), which produces such symptoms as palpitations (awareness of the heart beat), tachycardia (rapid heart rate), pallor, sweating, paresthesias (abnormal sensations of the skin), shakiness, and hunger. Moderate hypoglycemia affects the brain and may cause an individual to become confused and unable to make rational decisions. Impairment of the function of the brain and central nervous system occurs because the brain relies primarily on glucose for its metabolic functions. Severe cerebral hypoglycemia results from profound glucose deprivation and is characterized by disorientation, seizures, and loss of consciousness. Moderate or severe hypoglycemia may sometimes develop within a very short period of time.

Almost all diabetic patients run a risk of hypoglycemia, but it is far more prevalent in those who require insulin for their diabetes management.

DIAGNOSING HYPOGLYCEMIA

The diagnosis of hypoglycemia can be confirmed in those who develop symptoms suggestive of the disorder, in association with an abnormally low plasma glucose level, usually defined as 60mg or less/dl. However, because of individual differences, it is difficult to assign an exact number to the blood sugar level that will induce symptoms of hypoglycemia in an individual case.

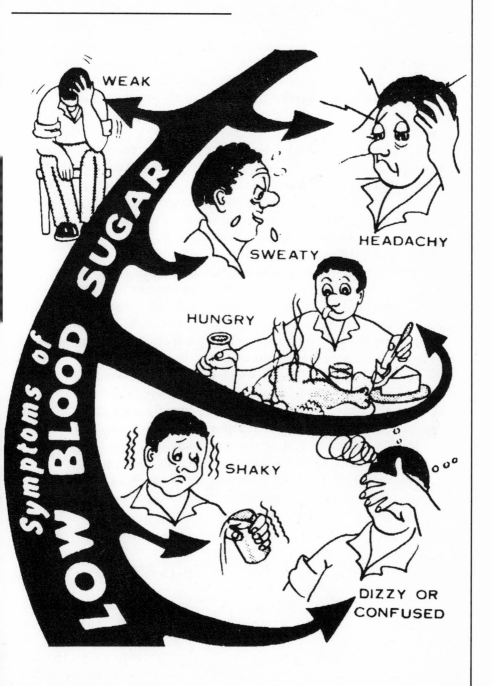

HYPOGLYCEMIA UNAWARENESS

The failure to develop symptoms of hypoglycemia when the blood sugar falls to levels that usually give rise to symptoms of hypoglycemia is called hypoglycemia unawareness. In some instances, the failure to "feel" symptoms of hypoglycemia results from neuropathy—nerve tissue damage—one of the long-term complications of diabetes (See Chapter 19, *Long-term Complications of Diabetes*).

Patients may also develop hypoglycemia unawareness following prolonged periods of repeated bouts of hypoglycemia. Avoiding even mild hypoglycemic episodes can sometimes help to restore hypoglycemia awareness. It is extremely important for those suffering from hypoglycemia unawareness to monitor their blood sugar closely. This may necessitate raising target fasting blood sugar levels from 80-120mg/dl (4.44 mMol/dl-6.67 mMol/dl) to 100-140mg/dl (5.55 mMol/dl-7.78 mMol/dl).

It is particularly vital to limit hypoglycemic episodes in children. The target blood sugar range may need to be kept between 100 and 200 mg/dl (5.55-11.1 mMol/dl). Children under seven years of age are often unable to recognize and respond to low blood sugar levels.

Epinephrine may be released, and hypoglycemia-like symptoms may also be experienced when the blood sugar falls rapidly, or when the blood sugar declines below the level to which the body may have become accustomed, even though the level attained may be within the normal range. This response, which is known as a "false" hypoglycemic reaction, results from the brain's glucose sensor reacting to sudden changes in the blood sugar level, which causes the release of epinephrine. Although physicians and patients usually focus on the clinical features—the signs and symptoms—of hypoglycemia when evaluating the condition, a blood sugar determination is necessary to confirm the diagnosis, monitor treatment and rule out "false" hypoglycemia.

TABLE 2
Symptoms of Hypoglycemia

A low blood sugar may cause any or all of the following symptoms, depending upon individual variations and the severity of the hypoglycemia. The diagnosis of hypoglycemia can be confirmed if the blood sugar level is less than 60 mg/dl (3.3 mMol/L).

MILD HYPOGLYCEMIA: Mild episodes cause the body to secrete epinephrine which gives rise to such symptoms as:

* Pallor (pale clammy skin — "cold sweat")
* Weakness and trembling
* Tachycardia (rapid heart rate)
* Palpitations (awareness of heart beating)
* Paresthesia (abnormal sensations of the skin)
* Shakiness
* Anxiety or panic
* Hunger
* Nausea

MODERATE HYPOGLYCEMIA: Moderate hypoglycemia is associated with symptoms caused by altered brain functioning, as a consequence of low blood sugar levels, which gives rise to such neurological symptoms as:

* Confusion & inability to concentrate and make rational decisions
* Lack of coordination
* Slurred speech and blurred vision
* Irrational behavior
* Extreme fatigue and sleepiness

SEVERE HYPOGLYCEMIA: Severe hypoglycemia represents a progression of the neurological symptoms associated with moderate hypoglycemia. Neurological malfunctioning deteriorates to the extent that assistance is required to obtain treatment. Symptoms associated with severe hypoglycemia include:

* Disorientation
* Automatic behavior
* Inability to arouse from sleep
* Loss of consciousness. If the unconscious patient does not receive prompt treatment, irreversible brain damage and even death can result.

NOTE: The symptoms of hypoglycemia do not necessarily progress in a linear fashion from those associated with mild hypoglycemia to those that are usually characteristic of severe hypoglycemia. When the decline in the blood sugar is gradual, it often fails to trigger the brain activated epinephrine alarm. In addition, some patients experience neurological symptoms characteristic of moderate hypoglycemia before they develop those associated with mild hypoglycemia from epinephrine release. Other patients may ignore mild symptoms attributable to epinephrine and experience those that result from the brain's deprivation of glucose as initial symptoms.

THE RELATIONSHIP OF HYPOGLYCEMIA TO THE TIME COURSE OF INSULIN ACTION

Patients should familiarize themselves with the properties of the type of insulin prescribed by their doctor and know its mode of action, as well as the timing of its peak activity.

Time Course of Action of Insulin Preparations:

Note: The typical time course of action of the various types of insulin is highly variable, being affected by such factors as the site of injection, physical activity following injection and skin condition.

1. **Very short-acting (Humalog) —**
   Therapeutic Action Onset : very rapid — within 15 minutes.
   Peak: About 45 minutes (30 to 60 minutes).
   Duration: 4 to 5 hours.
2. **Short-acting (Regular) —**
   Therapeutic Action Onset: 30 to 60 minutes.
   Peak: 2 to 6 hours. Duration: 5 to 7 hours.
3. **Intermediate-acting (NPH or Lente) —**
   Therapeutic Action Onset: 1 to 3 hours.
   Peak: 6 to 12 hours. Duration: 16 to 24 hours.
4. **Long-acting (Ultralente) —**
   Therapeutic Action Onset: 4 to 6 hours.
   Peak: 18 hours. Duration: 16 to 30 hours.
5. **Mixtures (70/30, 50/50) —**
   Therapeutic Action Onset: 30 minutes.
   Peak: 7 to 12 hours. Duration: 16 to 24 hours.

Hypoglycemic reactions tend to occur just before a meal or when injected insulin has its peak effect. Intermediate-acting insulins most often cause reactions in the late afternoon or just before the evening meal. Intermediate-acting insulin taken in the evening can cause reactions during the night or early the next morning. Humalog is a very fast acting insulin that can be taken immediately before eating. Regular insulin, however, should be taken 30 minutes prior to food. If regular insulin is taken immediately before or just after eating, a delayed hypoglycemic reaction could occur.

The majority of hypoglycemic episodes occur at night because the body's need for insulin decreases during the pre-dawn hours. It is at this time that the intermediate-acting insulins reach their peak action, causing the blood glucose to drop to low levels. Patients who have elected to follow an intensive insulin regimen, or those on the insulin pump, run a higher risk for hypoglycemic episodes than patients on conventional therapy.

TREATMENT OF HYPOGLYCEMIA

The goal of treatment of hypoglycemia is to normalize the blood sugar as rapidly as possible. Diabetics must always carry some form of carbohydrate, such as hard candy, with them at all times. They should not hesitate to initiate treatment after becoming aware of early symptoms suggestive of low blood glucose. Just as jet pilots are trained to recognize the early symptoms of anoxia (a lack of oxygen), diabetics must familiarize themselves with their own individual warning symptoms that occur when their blood sugar falls too low. Hypoglycemia may rapidly become severe enough to prevent determination of the blood glucose level. At the first sign of a possible low blood sugar reaction, even if in doubt, it is always safer to presume that the symptoms are caused by hypoglycemia and some form of carbohydrate should be taken. Even if it turns out that you do not have hypoglycemia, and your blood sugar is elevated, a small amount of additional sugar does no harm.

Mild Hypoglycemia Treatment

Mild hypoglycemia can generally be treated effectively by the ingestion of approximately 15 grams of carbohydrate. Following this simple measure, there is usually a fairly prompt response. Sources of 15 grams of carbohydrate include:

- 5 ounces Coke or 7-Up
- 1/2 cup of fruit juice
- 2 tablespoons of raisins
- 3 5-gram glucose tablets
- 1 cup of milk
- 7-1/2 lifesaver-type candies
- 3 teaspoons honey
- 6 ounces orange juice
- 3 ounces grape juice
- 6 ounces orange juice
- 5-1/2 ounces ginger ale

Moderate Hypoglycemia

Moderate hypoglycemia requires the ingestion of larger amounts of glucose to restore the blood sugar to normal. Thirty grams of glucose by mouth usually suffices. Following a response to the initial carbohydrate intake, patients should consume additional food. Blood sugar determination during treatment can serve as a guide for the necessity of additional carbohydrate intake. Some patients may continue to exhibit neurological symptoms for an hour or more after blood sugar levels have been restored above 100mg/dl (5.55 mMol/L).

Severe Hypoglycemia

Severe hypoglycemia requires rapid, and at times life-saving treatment. If a person is unconscious, never force them to eat or drink fluids. The most effective treatment is the intravenous injection of glucose (50cc of 50 percent). Glucagon vials are available for home treatment. The usual adult dose is 1mg. Complete instructions for their use are packaged with the glucagon vial. The expiration date on the glucagon vial should be checked periodically. It is a good idea to have family members practice injection technique using normal sterile saline so that they are ready and capable should the need arise. If a rapid response to the above measures is not forthcoming or if no glucagon for injection is available, call 911 immediately. If one vial of glucagon does not cause a satisfactory response, a second injection is not likely to improve the condition. Patients on oral medications should be aware that hypoglycemia may last for several hours, and even days in the case of chlorpropamide, a first generation sulfonylurea oral agent. Treatment of these delayed reactions requires constant blood glucose monitoring and intravenous infusion of a glucose solution, especially in older patients.

Patients who reside alone sometimes take too much carbohydrate to offset the symptoms of low blood sugar. Over-treatment can become a problem, causing the patient's sugar to rise to unacceptably high levels.

Hypoglycemia is a serious complication of diabetes, but with intelligent preparation, knowledge, and adherence to basic principles, it can be managed very well by the vast majority of diabetic patients.

CONDITIONS THAT CAN BE MISTAKEN FOR HYPOGLYCEMIA

Anxiety or panic attacks can cause symptoms that are similar to those of mild hypoglycemia. Both conditions are associated with the release of the hormone epinephrine from the adrenal glands. The former as a response to our ancient "fight or flight" mechanism and the latter from cerebral stimulation of the adrenal glands by the autonomic nervous system as the brain attempts to raise the blood sugar level by releasing this insulin antagonist hormone. Strokes and other conditions that are associated with a decreased oxygen supply to the brain can also be confused with hypoglycemia. The differentiation of DKA coma and hypoglycemia is shown in Table 3.

TABLE 3: COMPARISON OF DIABETIC COMA & INSULIN REACTIONS

	DIABETIC COMA	INSULIN SHOCK—HYPOGLYCEMIA— LOW BLOOD SUGAR	
	CLINICAL FEATURES	REGULAR INSULIN	LONG-ACTING INSULIN
ONSET	SLOW, DAYS	SUDDEN, MINUTES	GRADUAL, HOURS
CAUSES	IGNORANCE, NEGLECT INTERCURRENT DISEASE OMISSION OF INSULIN AND FOOD	OVERDOSAGE DELAYED, OMITTED, OR LOST MEALS EXCESSIVE EXERCISE BEFORE MEALS	OVERDOSAGE DELAYED, OMITTED OR LOST MEALS EXCESSIVE EXERCISE BEFORE MEALS
SYMPTOMS	THIRST FREQUENT URINATION HEADACHE NAUSEA VOMITING ABDOMINAL PAIN DIM VISION CONSTIPATION SHORTNESS OF BREATH	"INWARD NERVOUSNESS" WEAKNESS SWEATING HUNGER DOUBLE VISION, BLURRED VISION TINGLING SENSATIONS PATIENT MAY ACT DRUNK STUPOR, CONVULSIONS	FATIGUE WEAKNESS HEADACHE SWEATING SOMETIMES ABSENT DIZZINESS DOUBLE, BLURRED VISION PATIENT MAY ACT DRUNK STUPOR, CONVULSIONS
SIGNS	FLORID FACE RAPID BREATHING DEHYDRATION—DRY SKIN FEVER RAPID PULSE SOFT EYEBALLS ACETONE BREATH DROWSINESS, COMA	PALLOR SHALLOW RESPIRATION SWEATING PULSE NORMAL EYEBALLS NORMAL	PALLOR SHALLOW RESPIRATION SKIN MAY BE DRY PULSE NOT CHARACTERISTIC EYEBALLS NORMAL
BLOOD GLUCOSE	GREATER THAN 250 MG/DL	LESS THAN 60 MG/DL	LESS THAN 60 MG/DL
ACETONE DIACETIC ACID	POSITIVE POSITIVE	NEGATIVE NEGATIVE	NEGATIVE NEGATIVE
WHAT TO DO	CALL PHYSICIAN OR EMERGENCY HOSPITAL AT FIRST SIGN OF SYMPTOMS	IF PATIENT CAN SWALLOW, GIVE SUGAR IN SOME FORM—CANDY, SYRUP, COLA OR SIMILAR BEVERAGES THAT CONTAIN SUGAR, ORANGE JUICE, ETC. CALL A PHYSICIAN OR EMERGENCY HOSPITAL.	IF PATIENT CAN SWALLOW, GIVE SUGAR IN SOME FORM—CANDY, SYRUP, COLA OR SIMILAR BEVERAGES THAT CONTAIN SUGAR, ORANGE JUICE, ETC. CALL A PHYSICIAN OR EMERGENCY HOSPITAL.
TREATMENT RESPONSE	SLOW	USUALLY RAPID LATE	MAY BE SLOW OR

NOTE: EXCESSIVE DOSAGE OF SOME OF THE ORAL HYPOGLYCEMIC AGENTS OR OMISSION OF FOOD MAY CAUSE HYPOGLYCEMIA, AND THE SYMPTOMS MAY BE THE SAME AS THOSE SEEN WITH REGULAR INSULIN OR THE LONGER-ACTING INSULINS.

C H A P T E R
• 11 •

Oral Drugs for Diabetes

Oral Agents
Combination Therapy With Oral Drugs
Dosage Mechanism of Action, Advantages
& Disadvantages of the Oral Agents

What Type 2 diabetics eat is the single most important factor in their blood sugar control. For many, making healthy lifestyle changes—proper meal planning, moderate exercise and weight loss when necessary—may suffice to keep their blood sugar under satisfactory control. Lifestyle adjustments should be emphasized as the primary form of treatment of Type 2 diabetes. If the foregoing supportive measures are not adequate to attain target blood sugar levels, oral medications and/or insulin therapy is indicated.

Medications taken by mouth to treat diabetes are known as oral hypoglycemic agents. This is a misnomer because these drugs are not prescribed to cause hypoglycemia—low blood sugar. They are given to lower the blood glucose level to normal, or near normal levels.

The oral agents are not insulin; they are synthetic drugs that stimulate the pancreas to secrete insulin or to utilize the insulin produced by the pancreas more efficiently, by increasing sensitivity to insulin's physiologic actions.

Although the sugar lowering effect of some medications and certain herbs had been recognized for many years, it was not until World War II that sulfa drugs were developed specifically for their blood sugar lowering effects. These drugs soon became the treatment of choice for Type 2 diabetics who were unable to bring their diabetes under satisfactory control with diet, weight loss, and exercise programs. The sulfonylurea drugs belong to the class of oral agents known as insulin secretogogues—drugs that cause the beta cells of the pancreas to secrete insulin. They are of no benefit in Type 1 diabetes because Type 1's do not have functional beta cells. The sulfonylureas are most effective in treating Type 2 patients with fasting blood sugars below 225mg/dl. However, there is no universal agreement among diabetologists on this cutoff value.

The first generation sulfonylureas—Orinase®, Diabanese®, Dymelor®, and Tolinase®—are no longer widely prescribed. They have been replaced by the second and third generation sulfonylureas Glipizide (Glucotrol®, Glucotrol XL®), Glyburide (Diabeta®, Micronase®, and Glynase®) and Glimepiride (Amaryl®). These newer drugs are well tolerated and produce considerably fewer side effects and interactions with other drugs than their predecessors.

In recent years, new classes of oral agents that work well independently or in combination with one another have made a radical change in the treatment of Type 2 diabetes. The large number of new effective hypoglycemic agents with differing mechanisms of action have made it possible to achieve target blood sugar control in an increasingly higher percentage of Type 2 diabetics. In addition to the sulfonylureas, we now have Metformin (Glucophage®), an oral agent that belongs to the chemical class of drugs known as biguanides which work primarily by suppressing glucose production in the liver and increasing glucose uptake by the muscles. Another newcomer is drugs of the chemical class called thiazolidenediones that lower the blood sugar by reducing insulin resistance by enhancing insulin's action in muscle, fat and liver tissues. Prandin® is a new insulin secretogogue that belongs to the chemical group known as meglitinides. Prandin® stimulates pancreatic insulin release primarily in response to elevations of the blood sugar. When taken thirty minutes or less before eating, insulin response is generally limited to after-meal related blood sugar elevations, which are known as post-prandial "spikes." Therefore, it is effective in providing insulin when most needed. Acarbose (Precose®) is another new glucose lowering drug. It belongs to the category called Alpha Glucosidase Inhibitors. Acarbose helps to control post-prandial "spikes" in blood sugar by delaying carbohydrate digestion and absorption from the intestinal tract, thus promoting a more gradual and smooth absorption of glucose.

PRIMARY AND SECONDARY FAILURES
OF ORAL AGENT THERAPY

Many diabetics on oral agent therapy achieve satisfactory control of their blood sugar. Some, however, do not respond adequately to oral agent therapy, a condition called primary therapeutic failure.* With sulfonylureas, for example, ten to twenty per cent of those who initiate treatment of their diabetes with sulfonylureas respond poorly to the treatment. Others experience an initial satisfactory response, but over time the drug loses its effectiveness. Three to ten percent of patients taking sulfonylureas fail to respond satisfactorily each year. Eventually, approximately 50% of patients treated with sulfonylureas do not respond to this class of oral agents. The natural course of Type 2 diabetes is associated with a gradual deterioration of beta cell function—the ability to secrete insulin. This progressive failure of the insulin producing capacity of the beta cells may be responsible for many secondary failures. Others, undoubtedly, result from patients disregarding nutrition and exercise programs as well a non-compliance with taking medications regularly as prescribed.

Another cause of primary failure is the initiation of treatment in Type 2 diabetics who have had high blood glucose levels for a time before therapy is started. Patients whose blood sugars have been elevated for a prolonged period often develop glucose toxicity. As discussed in Chapter 1, *Diabetes Mellitus—An Overview*, glucose toxicity is the impairment of insulin production caused by the adverse effect chronically elevated blood sugar levels exert on pancreatic insulin production. Temporary control of the blood sugar with injections of insulin can normalize the blood sugar and break the glucose toxicity cycle, permitting responsiveness to oral agents to be regained. Maximum dose sulfonylurea therapy has also been used successfully to overcome glucose toxicity.

Type 2 diabetics may occasionally experience periods of decompensation of their blood sugar control in response to environmental stress factors such as an acute illness. During out-of-control periods it may be necessary to temporarily stop oral agent treatment and control the blood sugar with insulin. When the stress is no longer present, the patient can usually control his blood sugar with oral agents. The possibility of failure when using oral agents reinforces the importance of self-monitoring of blood sugar levels. (See Chapter 12, *Self-Monitoring of Blood Glucose.*)

---

*Primary failures are described as a blood sugar lowering response of 30mg/dl or less.

COMBINATION INSULIN AND
ORAL AGENT THERAPY

Combination insulin and oral agent therapy has grown in popularity over the past twenty years. Bedtime Insulin Daytime Sulfonylurea (BIDS) employs an intermediate acting insulin to control fasting elevations of the blood sugar and daytime sulfonylureas to prime pancreatic insulin secretion, to accommodate mealtime insulin needs. Currently, the term BIDO (Bedtime Insulin, Daytime Oral Medication) is employed to describe a regimen of bedtime insulin with daytime use of the newer oral agents. All classes of oral hypoglycemic medications may be used in combination with insulin.

DRUG INTERACTIONS

Many medications may augment or interfere with the blood sugar lowering effect of the oral agents. It is important, therefore, to inform your doctor of any prescription or over-the-counter medications that you may be taking. Sometimes, drugs that are harmless by themselves can interact to cause side effects. Beta blockers may mask the signs and symptoms of hypoglycemia and should not be prescribed for patients with diabetes.

Drugs that may increase the tendency of insulin or Oral Diabetic Medications to cause low blood sugar levels (Hypoglycemia) are:
- Alcohol
- Allopurinol (Zyloprim®)
- Beta blockers
- Clofibrate (Abifrate, Atromid-S®)
- Coumadin
- Monoamine oxidase inhibitors
- Probenecid (Benemid®)
- Salicylates
- Sulfonamides (rarely, e.g. Bactrim®)

Drugs that may cause high blood sugar levels (Hyperglycemia) are:
- Calcium channel blockers
- Corticosteroids
- Isoniazid

- Nasal decongestants (Sympathomimetics — Epinephrine-like drugs)
- Oral contraceptives (including Estrogens)
- Dilantin
- Rifampin
- Thiazide diuretics
- Nicotinic acid

Note: Drug interactions vary from person to person. Check your blood sugars more frequently whenever adding or discontinuing any medication.

ORAL HYPOGLYCEMIC AGENTS

CAUTION: Oral hyporglycemic drugs are contraindicated in pregnant or lactating women, those with significant liver or kidney disease (depending on the oral agent), and anyone who has experienced an allergic reaction to them.

INSULIN SECRETAGOGUES: Drugs that stimulate the pancreas to secrete unsulin

Sulfonylureas
Summary
Drug Class: Sulfonylureas
These oral hypoglycemic medications for Type 2 diabetes work by stimulating the beta cells in the pancreas to release more insulin.

Mechanism of action: All sulfonylureas work by stimulating pancreatic insulin production.

Adverse effects: May cause hypoglycemia. Skin rashes or other signs of allergy sometimes seen. Prolonged use may exhaust beta cell function in an already overworked pancreas. Excessive insulin production from these medications may cause weight gain.

New sulfonylurea drugs: May be taken alone or with other diabetes drugs, with appropriate diabetes meal planning and exercise. The newer second and third generation sulfonylureas can be taken at reduced frequency than older drugs in the class. They are better tolerated — cause fewer side effects. They are currently the drugs of choice in this category of oral agents.

FIRST GENERATION SULFONYLUREA DRUGS

Generic Name	Trade Name	Duration of Action
Tolbutamide	Orinase	6-12 hours. Metabolized by the liver and excreted in the urine, as are all the sulfonylureas.
Dose: 500mg-1500 mg/day		
Clorpropamide	Diabenese	Effect may last as long as 60 hours. Can increase secretion of anti-diuretic hormone resulting in water retention and abnormal lowering of sodium in the blood.

SECOND GENERATION SULFONYLUREA DRUGS

These drugs are more potent than the first generation sulfonylureas and therefore require lower doses and have fewer side effects. The long acting formulations—Glucotrol XL and Amaryl—are taken only once a day. Adverse reactions are seen in less than 2 percent of those taking these medications, an incidence less than half that of their predecessors.

Generic Name	Trade Name	Duration of Action
Glipizide	Glucotrol Glucotrol XL	12-24 hours
Dose: 5mg-20mg/day		
Glyburide	Diabeta Micronase Glynase (micronized glyburide)	12-24 hours
Dose: 1.25mg-20mg/day Glynase Dose: .75mg-12mg/day		

THIRD GENERATION SULFONYLUREA DRUGS

Generic Name	Trade Name	Duration of Action
Glimepiride	Amaryl	24 hours

Dose: Starting dose -1mg/day; usual maintenance dose: 1mg-4mg/day.

Maximum dose: 8mg/day. Once daily alone or with other diabetes medications. Reduced frequency of dosage can improve adherence.

Amaryl is insulin sparing and controls glucose without any significant increase in fasting insulin levels. It is indicated for use alone as well as second-line treatment in combination with insulin. Amaryl increases insulin sensitivity and patients taking insulin injections may be able to cut insulin dosage significantly. Amaryl binds to a different part of the sulfonylurea cell receptors than other drugs in this group. The clinical relevance of this mechanism has not yet been determined. The combined use of Amaryl and insulin may increase the potential for hypoglycemia.

BIGUANIDES

Summary
Drug Class: Biguanides.
Biguanides suppress glucose production in the liver and lower insulin resistance.
Mechanism of action: Help the body use insulin more efficiently. Decreases glucose production in the liver and increases glucose uptake in the muscle and fat tissue.
Side effects: Rarely, may accumulate and cause severe lactic acidosis, a dangerous metabolic condition. This usually occurs in patients who use alcohol (even low or moderate amounts), have kidney dysfunction, or liver impairment. May cause loss of appetite, stomach ache, nausea, or other GI symptoms.
Advantages: May cause small weight loss. Improves blood lipid profile. Does not cause hypoglycemia or weight gain when used alone. Does not stress pancreas through insulin overproduction.

Trade Name	Generic Name	Duration of Action
Glucophage	*Metformin*	*4-8 hours*

Dose: 500mg-2000mg/day (Rarely 2500mg/day). Taken with food to minimize GI side effects.
Note: Dosage above 2000mg/day does not improve therapeutic effects.
Side Effects: GI upset. A tendency that decreases over time.

Although Biguanides have been known to lower blood glucose since the nineteenth century and have been used extensively in Europe for the past forty years, Metformin is a relatively new drug to the U.S. market. Since its introduction in 1995, it has become a widely prescribed oral hypoglycemic agent. The biguanides have a totally different mechanism of action than the sulfonylureas. Rather than stimulating the production of insulin in the diabetic who may already have high insulin levels as well as insulin receptors on the cells that do not function normally, Metformin sensitizes the body's cells to insulin's effects by reducing the output of glucose from the liver and increasing muscle cell sensitivity to insulin. This physiologic action helps the body utilize its own insulin to work more efficiently. **Because it works without stimulating insulin secretion, it lowers the blood sugar without the risk of causing hypoglycemia when used alone.**

Biguanides were available in the United States in the 1970's as the widely prescribed drug, Phenformin®. This drug was less effective than Metformin and occasionally caused the serious and often fatal metabolic complication known as lactic acidosis. The occurrence of this serious side effect tarnished the drug's reputation and it was withdrawn from the U.S. market in 1977. Metformin can also cause lactic acidosis, but this can usually be avoided if patients are carefully screened for pre-existing kidney disease, liver disease, or congestive heart failure. Other patients at risk for lactic acidosis are moderate to heavy drinkers, those with chronic respiratory disease, and the elderly. The drug should not be used in those over 80 years of age unless kidney function is normal. Patients undergoing radio-contrast studies such as cardiac catheterization or vascular angiography, should be taken off Metformin temporarily because of the possibility of an untoward reaction to the dye, with a decrease in blood pressure as well as decreased excretion of the biguanide. Metformin may have some mild side effects. Between 10-30 percent of those taking the medication experience GI symptoms—nausea, vomiting, diarrhea, or loss of appetite. These symptoms usually subside over time. In order to reduce the incidence of side effects, Metformin should be taken with meals, starting with a small dose and gradually increasing it until the optimal dose is determined.

Extensive use in Europe has confirmed the benefits and safety of Metformin in Type 2 diabetes when proper screening and monitoring measures are employed. Metformin, either alone, or in combination with the sulfonylurea drugs, has proven to be quite effective in achieving glucose control. Metformin augments the effects of sulfonylureas and is often added to the treatment regimen when a sulfonylurea loses its effectiveness, or vice versa; a sulfonylurea may be added to Metformin if it is ineffective when used alone.

THIAZOLIDENEDIONES

Summary

Drug Class: Thiazolidenediones.
New class of drugs for Type 2 diabetes. Acts in muscles, sensitizes cells to insulin action, and reduces glucose production by the liver.

Avandia®:   (Generic: Rosiglitazone)
                Dose: 2-8mg daily. Usual dose, 4mg.
Rezulin®:   (Generic: Troglitazone)
                The first thiazolidenedione drug developed. It was
                withdrawn from the market in March 2000 because
                of rare, but sometimes lethal, liver toxicity.
Actos®:   (Generic: Pioglitazone)
                Dose: Starting dose 15-30mg per day. Maximum dose 45mg.

Mechanism of action: Lowers insulin resistance to injected or natural insulin and enhances insulin action primarily by facilitating glucose uptake in muscle and fat tissue with a lesser effect on insulin action in the liver. Approved for broad range of people with Type 2 diabetes.

Usage: Alone or in combination with sulfonylureas or insulin.

Side effects: Patients taking insulin may need to lower their insulin dose when taking Thiazolidenediones, to prevent hypoglycemia. Patients with congestive heart failure or liver disease may be poor Thiazolidenediones candidates because they may experience liver failure. Liver function tests must be monitored regularly when taking Thiazolidenediones. The newer drugs of this class such as Rosiglitazone and Pioglitazone are purported to have a much better safety profile than their predecessor Troglitazone, but patients liver function tesets must still be monitored. Patients on oral contraceptives may have lowered birth control protection when on this drug. Cholestyramine reduces the absorption of Thiazolidenediones by approximately 70 percent thus, co-administration of cholestyramine and Thiazolidenediones is not recommended.

Advantages: Does not "strain" the pancreas by causing excessive insulin production. Reduces insulin resistance. Insulin dosage may be reduced or eliminated. Reduces glucose production by the liver, improves blood lipid levels. No known drug interactions.

Disadvantages: High failure rate when used alone as monotherapy. Potential for causing liver damage.

ALPHA-GLUCOSIDASE INHIBITORS

Summary

Drug Class: Alpha-Glucosidase Inhibitors

These drugs work in the small intestine and inhibit enzymes that digest carbohydrates, thus delaying carbohydrate absorption, and thereby lowering post-meal glucose levels.

Mechanism of action: Delays carbohydrate absorption in the small intestine by slowing down the digestion of complex carbohydrates and sucrose, thereby lowering glucose levels after meals. Unique nonsystemic mode of action, delaying glucose absorption.

Usage: May be taken alone or with other diabetes drugs. Primarily with sulfonylureas or Metformin®.

Side effects: Does not cause hypoglycemia or weight gain when used alone. May cause liver damage. The most common side effects are cramping abdominal pain, diarrhea and flatulence (gas). This latter symptom may be particularly severe and lead to discontinuance of the medication. Although the GI symptoms may make patients feel uncomfortable, they are not a serious health concern.

Despite the fact that the drug is not absorbed from the intestinal tract, some of the products produced by intestinal breakdown of the medication do get into the bloodstream. These metabolites are believed to be responsible for possible liver damage. Liver function tests should be monitored every three months for the first year of therapy, and periodically thereafter. Liver toxicity is believed to be dose related and is uncommon at doses under 200mg per day. For those weighing less than 130 lbs., a maximum dose of 150gm is recommended.

Precose®:   (generic acarbose) available in 25mg, 50mg and 100mg tabs
Glyset®:   (generic miglitol) available in 25mg, 50mg and 100mg tabs

Dose: The recommended starting dose of Precose® and Glyset® is 25mg three times daily, with the first bite of each meal. Some patients may benefit from a starting dose of 25mg once daily to minimize gastrointestinal effects and permit identification of the minimal dose required to achieve adequate glycemic control. After 4 - 8 weeks on a regimen of 25mg three times daily, the dosage should be increased to 50mg three times a day for approximately 3 months. If the glycosylated hemoglobin is not satisfactory at that time the dose may be increased to 100mg three times daily, the maximum recommended dose. If no further reduction in post-prandial glucose or glycosylated hemoglobin levels is observed, consideration should be given to lowering the dose. Once an effective and tolerated dosage is established, it should be maintained. 100mg dose tid only for those who weigh more than 130 pounds.

NON-SULFONYLUREA INSULIN SECRETAGOGUES

MEGLITINIDES

Summary

Drug Class: Meglitinides.

A new class of drugs for treatment of Type 2 diabetes.

Mechanism of Action: Stimulates release of insulin from the pancreas.

Usage: Alone or in combination with other oral agents.

Side Effects: Generally similar and comparable to sulfonylurea drugs.

Advantages: Rapid onset of action in response to blood glucose level simulates body's natural release of insulin from the pancreas.

Prandin®:   (Generic: Repaglinide)
Dose: Taken just before or up to 30 minutes prior to meals. 0.5mg with mild elevations of blood sugar. 1-2mg when blood sugar is high. Dose may be doubled once weekly to a maximum of 4mg before meals. Increase dosage cautiously in presence of kidney disease.

Starlix ® :   (Generic Nateglinide)
Dose: Take 1 - 30 minutes before meals. 120mg three times daily. 60mg dose three times for those who are close to their HbA1c goal

Specific Types of fixed oral agent combination Therapy
Sulfonylureas & Metformin

When sulfonylureas prove to be ineffective in controlling the blood sugar when used alone, switching to Metformin will also usually prove to be ineffective. And vice versa; when Metformin is a primary therapeutic failure, sulfonylureas will also usually be ineffective. However, when these two medications are used together, they often achieve blood sugar control that was impossible to accomplish when either was used alone. The use of sulfonylurea and Metformin combination therapy has been the subject of extensive clinical studies documenting the safety and benefits of this therapy.

Thiazolidinediones & Metformin

Both of these drugs spare stimulation of the Type 2 diabetic's "tired and overworked" pancreas by improving the efficiency of the body's secreted pancreatic insulin. Thiazolidinediones (Rosiglitazone, Pioglitazone and Troglitazone) decrease insulin resistance, thereby increasing glucose uptake by the cells as well as reducing glucose output by the liver—the main defects associated with Type 2 diabetes.

APPROVE FIXED COMBINATION THERAPY WITH ORAL ANTI-DIABETIC AGENTS

1 - Metaglip   (Metformin and Glipizide)
Dosage of Metaglip must be individualized on the basis of both effectiveness and tolerance while not exceeding the maximum recommended daily dose of 20mg Glipizide/2000mg Metformin, with gradual dose escalation in order to avoid hypoglycemia (largely due to Glipizide) and to reduce GI side effects (largely due to Metformin) and to permit determination of the minimum effective dose for adequate control of blood glucose for the individual patient.

Metaglip for initial therapy - For patients with Type 2 diabetes whose hyperglycemia cannot be satisfactorily managed with diet and exercise alone, the starting dose of Metaglip is 2.5mg/250mg once a day with a meal. For patients with a fasting blood glucose (FPG) of 280mg/dL to 320mg/dL, a starting dose of Metaglip 2.5mg/500mg twice daily should be considered. The efficacy of Metaglip in those whose FPG exceeds 320ng/dL has not been established. Dosage increases to achieve adequate blood sugar control should be made in increments of one tablet per day every two weeks up to a maximum of 10mg/1000mg or 10mg/2000mg Metaglip per day in divided doses.

Metaglip as a second line therapy - For those not adequately controlled on either Glipizide (or another sulfonylurea) or Metformin alone, the recommended starting dose of Metaglip is 2.5mg/500mg or 5mg/500mg twice daily with the morning and evening meals. In order to avoid hypoglycemia, the starting dose of Metaglip should not exceed the daily dose of Glipizide or Metformin already being taken. The daily dose should be titrated in increments of no more than 5mg/500mg up to the minimum effective dose to achieve adequate control of blood glucose to a maximum dose of 20mg Glipizide/2000mg Metformin per day.

2 - Glucovance   (Glyburide and Metformin tablets)
Like Metaglip, the dosage of Glucovance must be individualized on the basis of both effectiveness and tolerance while not exceeding the maximum recommended daily dose of 20mg Glyburide/2000mg Metformin.

Glucovance as initial therapy - Recommended starting dose: 1.25mg/250mg once or twice daily with meals.
For patients with Type 2 diabetes whose hyperglycemia cannot be satisfactorily managed with diet and exercise alone, the recommended starting dose of Glucovance is 1.25mg/250mg once a day with a meal. As initial therapy in patients with baseline HbA1c greater than 9% or a FPG greater than 200mg/dL, a starting dose of Glucovance 1.25mg/250mg twice daily with the morning and evening meals may be used. Dosage increases should be made in

increments of 1.25mg/250mg per day every two weeks up to the minimum effective dose necessary to achieve adequate control of blood glucose. In clinical trials of Glucovance as initial therapy, there was no experience with total daily doses greater than 10mg/2000mg per day. **Glucovance 5mg/500mg should not be used as initial therapy due to an increased risk of hypoglycemia**.

Glucovance use in previously treated patients (second line therapy) - Recommended starting dose: 2.5mg/500mg or 5mg/500mg twice early with meals.

For patients not adequately controlled on either Glyburide (or another sulfonylurea) or Metformin alone, the recommended starting dose of Glucovance is 2.5mg/500mg or 5mg/500mg twice daily with the morning and evening meals. In order to avoid hypoglycemia, the starting dose of Glucovance should not exceed the daily doses of Glyburide or Metformin already being taken. The daily dose should be titrated in increments of no more than 5mg/500mg up to the minimum effective dose to achieve adequate control of blood glucose or to a maximum dose of 20mg/2000mg per day.

For patients previously treated with combination therapy Glyburide (or another sulfonylurea) plus Metformin, switched to Glucovance, the starting dose should not exceed the daily dose of Glyburide (or equivalent dose of another sulfonylurea) and Metformin already being taken. Patients should be monitored closely for signs and symptoms of hypoglycemia following such a switch and the dose of Glucovance should be titrated as described above to achieve adequate control of blood glucose.

AVANDAMET®: (Rosiglitazone and Metformin tablets)

Avandamet   tablets contain two oral antihyperglycemic drugs used in the management of Type 2 diabetes: Rosiglitazone and Metformin. The combination of Rosiglitazone and Metformin has been previously approved based on clinical trials in people with Type 2 diabetes inadequately controlled on Metformin alone.

Rosiglitazone is an oral antidiabetic agent, which acts primarily by increasing insulin sensitivity. Rosiglitazone improves glycemic control while reducing circulating insulin levels. Pharmacological studies in animal models indicate that Rosiglitazone improves sensitivity to insulin in muscle and fat tissue and inhibits glucose production by the liver. The selection of the dose of Avandamet should be based on the patient's current doses of Rosiglitazone and/or Metformin. The safety and efficacy of Avandamet as initial therapy for patients with Type 2 diabetes have not been established.

The following recommendations regarding the use of Avandamet in patients inadequately controlled on Rosiglitazone and Metformin monotherapies are based on clinical practice experience with Rosiglitazone and Metformin combination therapy.

* The dosage of antidiabetic therapy with Avandamet should be individualized on the basis of effectiveness and tolerability while not exceeding the maximum recommended daily dose of 8mg/2000mg.

* Avandamet should be given in divided doses with meals, with gradual dose escalation. This reduces GI side effects (largely due to Metformin) and permits determination of the minimum effective dose for the individual patient.

* Sufficient time should be given to assess adequacy of therapeutic response. FPG should be used to determine the therapeutic response to Avandamet. After an increase in Metformin dosage, dose titration is recommended if patients are not adequately controlled after 1 - 2 weeks. After an increase in Rosiglitazone dosage, dose titration is recommended if patients are not adequately controlled after 8 - 12 weeks.

For patients inadequately controlled on Metformin monotherapy: the usual starting dose of Avandamet is 4mg Rosiglitazone (total daily dose) plus the dose of Metfomin already being taken (see Table 2).

For patients inadequately controlled on Rosiglitazone monotherapy: the usual stating dose of Avandamet is 1000mg Metformin (total daily dose) plus the dose of Rosiglitazone already being taken (see Table 2).

Table 2. Avandamet starting dose

PRIOR THERAPY	Usual AVANDAMET	Starting Dose
Total daily dose	Tablet strength	Number of tablets
Metformin HCl*		
1000mg/day	2mg/500mg	1 tablet b.i.d
2000mg/day	1mg/500mg	2 tablets b.i.d.
Rosiglitazone		
4mg/day	2mg/500mg	1 tablet b.i.d.
8mg/day	4mg/500mg	1 tablet b.i.d.

*For patients on doses of Metformin HCl between 1000 and 2000mg/day, initiation of Avandamet requires individualization of therapy.

When switching from combination therapy of Rosiglitazone plus Metformin as separate tablets: the usual starting dose of Avandamet is the dose of Rosiglitazone and Metformin already being taken.

If additional glycemic control is needed: the daily dose of Avandamet may be increased by increments of 4mg Rosiglitazone and/or 500mg Metformin, up to the maximum recommended total daily dose of 8mg/2000mg.

No studies have been performed specifically examining the safety and efficacy of Avandamet in patients previously treated with other oral hypoglycemic agents and switched to Avandamet. Any change in therapy of Type 2 diabetes should be undertaken with care and appropriate monitoring as changes in glycemic control can occur.

Table 1.

Approved oral agent combinations for diabetes therapy

Key: Sulfonylureas (SU)	a-Glucosidase Inhibitors (AG)
Thiazolinediones (TZD)	Non-sulfonylurea secretagogues (non-SU)

DRUG	APPROVED COMBINATIONS

Sulfonylurea (SU)
   - Glyburide®
   - Glipizide®
   - Glimeperide®
	Insulin, Metformin, TZD, AG

Biguanid - Metformin®	Insulin, SU, non-SU, TZD

Thiazolidinediones (TZD)
   - Rosiglitazone
   - Pioglitazone
	nsulin, SU, Metformin

a-Glucosidase inhibitors (AG)
   - Acarbose®
   - Miglitol®
	SU

Non-sulfonylurea secretogogues (non-SU)
   - Repaglinide®
   - Nateglinide®
	Metformin

Insulins
   - Lispro, aspart®
   - Glargine
   - Regular
   - NPH
   - Lente
	SU, Metformin, TZD

GENERIC NAME	BRAND NAME	DOSAGE RANGE (mg/day)	DURATION OF ACTION (h)	DOSING FREQUENCY (per day)	EXCRETION
SULFONYLUREAS					
Tolbutamide	Orinase	500–3000	6–12	2–3 times	Kidney
Chlorpropamide	Diabinese	100–500	60	once	Kidney
Tolazamide	Tolinase	100–1000	12–24	twice	Kidney
Acetohexamide	Dymelor	250-1500	12-18	twice	Kidney
Glipizide	Glucotrol	2.5–40	12–24	twice	Kidney (Bile 20%)
Glipizide-GITS	Glucotrol XL	5–20	24	once	Kidney (Bile 20%)
Glyburide	Diabeta Micronase	1.25–20	16–24	twice	Kidney 50%, Bile 50%
Glyburide- (Micronized)	Glynase	0.75–12	12–24	twice	Kidney 50%, Bile 50%
Glimiperide	Amaryl	1-8	24	once	Kidney (Bile 20%)

Primary Action — Increases insulin secretion by beta cells.
Advantages — Effective in more than 50% of newly diagnosed diabetics. May be used alone or in combination with other oral agents or insulin.
Disadvantages — 5-10% annual failure rate. Can cause hypoglycemia, weight gain and elevated blood insulin levels.

BIGUANIDE					
Metformin	Glucophage	1000–2550	5-6	2-4 times	Kidney

Primary Action — Decreases glucose production in liver. Increases glucose uptake by muscles.
Advantages — Effective alone or as combination therapy with sulfonylureas or Rezulin. May cause weight loss or stabilization. Modest lipid lowering effect.
Disadvantages — GI distress in 30% of patients. Rare lactic acidosis. Not to be used in patients with liver or kidney impairment or dysfunction.

ALPHA-GLUCOSIDASE INHIBITOR					
Acarbose	Precose	150-300	6	2-4 times (with meals)	Not absorbed

Primary Action — Temporarily blocks enzymes that digest starches; thus helps to keep post-meal glucose levels from rising too high.
Advantages — Effective when used alone or in combination with sulfonylureas, Metformin or Rezulin. Does not cause hypoglycemia when used alone.
Disadvantages — May cause flatulence. Diarrhea and abdominal cramping particularly when first taken. If hypoglycemia develops when Acarbose is used in conjunction with another oral agent, sucrose (table sugar) is ineffective. If glucagon is not available, milk, which contains lactose or dextrose tabs, may be used.

GENERIC NAME	BRAND NAME	DOSAGE RANGE (mg/day)	DURATION OF ACTION (h)	DOSING FREQUENCY (per day)	EXCRETION
THIAZOLIDINEDIONE					
Rosiglitazone	Avandia	4-8	24	1-2 times	Bile
Pioglitazone	Actos	15-45	24	once	Bile

Primary Action — Decreases insulin resistance. Decreases glucose synthesis by liver and increases glucose uptake and utilization by muscles. Insulin sensitizers. Significantly reduces insulin resistance. Increases glucose uptake fat and muscle tissue. Reduces glucose output by liver.

Advantages — Particularly effective when used in combination with insulin or other oral agents. May be used alone. Favorable effect on blood pressure and lipid metabolism. Actos had most favorable effect on lipid metabolism.

Disadvantages — Potential for causing liver damage requires careful monitoring of liver enzymes. Increases risk for pregnancy in pre-menopausal women by stimulating ovulation and diminishing effects of oral contraceptives. May increase blood plasma volume causing edema. No cases of jaundice were seen with Avandia or Actos in pre-marketing studies. Post market studies show a very limited incidence of liver damage.

MEGLITINIDE DERIVATIVE (Insulin Secretagogue)

Repaglinide	Prandin	2-16	1-4	2-4 times (with meals)	Bile

Primary Action — Stimulates pancreas to secrete insulin in response to food intake. Increases insulin secretion by Beta cells, similar to sulfonylureas. Because it has a short half-life, its main effect is to lower post-meal blood sugar elevations.

Advantages — Stimulates insulin secretion only in response to dietary food intake. May be used in combination with Metformin (Glucophage). Less likely to cause hypoglycemia than sulfa drugs except when given to patients with liver disease.

Disadvantages — May interact with anti-fungal drugs, Erythromycin, barbiturates and Rezulin, causing decreased sugar lowering effectiveness. Must be taken with each meal.

C H A P T E R
• 12 •

Self-Monitoring of Blood Glucose (SMBG) & Laboratory Testing for Glycosylated Hemoglobin

Benefits
Finger-Stick Method
Equipment
Glycosylated Hemoglobin

W ithout monitoring the blood sugar, one cannot really evaluate diabetes control, the key to reducing long-term complications. Unless the blood sugar can be kept within an acceptable range, there is likely to be slow but steady damage to vital body organs. Some patients are under the mistaken impression that a blood sugar done in a doctor's office once every three or four weeks is adequate to assess control and prevent long-term complications. This concept is completely erroneous. Frequent monitoring of blood sugars is the only acceptable method of obtaining reliable data to evaluate diabetes control.

Self-monitoring of blood glucose (SMBG) enables a person with diabetes to determine if blood sugar levels are too high or too low. The development of SMBG is, perhaps, the most significant advance in the management of diabetes since the discovery of insulin. Every diabetic should take advantage of it. Blood sugar determinations help you to monitor your diabetes control to determine if adjustments in diet, insulin, or exercise are needed. Although SMBG may at first seem difficult, and adds to the expense of treatment, diabetes control has improved greatly since self testing became widely available.

SMBG enables you to become a full partner with your diabetic educator in the management and treatment of your diabetes. Home monitoring records help your doctor to evaluate your blood sugar control and reduce the risks of acute and long-term complications. SMBG enables you to participate fully in everyday activities and take charge of your life without underlying fear and apprehension. You will be able to recognize disruptions in your regular patterns and make adjustments to maintain satisfactory control, which will improve your sense of well being through more stamina and energy.

Type 1 patients certainly need to check their blood sugars regularly. In the past, SMBG was used by Type 2 patients primarily when monitoring changes in treatment or during periods of illness. We now know that long-term control of blood sugar levels is as important for Type 2 patients as it is for Type 1 if damage to body organs is to be prevented. Type 2 patients who require oral medication or insulin to control their diabetes should take advantage of the benefits self-monitoring has to offer.

Self-monitoring schedules vary; generally it is done daily. Patients taking insulin usually perform at least one additional test—either at lunch or dinner, or at bedtime. All patients should perform a one day profile including a fasting, after meals and bedtime tests, approximately every one or two weeks. If the finger stick blood sugar is over 240 mg/dl, the urine should be tested for ketones.Monitoring post-prandial (after meal) blood sugar levels gives valuable information, particularly in view of studies which have shown that post-prandial glucose levelsare more significant than fasting blood sugar levels as predictors of the long-term complications associated with diabetes.

Testing the urine for glucose has been shown to be unreliable for obtaining accurate information regarding blood sugar, because the renal threshold (the point above which the urine will contain sugar) varies from individual to individual. In children, the renal threshold is usually low. In older individuals, the renal threshold may run as high as 180 to 190 mg/dl. When the blood glucose rises to abnormally high levels, the kidneys lose the ability to recycle the sugar back into the blood stream and the sugar literally "spills" into the urine and is excreted. Although the renal threshold may vary from patient to patient, in general, the blood sugar is already too high when the urine tests are positive for glucose. For this reason, blood sugar analysis has been accepted as the only accurate way to evaluate the management of diabetes.

INTERPRETING BLOOD SUGAR READINGS

It is not a desirable practice to check the blood sugar and give a dose of regular insulin to "cover" a high reading. Checking the urine for ketones should alleviate any concern that high blood sugar heralds impending acidosis. Often, an elevated blood sugar is noted before breakfast and the diabetic patient may mistakenly take an injection of regular insulin to "cover" the elevated blood sugar.

The most common cause of a high blood sugar in the morning is related to the previous insufficient bedtime or before-dinner dose of long-acting (NPH or Lente) insulin. If this is the case, your diabetic educator or physician will adjust the bedtime dose to eliminate this problem.

An important entity to be aware of is the Somogyi Effect. This is a surge of counter-regulatory hormones to control hypoglycemia that occurs during the sleeping hours. This counter-regulatory mechanism may cause the blood sugar to soar—a rebound phenomenon that causes a marked rise in blood sugar. Those who experience a Somogyi reaction may be completely unaware of their nocturnal hypoglycemic episode. In the morning, when the blood is tested, a high level is noted, leading them to believe they may need more insulin with their evening dose. In fact, the reverse is true. People who experience high glucose levels in the morning need to test their blood sugar in the middle of the night to rule out a Somogyi Effect. This is easily done by keeping the test meter at the bedside and setting an alarm clock for 2:00 a.m. If blood glucose is falling or low, adjustments in the evening snack or insulin dose by your doctor may be in order.

A third cause of unexpected elevated blood sugars in the early morning hours is the Dawn Phenomenon. This may occur in both Type 1 and Type 2 patients. It is characterized by reduced tissue sensitivity to insulin developing between 5:00 a.m. and 8:00 a.m. This is believed to be related to spikes of growth hormone released during the night, which depress insulin activity. Again, this problem should be discussed with your physician. You may need to eat less food the night before or at breakfast. Perhaps a change in insulin dosage is in order. Notify your doctor for guidance.

Stressful life situations, too, can cause hormones to be released that can raise the blood sugar significantly. Stress is often responsible for otherwise unexplained swings in blood sugar. If an adjustment of insulin is indicated, two basic facts regarding insulin action must be considered. Regular insulin acts for about 4-6 hours after being administered, reaching its peak action in 2-4 hours. Intermediate-acting insulin (NPH or LENTE) continues to have its effect on blood sugar for 10-12 hours and has a peak activity about 6-8 hours after injection. By understanding these two fundamental facts about the action of insulin, excellent control can usually be obtained. **Always consult with your doctor if you think a change in your insulin is in order.**

Late afternoon blood sugar represents the action of intermediate insulin taken before breakfast. If the high blood sugar is persistent at a given hour, the patient must consult his doctor to make changes in the intermediate or long-acting insulin (or mixtures of insulin) rather than "treating" the high blood sugar with a dose of fast-acting regular insulin. *So-called "spikes" of sugar do not require treatment immediately with regular insulin.* If each spike is treated with insulin in this manner, the patient may find himself on a self-imposed rollercoaster ride with the sugar going up and down and out of control.

For patients using only one dose of insulin daily to control their blood sugar, before meal and bedtime testing will usually provide their doctor with adequate information to properly adjust insulin dosage.

Many physicians recommend different regimens for checking the blood sugar, depending on food intake, snacks, physical activity, school or work hours, etc.

The main goal is to keep your blood sugar within the range prescribed by your diabetic educator or physician.

For those patients who do not require insulin injections, the morning test can be helpful in estimating rises in blood sugar during the night time hours. Another finger stick an hour after dinner gives information regarding the blood sugar levels during the day.

EQUIPMENT

SMBG is now easier, essentially painless and more convenient than ever before. Thanks to the recent advances in the technology of glucometers the modern computerized hand held meters can determine the blood glucose level in less than two minutes thus enabling patients to take remedial action for unanticipated changes in the blood sugar level.

Pain is now also minimized with lancets that are made to accommodate varying thickness of skin. A laser beam has been developed that painlessly breaks the skin of the finger. The skin of the arm and thigh has fewer pain sensitive endings and these areas are utilized by the newly developed all-in-one lancets and monitors. A wristwatch style meter can detect the blood sugar through the skin and periodically report the blood sugar level. Should the blood sugar fall too low or rise too high an alarm sounds. The modern meters store results which can then be down loaded into a computer and E-mailed to the treating physician as required. There are also meters designed to accommodate people with special problems such as low visibility. Modern meters are quite accurate, but patient error in using the devices should be checked periodically in their physician's office by performing a test at the same time as the treating physician's laboratory. Inaccurate readings may result from dirty meters, outdated strips, inadequate blood or improperly calculating the meter for the tests strips employed, dirt or other substances, alcohol on the finger or a meter that is not at room temperature which can give a false reading.

The modern are pocket-sized meters have a digital readout on a small screen. If you are using a meter, follow the manufacturer's directions carefully. Most meters rely on color changes that occur when glucose comes in contact with a chemical reagent impregnated on a test strip. When the strip is inserted into the meter, the device electronically measures the color intensity, which correlates with the blood glucose level. Some of the newer models work by a process that is based on electrode sensor technology. Capillary action at the end of the test strip draws a small amount of blood into the reaction chamber and a reading is produced by an electric current which flows to the sensor. Because no blood comes in direct contact with the internal mechanism, it is not necessary to periodically clean any internal parts of meters that utilize this technology. Some meters can store the results of a large number of tests in computer memory and provide your doctor with a printed readout of the results. Common mistakes when utilizing these devices include incomplete coverage of the testing pad with blood (when required) and negligence in cleaning the meter (when required). Special glucose "control solutions" allow you to test the accuracy of the meter from time to time.

Tests with the new meters have shown them to be accurate within 10percent of commercial laboratory determinations. Generally, laboratory tests for blood sugars run about 10 percent higher than meter tests. Meter tests are performed on whole blood (plasma + red blood cells). Commercial laboratory determinations are performed on blood plasma—the liquid portion of the blood that remains after centrifuging the red cells to the bottom of the test tube. Other factors may also play a role in causing a variation in results. If the plasma is not separated from the whole blood in the laboratory fairly promptly, glucose in the blood begins to decompose and the laboratory results will be erroneously low. Comparing results between two properly functioning meters can also give different results. Some meters are designed to report results as though the sample was blood serum, while others are programmed to report values that correspond to glucose in whole blood. Most meters are well functioning devices. Problems most commonly arise from unreliable meter test strips, which may have been exposed to heat, humidity or cold.

Many different brands of meters are currently available. They are all capable of giving accurate information and good service. Some are more convenient—user friendly—while others are more complex and expensive.

Ask your doctor or diabetic educator what they recommend. If they have no personal preference you must decide for yourself which one of the products best suits your needs. Shop around before you purchase a meter. Look for a diabetes-supply house or pharmacy that will provide personal instruction in operating the instrument. When purchasing a meter, also consider test strip costs and availability.

Records of your blood sugar results should be kept and shown to your doctor during your regular visits.

EVALUATION OF LONG-TERM BLOOD SUGAR CONTROL

The Hemoglobin A₁c Test

Many diabetics mistakenly believe that a daily do-it-yourself blood sugar test is all that is required to evaluate blood sugar control. They are wrong. The daily tests provide helpful information, but tell you only about the blood sugar level at the present moment. The glycosylated hemoglobin, also called glycated hemoglobin or hemoglobin A1c (HbA1c) test serves as an indicator of long-term glucose control.

Hemoglobin, an iron containing protein pigment, is the oxygen-carrying component within the red blood cells that transports oxygen from the lungs to all parts of the body and removes carbon dioxide formed by body metabolism. Red blood cells have a life span of approximately four months. As the red blood cells mature and die, the body constantly forms new ones. At any given moment, a sample of blood will represent a collection of newly formed red blood cells, middle-aged and dying cells.

Most of the hemoglobin in the red blood cells exists in a form called Hemoglobin A. Normally, a small amount of Hemoglobin A is converted into a different form called Hemoglobin A₁c or glycosylated hemoglobin. This occurs when glucose attaches itself irreversibly to the hemoglobin inside the red blood cell. This chemical union is sometimes written in an abbreviated symbolic form, HbA₁c. The amount of glucose that becomes glycosylated depends on the amount of glucose in the blood. High levels of blood glucose sustained over time allow more glucose to become bonded to hemoglobin molecules. Thus, the percentage of hemoglobin that is glycosylated is directly related to the *time* it has been exposed to a given concentration of glucose. The practical significance of the HbA₁c is its ability to assess long-term glucose control by averaging out the peaks and valleys of blood sugar fluctuations. The HbA₁c level provides information that helps to estimate the average blood glucose level over the three month period prior to the test. Obviously, the HbA₁c level provides a better index of blood sugar control than daily or random examinations.

HbA₁c is expressed as a percentage of the total hemoglobin that has glucose attached. The normal range for the HbA₁c test is 6 percent or less. However, some diabetologists will accept somewhat higher levels (6% to 8%)

when patients begin with unusually elevated levels and find it very difficult to achieve 6 percent HbA1c levels.

An average blood sugar over a several month period of 120 mg/dl would correspond approximately to a HbA1c of 6 percent. A reading of 150 mg/dl over the same period would show a reading of about 7 percent, and 180 mg/dl would be associated with a reading in the 8 percent range. Readings between 6 percent and 7 percent are satisfactory. Readings of 8 percent or higher are considered undesirable and unacceptable.

Becton Dikinson and Co. has developed a home test kit for hemoglobin A1c that can be purchased at your local pharmacy. Two drops of blood are applied to a test strip which is then mailed to the laboratory. Results are reported to you in seven to ten days.

THE FRUCTOSAMINE TEST

The fructosamine test is a measurement of the glycation of a protein in the blood that has a shorter half-life than hemoglobin. This test can serve as an indicator for the average blood glucose level during the two to three week period prior to the test. It is particularly useful for monitoring patients with gestational diabetes and for evaluating the affect of treatment changes on glucose control. The fructosamine test can be performed quite rapidly and is less expensive than the HbA1c test. A home test kit is available for patients who wish to self-monitor their fructosamine level. In the Type 2 diabetic who takes insulin, the fructosamine test and the HbA1c level generally provide equivalent results in patients who have been stabilized.

C H A P T E R
• 13 •

Patterns of Control & Sick Day Care

Information Gleaned From Careful Records in Diary Form
When to Call Your Doctor
Sick Day Rules

T he goal of a diabetes control program is to keep blood glucose levels as close to "normal" as possible. As repeatedly emphasized throughout this book, good control reduces the risk of future diabetes complications.

Control is achieved by balancing a number of things in your life: food intake with energy expenditure (exercise/activity) and medication (if you are on insulin or oral agents). Your body and your diabetes needs change as you grow older, as your lifestyle changes, and even as you face a new activity, such as a vacation. The balance of your diabetes control plan may be upset by these changes and adjustments in food intake, exercise, and sometimes, medication, may be in order.

Control is not absolute, nor is it perfect. No one, not even the most experienced diabetes expert, can achieve perfect control of blood glucose. There will be times when some blood glucose levels are high or low. Self-monitoring of blood glucose that reveals an elevated blood sugar or one that is too low can alert you to a potentially dangerous situation, but only by documenting day-by-day changes can you gain insight into their cause. What you want to do is to be as close to satisfactory control as possible, most of the time. You also want to know when the *patterns* of blood glucose are above or below normal for a period of time. And, you want to be able to find, if possible, what causes these high or low glucose levels, so you can take action to reduce or get rid of the causes.

For you to practice *pattern* control, you need some basic tools:

• You need a diary in which you can record glucose measurements, exercise, food intake, medication, feelings and events.

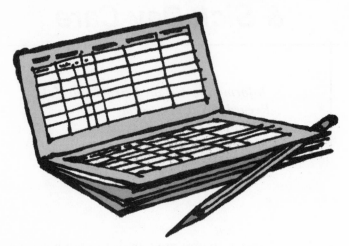

• You need a method of measuring glucose:
  1. blood glucose monitoring meter.
  2. glucose test strips
  3. ketone test strips.

You need instructions from your physician and diabetic educator on how and when to make adjustments in food, medications, and exercise, based on glucose measurements.

You need to practice *pattern* control on an ongoing basis—day by day, month by month. You will need to do regular, frequent glucose monitoring to develop information about your glucose level patterns. A single, once-a-week glucose test won't give you much information about how your glucose levels have been changing during the previous seven days. A *single* test doesn't show you a pattern, either.

When you make adjustments based on analysis of patterns, you need to be patient and realistic about the results you expect. Sometimes you can get back in good control immediately, but sometimes it may take quite a while.

HOW TO DO PATTERN CONTROL

Monitor your glucose frequently and regularly. Your monitoring schedule should be set when you discuss your management plan with your doctor or educator.

Record all test results in your diary. Take care to record these results accurately.

Write down information about food, exercise, medication and feelings.

Check your diary every day. If you have a very high or a very low reading, repeat the result and, if there is no change, call your doctor or educator.

Review the diary every three to four days. Note if there is a pattern of very high or very low sugar levels for the same time every day.

A. **Match the time with other factors such as meal time, exercise, medications or special events.**
B. **Determine if something out-of-the-ordinary occurred at these times, such as illness or severe stress.**

To be effective, pattern control requires you to record as much information as possible in your diary and record it as accurately as you can. Observations of this type will aid your physician in making appropriate changes in your regimen.

HOW THE PATTERN CONTROL WORKS

Let's suppose that two hours after the noon-time meal, for the past three days, your blood glucose has been over 200 mg/dl. In the past, they have rarely gone over 175 mg./dl in the afternoon. Your review of the PATTERN in your diary indicates that something is amiss in your control program and you know that you have to do three things to bring your blood glucose levels down into your normal range. Your choices are:

• Reduce the quantity of food for your lunchtime meal.
• Increase the time you spend on your after-lunch walking session.
• Increase (with your doctor's permission) the dose of anti-diabetic medication.

Remember, a single, high, post-meal glucose measurement may not need to be acted upon. However, a pattern of high, post-meal measurements requires changes in your management program.

Adjusting food, medication, or exercise (or a combination of these) should be decided when you discuss your program with your doctor.

Following is another example of pattern control. Let's suppose that your before-dinner blood glucose readings are in the 50-90 mg/dl range. Your review of the diary shows that you were eating the same meals and injecting the same amount of insulin each day. However, you see in your diary that on Monday, Wednesday, and Friday you participated in a new aerobic exercise program.

That pattern of low glucose readings seemed to be linked to your new exercise program. Clearly, something needs to be done to adjust to this beneficial activity without causing an insulin reaction.

Your physician may respond by recommending a larger mid-day meal, rather than changing the insulin dosage. Or, he may recommend a fruit or cheese snack before your exercise. (Carrying a candy or fruit-juice "emergency" snack with you when exercising can help prevent a hypoglycemic reaction. See Chapter 10.)

ANOTHER EXAMPLE OF PATTERN CONTROL

If the "before breakfast" glucose changes from normal to "low," that is a signal that you need to:

• Eat a bed-time snack or change the contents of your night-time snack.
• Change the dosage of the evening insulin dosage, (with your doctor's supervision).

Remember, a single low blood sugar determination may not be significant, but a pattern of low blood sugars is a clue that changes have to be made.

WHEN TO CALL YOUR DOCTOR

Call Your Doctor When:
• Any illness persists for several days
• Vomiting or diarrhea last for six hours or more
• Urinalysis for ketones shows moderate to large amounts present
• You take insulin and your blood sugar remains over 240 mg/dl despite several additional doses of regular insulin per a preplanned schedule from your doctor
• You develop hypoglycemia—blood sugar level lower than 60 mg/dl (3.3 mmol/dl)

- You have any signs of diabetic ketoacidoses
- You develop any signs of hypoglycemia
- You have Type 2 diabetes and take oral agents, and your preprandial blood sugars are over 240 mg/dl for 24 hours
- You have any signs or symptoms of hyperosmolar non-ketotic syndrome
- You have signs of extremely high blood sugar: dry mouth, dehydration, confusion or other symptoms of deterioration of mental competence

SICK DAY RULES

One of the questions commonly asked by diabetics is, "How does my diabetic program change during an illness?" The following answers most of the queries that arise during sick days:

MEALS: Stay on your regular meal plan if at all possible. In addition, drink lots of fluids—1/2 cup of calorie-free broth or water every hour during the time you are awake. If you are unable to eat regular meals, try to drink fluids containing 10g of carbohydrates *every* hour you are awake. (Drinks with 10g of carbohydrates include ½ cup regular soda, ginger ale, orange juice, or ½ cup of apple juice.)

MEDICATION: If you inject insulin, stay on your regular schedule even if you are unable to follow your regular meal plan. You may have to increase the dosage of insulin during the illness, so check with your doctor in advance to see how much and when to make an adjustment. Measure your blood glucose before making a dosage change to avoid an insulin-induced low blood sugar reaction.

If you are not taking insulin, you should also stay on your oral hypoglycemic pill to control your diabetes. Do not stop your medication even if you must change your food intake. The illness itself may be *raising* your blood sugar. Certain medications given to treat your illness may have an adverse effect on your blood sugar. This must be checked with your physician.

MONITORING: If you inject insulin, monitor your glucose levels every four hours if possible, and test your urine for ketones at intervals to avoid ketoacidosis. Call your doctor immediately if your blood glucose is very high or if you have moderate to large amounts of ketones in the urine. It is important to report vomiting episodes to your physician before dehydration occurs. If your condition worsens and you cannot reach your doctor, you should go to the nearest hospital emergency room for further advice and treatment.

It is important to continue to keep a close record of your status and additional insulin doses until you are feeling better and your glucose returns to normal.

During an illness, diabetic patients may have gastrointestinal symptoms that may cause loss of appetite, nausea, vomiting, change in bowel habits and dehydration. This may cause some patients to alter their insulin dosage for fear of low blood sugar and symptoms of hypoglycemia. It is very important *not* to change insulin or oral medications without specific advice from your doctor or diabetic educator. The reason for this is that the illness itself may be contributing to stress, causing elevation of blood glucose.

It is equally important to take enough food in the form of carbohydrate (starch or sugar) to maintain nutrition and offset any possibility of a hypoglycemic reaction caused by your usual insulin dosage regimen.

The following list of foods can substitute for each serving of starch, milk, or fruit that continue to be necessary during illnesses that have adverse effects on the gastrointestinal system:

- ½ cup of hot cereal or 1 slice of bread or toast
- 1 cup of plain yogurt or ½ cup of ice cream
- 1 cup of clear soup or ½ cup of egg nog
- 6 saltine crackers or 1/3 cup of tapioca
- 1/3 cup of fruit juice, such as grape juice, apple or cranberry juice
- 2 teaspoons of honey or 2 ½ teaspoons of sugar in a suitable liquid
- 3/4 cup of a cola drink (non-diet) or 1/3 cup regular jello

Remember that many medications can affect the blood sugar level. However, your doctor has a wide variety of drugs in his therapeutic arsenal that can bring you comfort and relief without causing marked changes in your diabetic status.

By observing these simple rules and keeping in close touch with your physician, you can maintain good control of your diabetes even in the face of unpleasant and debilitating illnesses.

C H A P T E R
• 14 •

Intensive Management of Diabetes

Affect on Vision
Renal Function
Nerve Tissue
Cardiovascular Disease

The Diabetes Control and Complications Trial (DCCT) is a clinical study conducted from 1983 to 1993 by the National Institute of Diabetes and Digestive and Kidney Diseases (NIDDK). The study showed that keeping blood sugar levels as close to normal as possible slows the onset and progression of eye, kidney, and nerve diseases caused by diabetes. In fact, it demonstrated that *any* sustained lowering of blood sugar helps, even among those with a prior history of poor control. The study compared the effects of two treatment regimens: standard therapy and intensive control on the complications of diabetes.

Intensive therapy included not only dietary control and frequent visits to the clinic, but had as its main goal the maintenance of blood glucose as close to normal as possible: between 70-120mg/dl before meals, under 180mg/dl after meals, and above 65mg/dl at three a.m. to avoid hypoglycemia. Attempts were made to keep the HbA1C below 6.1 percent. The patients were instructed to monitor blood glucose by finger-stick method four times daily.

How Did Intensive Treatment Affect Diabetic Eye Complications?

All DCCT participants were monitored for diabetic retinopathy, an eye disease that affects the retina, the light-sensing tissue at the back of the eye.

According to the National Eye Institute, one of the National Institutes of Health, as many as 24,000 persons with diabetes lose their sight each year. In the United States, diabetic retinopathy is the leading cause of blindness in adults under age 65. (See Chapter 19, *Long Term Complications of Diabetes.*)

Eye photographs were taken every six months to determine presence or absence of retinopathy. Fifteen percent of the intensive managed care patients sustained retinopathy while fifty percent of those subjects under conventional therapy were found to have retinopathy.

How Did Intensive Treatment Affect Diabetic Kidney Disease?

Participants in the DCCT were tested to assess the development of diabetic kidney disease (nephropathy). Findings showed that intensive treatment prevented the development and slowed the progression of diabetic kidney disease by 50 percent.

Diabetic kidney disease is the most common cause of kidney failure in the United States and the greatest threat to life in adults with Type 1 diabetes. After having diabetes for 15 years, one-third of people with Type 1 develop kidney disease. Diabetes damages the small blood vessels in the kidneys, impairing their ability to filter impurities from blood for excretion in the urine. Persons with severe kidney damage may require a kidney transplant or rely on dialysis to cleanse their blood.

How Did Intensive Treatment Affect Diabetic Nerve Disease?

Participants in the DCCT were examined to detect the development of nerve damage (diabetic neuropathy). Study results showed the risk of nerve damage was reduced by 60 percent in persons on intensive treatment.

Diabetic nerve disease can cause pain and loss of feeling in the feet, legs, and fingertips. It can also affect the parts of the nervous system that control blood pressure, heart rate, digestion, and sexual function. Neuropathy is a major contributing factor in foot and leg amputations among people with diabetes.

How Did Intensive Treatment Affect Diabetes-Related Cardiovascular Disease?

DCCT participants were not expected to have many heart-related problems because their average age was only 27 when the study began. Nevertheless, they underwent cardiograms, blood pressure tests, and laboratory tests of blood fat levels to look for signs of cardiovascular disease. The study proved that volunteers on intensive treatment had significantly lower risks of developing high blood cholesterol, a cause of heart disease. The risk was 35 percent lower in these volunteers, suggesting that intensive treatment can help prevent heart disease.

The average HbA1c for the conventional therapy group was 9.0, compared to 7.0 for the intensive management subjects.

What are the Risks of Intensive Treatment?

In the DCCT, the most significant side effect of intensive treatment was an increase in the risk for low blood sugar episodes—severe hypoglycemia. Because of this risk, DCCT researchers do not recommend intensive therapy for children under age 13, people with heart disease or advanced complications, older adults, and people with a history of frequent severe hypoglycemia.

Adverse effects of intensive therapy included a rather marked increase in weight in some patients, probably secondary to decreased loss of sugar in the urine due to better control, and also, an increase in food intake whenever signs or symptoms of hypoglycemia were experienced. For this reason, intensive management may not be appropriate for people with diabetes who are more than moderately overweight.

The most significant side effect of strict control of the blood sugar was the increased frequency of serious hypoglycemic episodes. The data showed a three-fold increase in serious hypoglycemic attacks when compared to those patients who remained on conventional treatment.

Hypoglycemia was considered "serious" when one of the following occurred:

1. Loss of consciousness
2. Seizure
3. Confusion requiring assistance from an outside source with immediate institution of carbohydrate or glucagon therapy

The main reasons given for choosing intensive management despite the inconveniences demanded by the regimen are as follows:

1. Difficulty in stabilizing blood sugars, causing marked variations in glucose ranging from high to low even after attempts to standardize food intake, exercise, and insulin dosage.
2. A strong desire to lower the risk of kidney, eye, nerve tissue, and cardiovascular complications.
3. An unpredictable lifestyle or occupation that makes it almost impossible to follow the same routine from day to day.

As noted, intensive therapy sets stringent goals such as fasting blood sugar 70-111mg/dl, pre-lunch and pre-supper values of 70-120mg/dl and levels of 180mg/dl one hour after meals. To avoid hypoglycemia, the blood sugar should be over 65mg/dl around 3 a.m. Also, the goal of keeping the glycohemoglobin levels within near normal range requires constant adherence to the regimen advised by the physician and diabetic educator.

There are various methods of dosing and scheduling insulin that are determined by the philosophy of the individual doctor and patient's response to different schedules. Administering regular insulin before each meal and an injection of NPH at bedtime has worked well for some patients. An alternative method is to give regular insulin before meals and one daily injection of Ultralente. A mixture of regular and NPH insulin before breakfast, regular insulin before dinner, and an injection of NPH insulin at bedtime, has also worked well for some patients.

The above regimens of insulin dosage do not take into account changes in diet, exercise, stress and other variables that will upset the predominant regular insulin dose routine.

The need to test the urine for ketones remains important not only with conventional diabetic management, but also on the intensive management program.

If you wish to follow an intensive management regimen, your physician will draw a plan for you that will recommend the insulin dosage to be injected, depending on blood glucose levels. Target blood glucose control goals with an intensive regimen will be as close to those of non-diabetics as is reasonably safe. You will want your blood sugar to be as close to normal as possible without causing excessive hypoglycemia. Careful home monitoring records must be kept to aid your physician or diabetic educator to elicit a pattern of behavior and food intake. Their relationship to your blood sugars and glycohemoglobin results will determine variations in insulin and diet changes.

The diet plans prescribed by your doctor, and given to you by a dietitian, will be tailored to your particular needs and take into account your height, weight, daily activity, exercise, lifestyle and other factors. The U.S.D.A. dietary goals recommend a variety of foods daily; maintenance of desirable weight; a diet low in fat, particularly saturated fats and cholesterol, high in vegetables, fruits and grain products; and limited use of sugar, salt, and alcohol.

When a diabetic patient makes the decision to accept the discipline, skill, and responsibilities of intensive insulin control, either by frequent daily injections of insulin or by using the insulin pump, he is making a decision that will lower the risk of diabetic complications and remove much of the fear and apprehension that often accompany the disease.

To qualify as a candidate for intensive diabetic therapy you must:

1. Be under the care of a medical team that can provide the expertise to evaluate and treat your diabetes with regular follow-up supervision.
2. Be knowledgeable about diet and weight control and have the dedication to follow the meal plan designed to avoid the weight gain that is frequently associated with intensive care.
3. Be willing to test your blood four or more times daily—indefinitely.
4. Be willing to accept the increased risk for hypoglycemic reactions.
5. Learn how to treat—or preferably—avoid hypoglycemic reactions.
6. Become knowledgeable, under the guidance of your treatment team, about adjusting insulin dosage to accommodate changes in lifestyle activities, including taking three or more insulin injections a day or keeping a subcutaneous plastic tube permanently in place to accept insulin delivery from a pump device.
7. Have the financial means or insurance to cover the added cost this regimen entails.

You are not a candidate for intensive treatment if:

1. You have heart disease or other medical conditions that could be adversely affected by a severe hypoglycemic reaction.
2. You have a history of severe hypoglycemic reactions requiring injection of glucagon or treatment in the hospital emergency room.
3. You are under seven years of age.
4. You have a drug or alcohol problem and/or you are unable to make reasonable treatment decisions in the management of your diabetes.
5. You suffer from debilitating arthritis or have a visual impairment that would interfere with your ability to perform the routine procedures required for intensive management.

DCCT researchers estimate that intensive management doubles the cost of managing diabetes because of increased visits to health care professionals and the need for more frequent blood testing at home. However, this cost is offset by the reduction in medical expenses related to long-term complications and by the improved quality of life of people with diabetes.

For the proper use of the insulin pump, the role of exercise, and the intensive management of diabetes in pregnancy, refer to the specific chapters on these subjects.

THE UNITED KINGDOM PROSPECTIVE DIABETES STUDY (UKPDS) 1977-1998

The UPKDS was a twenty year, prospective, randomized clinical study of 4,209 Type 2 diabetics, which compared the effects of intensive therapy designed to achieve tight blood sugar control to conventional therapy on the long-term complications of diabetes. Sulfonylurea drugs or insulin were found to be equally effective in reducing microvascular complications, primarily retinopathy and microalbuminuria (indicative of nephropathy). The study demonstrated that agressive control of blood pressure did reduce the incidence of strokes and progression of retinopathy as well as overall diabetes related mortality. Although the study left some questions unanswered, it clearly demonstrated that Type 2 patients could avoid or delay the progression of many of the long-term complications of Type 2 diabetes.

C H A P T E R
• 15 •

The Insulin Pump

Advantages Over Conventional Treatment
Description of Equipment & Maintenance
Getting Started

T he Diabetes Control and Complications Trial (DCCT) clearly demonstrated the link between the poor control of diabetes and the eventual development of chronic and disabling complications, including heart disease, neuropathy, visual loss and kidney disease. (See Chapter 14, *Intensive Management of Diabetes*.)

Present day treatment of Type 1 diabetes includes home glucose monitoring, mixed insulins taken at least two times a day, strict adherence to nutrition and proper hygiene, and adequate exercise.

Despite dramatic progress in the development and availability of new forms of insulin, tight control is rarely achieved. Patients who cannot achieve "rigid" control with standard treatment measures can avail themselves of a battery operated insulin infusion pump, an alternative form of treatment that more closely mimics the body's normal release of insulin to synchronize changing requirements. The pump is ideally suited for those who wish to maintain tight control of their diabetes with an intensive treatment regimen.

The pump offers advantages over multiple daily injections of Regular insulin by allowing some freedom from rigid estimations of food intake, sleep, and exercise schedules.

Pump devices provide a constant infusion of "basal" insulin, and are devised to inject a "bolus" of insulin to match carbohydrate consumption at mealtimes. They also permit an adjustment of insulin dosage immediately in response to finger-stick glucose determinations. Pumps offer the optimal regulation of the blood sugar presently available. Currently, pumps are manufactured by two companies, Mini Med and Diseetronic Medical Systems.

Settings are based on frequent finger-stick blood glucose determinations. The pump delivers a continuous amount of insulin at a "basal" rate of 0.5 to 2 units per hour, simulating the body's normal around-the-clock secretion of insulin. The patient is able to program a lower basal rate at night when blood glucose levels tend to be lowest, and a higher rate during the three to four hours before breakfast when the blood sugars have a tendency to rise (the "dawn" phenomenon). Pumps are equipped with safety features that warn the user if the insulin level is low or absent, the batteries are low, or the pump is malfunctioning. To guard against the distinct danger of hypoglycemia, which could occur if too much insulin were accidentally released by the pump, an automatic shut off valve is a standard feature of the currently available pump models.

The most important reason for an insulin dependent diabetic to "go on the pump" is to prevent or delay the serious long-term complications of diabetes, avoid wide fluctuations in blood sugar, provide flexibility in time and size of meals, and easily compensate for increased levels of physical activities. Those who use the pump believe they are availing themselves of the state-of-the-art technique that closely simulates nature's own way of regulating glucose metabolism. Special instructions are needed for showering, bathing, sleeping and sexual activity. The patient can be "off the pump" for varying periods of time, provided he takes the necessary precautions and is well-versed in his diabetes management.

Carbohydrate, fat, and protein all have impact on blood sugar levels; however, the effect of fat and protein is delayed. Carbohydrate intake is the major factor raising blood glucose levels. Patients are instructed to program the insulin pump, depending on the amount of carbohydrate consumed, intensity of physical activity, finger-stick blood glucose levels and usual daily needs.

Pumps are worn outside the body, weigh less than four ounces, and are about the size of a pager. A length of plastic tubing connects the pump (containing a reservoir of insulin) to a fine needleless infusion catheter that remains in place under the skin of the abdomen.

The main advantage of pump therapy is that it allows the patient to achieve a degree of metabolic control improbable with conventional therapy. The most reliable index of the efficacy of this form of treatment is the level of glycosylated hemoglobin (HbA_1c) and other parameters of satisfactory glucose control such as improvement in blood lipids.

There are special considerations associated with pump therapy that must be acceptable to the patient before he/she can be considered a serious candidate for this alternative to multiple daily injections of insulin.

To be considered as a candidate for the pump, a diabetic patient must:

1. Have the discipline, skill and determination to perform finger-stick blood determination testing four or more times a day.
2. Be willing to tolerate the inconvenience of wearing the pump.
3. Accept the burden of making adjustments in the microprocessor of the pump depending on food intake, physical activity, stress, travel and other unforeseen radical changes in everyday activities.
4. Use conscientious sterile technique.
5. Have family and peer support.
6. Have the resources for the substantial initial financial outlay (over $4000) to purchase the pump and ability to achieve the proper education to use it.
7. Be aware that infection of the infusion site, serious enough to require antibiotic medication, may occur periodically. The incidence of this side effect can be reduced by changing the infusion site every two or three days.
8. Realize that monitoring blood sugar closely is mandatory because a malfunctioning or pump failure will stop insulin delivery, causing a rapid rise of blood glucose and the possibility of ketoacidosis.

Patients on the pump have to concern themselves with maintaining batteries, checking the infusion catheters, carrying out meticulous skin care and staying in close touch with their physician and diabetic educator for changes required for "sick days," emergencies such as unusually high or low blood sugars and radical alterations in life style. Fortunately, modern pumps are electronic marvels. They beep when clogged, signal when batteries are low, and have built-in fail-safe mechanisms to prevent an accidental overage.

The fine control afforded by the pump seems to offer the type of blood glucose control required to prevent the destructive effect of elevated blood sugars. However, even after a substantial investment of money and time with trainers in the use of the pump, there is a moderately high "drop-out" rate.

GETTING STARTED

The medical team, specially trained in pump therapy, will begin the pump-diabetic patient on a temporary basal rate, food intake, and insulin reduction rate. Each formula is based on height, weight, and lifestyle. After experimentation with the beginning formula provided by the diabetic instructor, the patient calculates how his body is reacting to the prescribed diet, insulin and exercise regimens. There will be times that the sugar appears out of control, causing frustration and disappointment.

If the pump is not functioning correctly, an alarm will sound. Occasionally, the batteries will need to be changed or the tube may be dislodged from its place beneath the skin. A visit to the doctor will help in getting back "on track."

The normal non-diabetic eats three meals a day and returns his blood glucose level to normal within three hours. This means that the body is exposed for only nine hours out of twenty four to elevated blood glucose. Without the meticulous control provided by the pump, the diabetic's post-meal sugars would be "high" at least twelve to fourteen hours a day, contributing over many years to the progressive degenerative changes involving the eyes, kidneys, cardiovascular system and nerve tissue.

Starches are complex carbohydrates that will raise the blood sugar within a two hour period after eating. This requires enough insulin to bring the sugar to near normal as rapidly as possible. This can be done with greater facility with the pump. Protein does not impact the blood sugar as rapidly as carbohydrate because only about 58 percent is converted into glucose after digestion and its glucose raising effect may be prolonged until 4-6 hours after eating.

Only 10 percent of fat is generally converted into sugar; therefore larger amounts of fat are required to have any significant effect on blood sugar. Additionally, fat takes as long as 10-12 hours to manifest its effect. The blood should be checked two hours after a complex meal consisting of varying amounts of carbohydrate, protein and fat. A reducing dose of insulin should be administered via the pump if indicated by the results of the test. The basal rate can also be changed if the blood sugar remains elevated, indicating a rise due to the protein and fat content of the meal. Patients will learn by practice how much insulin is necessary to maintain blood sugar in the 120 mg/dl level by manipulation of the amounts of insulin delivered by the pump. Blood sugar levels as high as 160 mg/dl can be tolerated without drastic changes in the usual insulin regimen.

The basal rate (the amount of insulin needed per hour to maintain an acceptable blood glucose) can be determined by experimentation and close cooperation with the diabetic educator and physician. Some patients require one unit of insulin for every 10 grams of carbohydrate. Others may need .05 units or 1.5 units. This can only be determined by careful record keeping and frequent comparisons of food intake and insulin requirements. One cannot expect 100 percent accuracy by this method. Therefore, constant guidance by your instructor is mandatory. The ideal formula for obtaining the correct balance of food and insulin while on the pump demands understanding the carbohydrate/insulin ratio, deliberate diet planning and exercise routines. If these vary to any significant extent, the change in blood glucose and insulin requirements will become apparent within a short period of time.

Once you have estimated your basal rate and required boluses of insulin before meals, you may dispense with some of the finger-stick tests. It is important to rotate sites of finger-stick pricking to avoid sore fingers.

If blood glucose levels are unexplainably high when using the insulin pump, the following factors must be checked:

- Was the pump primed with insulin when a new cartridge was inserted?
- Has the insulin been stored properly? Has it expired?
- Is the needle properly positioned in place or is insulin leaking around the needle?
- Are there any signs of infection around the injection site?
- Is the basal rate properly set? Is there an adequate amount of insulin in the cartridge?

There are many patients who have mastered the use of the pump who agree with their diabetologists that they have achieved the reward of optimal diabetic control as well as a more flexible lifestyle. This in turn gives them confidence and the satisfaction of knowing that the special demands of living with the pump are well worth the effort.

C H A P T E R
• 16 •

Obesity and Diabetes

How Obesity is Measured
Causes of Obesity
Importance of Weight Control
Treatment of Obesity

The vast majority of diabetics have Type 2 diabetes (85-90 percent). The relationship of obesity to Type 2 diabetes has been clearly established. Medical research has also shown that the susceptibility to disease and early mortality is considerably higher among those who are significantly overweight. *An amazing fact is that weight reduction would allow 75 percent of Type 2 diabetics to discontinue their oral medications and would lower the blood pressure of most hypertensives.*

Obesity, which is epidemic in America today, may be defined simply as an excess accumulation of body fat. The exact physical criteria of obesity are not always clear. Variations exist between different cultures, ethnic groups, and even historic time frames. In Western nations, and particularly in the United States, the idealized image for both men and women includes a slender appearance. This concept has been abetted by the fashion world with the aid of an American diet market that records billions of dollars in gross sales annually from such weight loss related activities and products as low calorie foods and soft drinks, diet books, appetite suppressant drugs, medical and non-medical weight loss "clinics," and health spas. Unfortunately, the results of this tremendous expenditure has not slowed the increased incidence of either obesity or diabetes.

The vast majority of people with Type 2 diabetes are obese when first diagnosed. Fifty percent of the American population is considered obese by the currently accepted standards of measurement. Twenty-five to thirty percent have significant obesity—usually defined as 20 percent above the upper normal limit of the theoretical ideal weight as given on the generally accepted actuarial weight charts.

HOW IS OBESITY MEASURED?

"Obesity" is one of those words that has one meaning to the public and a more precise one to the medical world. To most people, to be obese means to be considerably overweight. To doctors and scientists, however, a person can be classified as obese even if the degree to which he or she is overweight is not very great. "Overweight" refers to body weight in excess of the normal range that includes all tissues—muscle, bone, and fat—as well as water. **"Obesity" refers specifically to having excess body fat.** One can be overweight without being obese: a body builder who has a large muscle mass, for example, would be classified as overweight according to the tables, although he or she is not obese. **For practical purposes, however, most people who are overweight are also obese.**

Everyone needs a certain amount of body fat for stored energy, heat insulation, shock absorption, and to support organs and other functions. As a rule, women have more fat than men. Doctors generally agree that men with more than 25 percent body fat and women with more than 30 percent body fat are obese. Measuring a person's body fat precisely, however, is not easy. The most accurate method is to weigh a person under water, an impractical procedure limited to laboratories with sophisticated equipment.

There are two simpler, but less reliable, methods for estimating body fat. One is to measure skinfold thickness with a special type of caliper in several parts of the body. The second involves sending a harmless electric current through a person's body (bio-electric impedance analysis). Both methods are commonly used in health clubs and in commercial weight-loss programs, but results should be viewed skeptically.

Because measuring a person's body fat is not easily performed, doctors often rely on other means to diagnose obesity. Two widely used measurements are weight-for-height tables and body mass index. While both measurements have their limitations, they are reliable indicators that someone may have a weight problem. They are easy to calculate and require no special equipment.

Weight-for-Height Tables

Most people are familiar with weight-for-height tables. Doctors have used these tables for decades to determine whether a person is overweight.

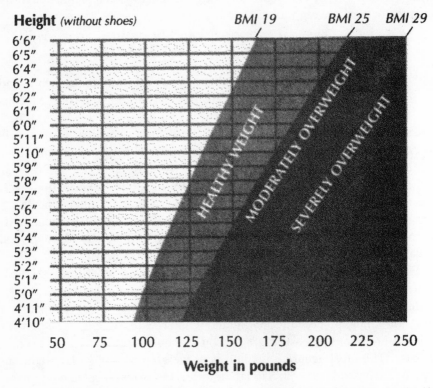

From the Dietary Guidelines for Americans, a pamphlet printed jointly by the U.S. Departments of Agriculture and Health and Human Services. This table has a wide range for what the pamphlet designates as "healthy" or "suggested" weights. In this table, the higher weights generally apply to men, who have more muscle and bone.

One problem with using weight-for-height tables is that doctors disagree over which is the best table to use. Many versions are available, all with different weight ranges. Some tables take a person's frame size, age, and sex into account; others do not. A limitation of all weight-for-height tables is that they do not distinguish excess fat from muscle. Still, weight-for-height tables can be used as general guidelines.

Body Mass Index (BMI)

Body mass index (BMI) is a new term to most people. However, it is the measurement of choice for many physicians and researchers studying obesity. BMI uses a mathematical formula that takes into account both a person's height and weight. BMI equals a person's weight in kilograms divided by height in meters squared. ($BMI = Kg/m^2$). The table printed here has already done the math and metric conversions. To use the table, find the appropriate weight in the left-hand column. Move across the row to the given height. The number at the point of intersection is the BMI for that height and weight.

BODY MASS INDEX (BMI), kg/m²						
			Height (feet, inches)			
Wt (lbs)	5'0"	5'3"	5'6"	5'9"	6'0"	6'3"
140	27	25	23	21	19	18
150	29	27	24	22	20	19
160	31	28	26	24	22	20
170	33	30	28	25	23	21
180	35	32	29	27	25	23
190	37	34	31	28	26	24
200	39	36	32	30	27	25
210	41	37	34	31	29	26
220	43	39	36	33	30	28
230	45	41	37	34	31	29
240	47	43	39	36	33	30
250	49	44	40	37	34	31

In general, a person age 35 or older is obese if he or she has a BMI of 27 or more. For people age 34 or younger, a BMI of 25 or more indicates obesity. A BMI of more than 30 usually is considered a sign of severe obesity. The BMI measurement poses some of the same problems as the weight-for-height tables. Doctors don't agree on the exact cutoff points for "healthy" versus "unhealthy" BMI ranges. However, like the weight-for-height table, BMI is a useful general guideline.

The BMI, however, does not tell the whole story. It does not provide information on a person's percentage of body fat. Where fat is stored—the type of fat distribution—is also important. The so-called "apple" shape, with greater girth to the abdomen than the hips, is caused by fat deposits deep within the abdomen—beneath the muscle and between the abdominal organs. Even thin "apples" run the same risk as obese "apples" because this type of fat poses a special risk for cardiovascular disease and diabetes. This so-called visceral, or intra-abdominal, fat usually results from an inherited genetic predisposition.

Men generally are more prone to this problem than women. Alcohol (the "beer belly"), smoking and stress also increase the likelihood of visceral fat deposits.

Visceral fat is deadlier than the ordinary fat which is deposited beneath the skin throughout the body. Both types of fat contain glycerol and fatty acids. However, the metabolism of the visceral fat is more active, releasing and picking up fatty acids from the bloodstream at a high rate. It is believed that the elevated levels of fatty acids increase LDL-cholesterol synthesis in the liver.

Exercise-induced weight loss has a remarkable effect on visceral fat. Even a loss of only ten to twenty pounds can produce a significant decrease in insulin resistance as well as reducing the overall risk for cardiovascular disease.

Stress also plays a role in visceral fat deposition. Emotional stress prompts the adrenal glands to secrete the hormone cortisol, which promotes fat deposition. Furthermore, cortisol induced fat deposition is most likely to occur within the abdominal cavity. Thus, stress not only raises blood sugar levels, but also adversely affects lipid metabolism.

WHAT CAUSES OBESITY?

In scientific terms, obesity occurs when a person's calorie intake exceeds the amount of energy burned—from eating more than is needed to meet the body's energy needs. What causes this imbalance between calorie consumption and burning is unclear. There are no simple explanations for obesity nor are there simple solutions. Evidence suggests obesity often has more than one cause. Genetic, environmental, psychological and other factors all may play a part.

The human body has approximately 35 billion fat cells that serve as storage depots. When the caloric content of your diet is greater than your immediate needs, the excess is converted into fat and stored away for future use. The body has an almost unlimited capacity to store fat. When you cut back your daily caloric intake by 500 calories, you will lose 1 pound per week. While rapid weight loss may be exciting, losing weight slowly and steadily—one or two pounds per week—is the safer and more effective way to shed pounds.

Genetic Factors (Leptin)

Obesity tends to run in families, suggesting that it may have a genetic cause. However, family members share not only genes but also diet and lifestyle habits that may contribute to obesity. Separating these lifestyle factors from genetic ones is often difficult. Still, growing evidence points to heredity as a strong determining factor of obesity. In one study of adults who were adopted as children, researchers found that the subjects' adult weights were closer to their biological parents' weights than that of their adoptive parents. The environment provided by the adoptive family apparently had less influence on the development of obesity than the person's genetic makeup.

Leptin, a newly discovered hormone has shown remarkable effects on hereditary obesity in laboratory animals. We now know that certain mice, as well as humans, have hereditary deficiencies of leptin, predisposing them to obesity. This hormone acts in an area of the brain called the hypothalamus, to control appetite as well as energy expenditure.

A recent article in the *New England Journal of Medicine* described a nine year old girl with excessive weight gain and obesity in association with very low levels of leptin. (This patient also had two cousins with undetectable leptin levels in their blood.) She was treated with injections of leptin over a twelve month period during which time she lost 16.4 kg at the rate of 1-2 kg per month. A marked change in the patient's eating behavior and loss of fatty tissue occurred in association with her weight loss.

Continued intensive research with leptin may lead to further understanding of the genetic causes of obesity and insulin resistance, and open doors to new effective treatments for obesity.

Nevertheless, people who feel that their genes have doomed them to a lifetime of obesity should take heart. As will be discussed later, a genetic predisposition to obesity can be countered.

Environmental Factors

Although genes play an important role in some cases of obesity, a person's environment also plays a significant role. Environment includes lifestyle behaviors such as what a person eats and how active he or she is.

Americans tend to consume high-fat diets, often putting taste and convenience ahead of nutritional content when choosing meals. Most Americans also don't get enough exercise.

People can't change their genetic makeup, of course, but they can change what they eat and how active they are. Some people have been able to lose weight and keep it off with the help of a nutritionist by:

- Learning how to choose more nutritious meals that are lower in fat.
- Learning behavior modification such as shopping habits and recognizing environmental cues (such as enticing smells) that may make them want to eat when they are not hungry.
- Learning techniques of portion control.
- Becoming more physically active.
- Learning how to choose more nutritious foods that are lower in fat.
- Minimizing the simple sugar content of the diet.
- Learning how to prepare food to save calories without sacrificing taste.

Psychological Factors

Psychological factors also may influence eating habits. Many people eat in response to negative emotions such as boredom, sadness or anger.

While most obese people have no more psychological disturbance than normal weight people, about 30 percent of the people who seek treatment for serious weight problems have difficulties with binge eating. Binge eating episodes are characterized by eating large amounts of food with loss of control over how much they are eating. Those with a severe binge eating disorder may have more difficulty losing weight and keeping the weight off than people without binge eating problems. Special measures, such as counseling or medication, to control binging can help to successfully manage this problem.

OTHER CAUSES OF OBESITY

In review, obesity is caused by consuming more calories than the body expends to meet its physiological needs or not expending enough energy to burn up the caloric content of the diet which exceeds the body's needs. Additional elements that are more obscure but that have been shown to play important roles in obesity are:

1. Individual variations in the "appetite control center" in the hypothalamic area of the brain that functions as a sort of satiety thermostat. These variations may be genetic or acquired.

2. The level of fat in the diet itself. Weight loss is facilitated by diets low in

fat even though the total caloric intake may be the same as a comparable diet with a higher fat content. Over the past eighty years the typical American diet has changed. Currently diets contain decreasing amounts of complex carbohydrates and increased amounts of fat. This is a consequence of lifestyle changes which have moved away from nutritious home meals high in complex carbohydrates, to high caloric, high fat, often pre-packaged, or "fast food" items.

3. Eating patterns can contribute to obesity. Skipping breakfast and consuming most of the daily caloric intake with the evening meal can lead to obesity. People who skip meals burn fewer calories than those who divide their daily intake into three or more separate meals.

4. Chronic dieting! Chronic dieting has been shown to lead to a reduction in basal metabolic rate. Chronic dieters have basal metabolic rates 10-20 percent below normal. Additionally, because the metabolic rate and caloric needs decline with weight loss, the task of shedding weight becomes more difficult the longer one is on a diet. When normal caloric intake is resumed, weight gain actually occurs easier than before.

5. Obesity itself. Data from the National Health and Nutrition Examination Survey substantiated   the claim of many obese people who insist they do not eat more than their lean counterparts. The results showed an inverse relationship between BMI and mean caloric intake required to maintain weight. Obese people tend to be less active than non-obese people. If caloric intake remains unchanged, increased activity or exercise is the only way to lose weight. Modest increases in physical activity seem to suppress appetite. However, marked increases of physical activity may stimulate appetite and caloric intake, although usually not to the extent of the additional calories expended.

6. Aging and accompanying inactivity. Basal metabolic caloric requirements gradually decrease with age, although appetite may remain unchanged as we grow older. A continued unchanged caloric intake without increased physical activity and exercise to burn any excess fuel beyond metabolic needs tips the balance toward obesity.

Some rare disorders can cause obesity. These include hypothyroidism, Cushing's syndrome, and certain neurologic problems that can lead to overeating. Certain drugs, such as steroids and some antidepressants, may cause excessive weight gain. Your doctor can determine if you have any of these conditions, which are believed to be responsible for only about one percent of all cases of obesity.

WHAT ARE THE CONSEQUENCES OF OBESITY?

Health Risks

Obesity is not just a cosmetic problem. It's a health hazard with a legion of dangers, many of which are life threatening. Someone who is 40 percent overweight is twice as likely than an average-weight person to die prematurely. (This effect is seen after 10 to 30 years of being obese). Obesity has been linked to serious medical conditions, including not only diabetes, but heart disease, high blood pressure, and stroke. It is also associated with higher rates of certain types of cancer. Obese men are more likely than non-obese men to die from cancer of the colon, rectum, and prostate. Obese women are more likely than non-obese women to die from cancer of the gallbladder, breast, uterus, cervix, and ovaries. Other diseases and health problems linked to obesity include:

- Gallbladder disease and gallstones.
- Osteoarthritis, a disease in which the joints deteriorate, possibly as a result of excess weight on the joints.
- Gout (another disease affecting the joints).
- Varicose veins.
- Blood clots in the deep veins of the lower extremities.
- Dyslipidemia (elevated levels of cholesterol and triglycerides in the blood).
- Pulmonary problems, including sleep apnea, in which a person can stop breathing for a short time during sleep.
- High blood pressure and heart disease.

Doctors generally agree that the more obese a person is, the more likely he or she is to have health problems. Even a loss of only 10 or 15 pounds can have a significant affect on blood glucose levels. After successful weight reduction, there is marked improvement in glucose tolerance and many Type 2 diabetics see their blood glucose levels return to normal.

Psychological and Social Effects

One of the most painful aspects of obesity may be the emotional suffering it causes. American society places great emphasis on physical appearance, often equating attractiveness with slimness, especially in women.

Many people assume that obese people are gluttonous, lazy, or both. However, more and more evidence contradicts this assumption.

Obese people often face prejudice or discrimination at work, at school, while looking for a job, and in social situations. Feelings of rejection, shame, or depression are common.

WHICH DIETS REALLY WORK?

A whole spectrum of "weight control" advice is offered in newspaper articles, television commercials, and magazines. Most fad diets lack scientific justification for their claims. Some are nutritionally unsound, lacking in essential nutrients, and potentially dangerous. Anecdotal testimonials from those who have used a weight control program with good results are of no scientific value. Even diets that are unsound physiologically often enjoy great popularity and do not lack enthusiastic supporters ready to proclaim their merits. Furthermore, chronic use of low calorie diets may actually lead to "binging."

Over the short term, results may be achieved with almost any approach that focuses attention on diet and exercise, particularly in a group setting where peer pressure and encouragement from an advisor help to motivate an individual to restrict caloric intake and to increase caloric expenditure with an exercise regimen. However, the only success that counts is long-term success. And long-term success can be accomplished only with lifestyle modifications that the dieter is willing to incorporate into his/her life on a permanent basis.

Many diets, particularly those that cause a rapid weight loss, achieve their dramatic initial results because of water loss. For every gram of stored glycogen or protein that is hydrolyzed for energy, three grams of water are released. This explains the initial "success" of many commercial weight loss programs. Two-thirds of this weight loss is water, not fat. Following prolonged dieting, physical changes occur in the body that promote sodium and fluid retention. When caloric intake is again increased, rehydration associated with a rapid weight gain occurs.

Severe calorie restriction diets should never be recommended unless there is some medical emergency such as markedly impaired cardio-pulmonary function, poorly controlled diabetes, poorly controlled high blood pressure, and perhaps "sleep apnea." *A general rule for safe dieting is to not restrict caloric intake below 10 calories per pound of body weight a day.*

THE PHYSIOLOGY OF NUTRITION

Understanding the basic physiology of nutrition enables one to make informed decisions about the dietary management of obesity.

Carbohydrates come in two forms: simple carbohydrates (such as sugar) and complex carbohydrates (fruits, vegetables, and grains).

Complex carbohydrates must be broken down to their simple sugars by enzymes in the gastrointestinal track before they can be utilized for energy or stored for later use. The excess remaining beyond immediate needs is converted to glycogen and stored primarily in the muscles and liver. Some may be converted to fat and stored in fatty tissue.

Simple carbohydrates (candy, for instance) are rapidly absorbed into the bloodstream, causing a brisk rise in blood sugar. This rapid rise in the non-diabetic is often followed by a dip in the blood sugar level, causing a recurrence of hunger. With diabetes, the rise in blood sugar is more sustained.

The complex carbohydrates take a longer time to break down into simple sugars and therefore enter the bloodstream at a slower rate with less impact on the blood glucose level.

Proteins are the building blocks of all of the organs and muscles of the body and are complex molecules made up of long chains of amino acids. Dietary proteins must be broken down to their amino acid constituents by digestive enzymes before they can enter the bloodstream. Amino acids are essential raw materials needed for the repair, maintenance, and growth of body tissues. Excess amino acids beyond the body's immediate needs can be converted into glucose for fuel or into fat for storage. Nitrogen containing by-products are produced from these metabolic conversion processes. These nitrogenous wastes are excreted by healthy kidneys. If there is renal disease or insufficiency, these nitrogen products build up in the blood and cause a serious medical condition called uremia.

Fat plays an important role in normal metabolism and is essential for survival. It supports the internal organs of the body as well as insulating them. Fat is also an important constituent of the outer membranes of cells. Fat is an efficient form of energy storage for the body, which makes it easy to accumulate and difficult to remove. Only by reducing caloric intake below body requirements will the body utilize stored fat for energy. To lose one pound of body fat per week, dietary caloric intake must be 500 calories per day less than needed.

Fat supplies nine calories per gram, whereas carbohydrate and protein provide only four calories per gram. Most tissues will use or prefer to use carbohydrates to provide their energy needs.

The American Diabetes Association (ADA) diet is simply a well-balanced diet that meets the nutritional needs of the diabetic as well as the non-diabetic. The standard ADA diet has been modified in recent years by reducing the fat content and increasing the fiber content, as research has shown the benefits of these changes for improving blood lipid levels as well as decreasing the odds against certain cancers.

To achieve long-term weight loss requires a change in dietary habits. The advice and guidance of a trained dietician combined with long-term follow-up can improve the odds of success. Eating habits and behavioral characteristics have to be altered and maintained in conjunction with a well-planned exercise regimen. Obesity is a chronic disease which requires long-term support and guidance to be treated successfully.

Many obese individuals give a history of being slender until middle age, when creeping weight gain began. Progressive weight gain of approximately five to ten pounds per year continues in those who are destined to become obese.

A plethora of contradictory dietary advice has left many people confused about weight loss regimens. There are only three different types of food stuffs; therefore, all diets are a result of various combinations of proteins, carbohydrates, and fats. High fiber content in the diet, derived from complex carbohydrate—vegetables, legumes, and whole grains—is beneficial because it adds bulk and the advantage of requiring a longer time to be chewed, thus prolonging the meal. Additionally, the fiber may contribute to the sense of satiety without adding calories by retaining water, which swells the fiber, producing a greater sense of fullness. In other words, some foods are more filling than others, even though they may contain the same number of calories. Many people complain that high-fiber diets are bland and tasteless. However, dieters can learn to prepare palatable high fiber complex carbohydrate meals from their dietician or from any of the many high fiber cook books available in book stores.

Formula diets depend on limited quantities of nutrients, often in the form of canned liquids, which are designed to contain minerals and vitamins in a protein-rich formula. These types of products are probably most useful when the formula is substituted for breakfast and/or lunch in conjunction with a low calorie evening meal. Some patients need the rigidity and discipline of a very specific restricted diet plan for long-term success.

ANORECTICS (APPETITE SUPPRESSING DRUGS)

Phenylpropanolamine and ephedrine are the main over-the-counter diet medications currently available. These drugs are only minimally effective as anorectics and carry the side effect risk of elevation of blood pressure, which can cause cardiovascular events, including strokes.

For many years, drug treatment for obesity included amphetamines. These drugs were potent anorectics, but had undesirable side effects including elevation of blood pressure, a rapid heart rate, nervousness, sweating, anxiety, and a marked propensity to cause addiction. They are no longer recommended nor are they approved for the treatment of obesity.

Serotonin is a naturally occurring substance that plays a key role in transmitting messages in the brain. Anorectic drugs that work by altering serotonin activity are called serotonin re-uptake inhibitors. Drugs in this class have proven effective, at least in the short term, in promoting weight loss. The serotonin re-uptake inhibitors are recommended only for people with significant obesity—those with a BMI of 30 or higher, or 27 or higher if there are associated health risk factors such as diabetes, high blood pressure or dyslipidemia.

The only serotonin re-uptake inhibitor currently on the market is Sibutramine (Meridia®). Like its predecessors, this drug is recommended only for those with a BMI greater than 30, or 27 if additional risk factors are present. The main significant side effect of Meridia® is seizures. Any serotonin activity altering drug has the potential to impair judgment, thinking and motor skills. It also increases the risk of developing primary pulmonary hypertension (PPH), a serious and often fatal disorder. This illness occurs in the general population at a rate estimated to be one or two cases per one million persons yearly. There does not appear to be a significant increase in the incidence of PPH in those who take the drug for short periods—three months or less. However, longer use increases the risk. The longer one stays on the drug, the greater the danger of this dreaded complication. Admittedly, the incidence of PPH is very low, even with the serotonin re-uptake inhibitors. However, if you are the one afflicted with PPH, your weight loss program could prove to be a fatal therapeutic misadventure. It is wise to limit the use of any of the anorectics. Those who choose to go on anorectic drugs must remain on guard against PPH, and report any signs of its development to their physician. The initial symptoms are usually shortness of breath, angina (chest discomfort from coronary artery insufficiency), fainting and sometimes lower extremity edema (swelling of the legs). Unfortunately, once symptoms become apparent, treatment is not always successful.

The main question to be decided is, "Are anorectic drugs effective in the long-term for most people?" Obese adults who seek medical help for weight loss, who are given dietary management instruction and anorectic medication, do lose more weight than those treated with placebo and diet, at least in the short-term. *The difference in weight loss between the drug treated patients and those receiving placebo and dietary instruction is, however, only minimal and often only a fraction of a pound per week.* The rate of weight loss is greatest in most trial studies for both drug and placebo treated subjects during the first few weeks and usually decreases in succeeding weeks.

The average weight loss with various anorectic drugs varies from trial to trial and is undoubtedly influenced by such factors as the specific dietary regimen prescribed, the patient's physician or nutrition counselor relationship, and the population group under study.

LONG-TERM STRATEGIES

Obesity usually develops gradually over the years. Successful treatment must also be long-term and involves changes in eating habits and lifestyle that promote gradual weight loss. Losing pounds is just the beginning. Adherence to a new regimen to insure maintenance of the pounds shed requires you to be prepared to follow an intelligent approach to nutrition and physical activity that will remain with you for the rest of your life.

Before making a serious commitment to a weight reduction diet and exercise program, you should have a complete medical exam by your physician. He will check your heart, blood pressure, and look for any contraindications to your anticipated exercise and dietary regimen. In the beginning, you will feel satisfaction as your weight declines. If you relapse, you may feel anguish and depression. Be prepared for these mixed emotions. Conquering your obesity and lowering the risk for all the possible medical disorders associated with excessive weight will raise your self-esteem and bring about a "good feeling" that you may not have had for years. There will be no more self-pity, resentment, or guilt feelings toward food, and most importantly, your diabetes will be much easier to control as insulin resistance declines and blood sugar levels decrease and possibly return to normal.

It is difficult to achieve normal body weight without a great deal of introspection, self-discipline, motivation, and reinforcement of self-esteem. One must realize that obesity is a chronic disease not unlike high blood pressure or diabetes.

Attempting to lose weight with the latest "fad" diet will not work. Skipping meals and "bingeing" later will not work. If you are obese you must accept an intelligent, nutritious diet plan, adopt a daily exercise routine, and remain on this regimen for the rest of your life. Your health and your appearance will make it all worthwhile.

C H A P T E R
• 17 •

Benefits of Exercise

Beneficial Effects on Metabolism
Medical Clearance for Exercise
Appropriate Exercise Programs

A lthough most people are aware that regular exercise is important, in today's society, especially in "advanced" western nations like the United States, the general population has become more sedentary— riding in cars to school or work, sitting at desks, using elevators instead of stairs, and relying on an ever expanding number of labor-saving applicances to make life easier. And let's not forget the couch potato sitting in front of the television, munching on snacks and operating the remote control.

More than half of all Americans are overweight. As we saw in Chapter 16, *Obesity and Diabetes*, non-diabetic obese persons may have normal or even elevated blood insulin levels, but physiologically there is a relative lack of insulin because of the increased insulin resistance associated with obesity. Inasmuch as insulin resistance is the main metabolic defect in Type 2 diabetes, obesity sets the stage for the development of diabetes in those predisposed to the disease, and it contributes to the severity of the disorder in those who have diabetes.

While diet and achievement of normal body weight is often considered the main lifestyle modification goal in the treatment of Type 2 diabetes, the other equally important half of the lifestyle equation is exercise and physical training.

Physical activity has a direct beneficial affect on insulin cell receptors—receptor affinity and numbers—thus helping to overcome insulin resistance. Aerobic exercise, the kind that gets your heart beating more rapidly and your breathing deeper, has benefits for everyone, but it is especially important for the diabetic, in whom it plays a critical role in improving glucose regulation. *Physical activity alone, even in the absence of weight loss, can significantly improve glucose tolerance.*

Other benefits of exercise, besides aiding in weight loss or maintaining weight, include increasing the energy level, lowering high blood pressure, increasing the efficiency of the respiratory and cardiovascular system, and raising the HDL-cholesterol. Aerobic exercise strengthens heart muscle and improves the blood lipid profile which helps to fight cholesterol plaque build-up. It also decreases irritability of the nerves controlling the heart rhythm. A daily exercise routine reduces stress and imparts a sense of well being that many patients feel is important in their everyday activities.

A regular exercise regimen combined with a healthy diet has enabled many Type 2 diabetes patients to discontinue taking their diabetes control medications or has, at least, been responsible for a marked reduction in the dosage needed to control their blood sugar.

MEDICAL CLEARANCE FOR EXERCISE

Before beginning an exercise program, a thorough check-up, including a cardiovascular assessment by your doctor, is necessary. He will evaluate your physical status and prescribe the proper amount and types of exercise on an individual basis. An examination of your heart, eyes, feet, circulation, and kidney function will be done before permitting you to start on a rigid regimen of physical activity.

If you have had diabetes for more than seven years, are over 35 years of age, have a family history of heart disease, or are planning a strenuous exercise program, the doctor will recommend a treadmill stress test. The routine electrocardiogram (ECG), done lying down at rest, may not reveal important cardiac abnormalities that only become apparent when extra work demands are made of the heart. However, a stress ECG (which monitors the heart while running on a motorized treadmill) may reveal abnormal rhythms or evidence of coronary artery blood flow insufficiency that would have otherwise gone undetected. A thallium stress test provides even more information about the status of the coronary arteries than an ordinary stress test. Radioactive thallium is injected into the circulation to aid detection of poorly oxygenated heart muscle.

Once your doctor's evaluation and recommendations for any restrictions, as well as the type of exercise that is suitable for you are concluded, you may embark on your physical activity program. A daily record of oral hypoglycemic medications or insulin doses should be kept when you begin your exercise regimen. Select an aerobic activity. Walking, swimming, dancing, bicycling and low impact aerobics are examples of aerobic activities that do not place undue stress on the joints. Patients with peripheral neuropathy are advised to avoid jogging because they may be insensitive to blisters or cuts that may develop on their feet. In patients with autonomic neuropathy, strenuous exercise must be avoided because the heart rate and blood pressure may not respond normally to exercise.

If you have proliferative retinopathy your diabetologist or ophthalmologist can instruct you in the types of activities permitted. You should avoid jarring exercise that can raise the blood pressure, such as weight-lifting or racquetball, which can cause serious damage to the eyes.

EXERCISING SAFELY

It is important to wear the proper shoes or athletic sneakers and cotton socks when exercising to avoid any blisters, corns, or calluses. Walking, running, or jogging can be associated with thickening of the outer layers of the skin of the feet (hyperkeratosis), giving rise to callouses. Also, because perspiration and dirt can be the nidus for blisters or infection, a thorough examination of the feet should be a part of your pre-exercise routine. Comfortable clothing and an I.D. bracelet should be carried in a convenient place and, of course, a readily available quick source of carbohydrate is essential.

Exercise should be done on a regular basis (at least three times a week), blood glucose levels should be monitored when necessary (a snack should always be available), and shoes and clothing must be selected carefully. (See Chapter 22, *Care of the Feet*) Remember to maintain an adequate fluid intake, depending on the environmental temperature and the activity in which you are engaged. Always begin your exercise program with a gradual warm-up period for at least 5 minutes. The warm-up period helps to increase the circulation to the heart gradually. Stretch the muscles to help prepare them for physical activity and thereby reduce the chances of injury that can occur if you begin exercising before your muscles are relaxed. Jogging in place or doing calisthenics for a few minutes are effective warm-up activities. If you have not been active for some time, begin your exercise program progressively with five to ten minutes of activity three or four times a week, and work up gradually to sessions of thirty minutes or more. In this manner, you can increase your endurance with minimal risk of injury.

MONITORING BLOOD SUGAR BEFORE, DURING AND AFTER EXERCISE

Hypoglycemia has a tendency to develop during exercise. When beginning your exercise regimen, glucose monitoring is essential to evaluate minor or major changes that result from burning additional calories during physical activity. With strenuous exercise, the heart rate, blood pressure and the cardiac output rise. The amount of fuel used and calories burned increases considerably. The glucose in the bloodstream can be used up rapidly during periods of aerobic physical activity. The body then turns to glycogen stores for additional glucose to supply additional energy. As exercise continues, glucose and free fatty acids are used as fuel. Increasing carbohydrate intake is the most rapid and convenient way to maintain the blood sugar in a satisfactory range during exercise. If the physical activity remains fairly similar from day to day, and finger-stick blood sugars are obtained before and after exercise for several days, the diabetic patient, with the guidance and advice of his physician, soon finds the correct amount of carbohydrate and insulin dosage required to stay well regulated. Those using the pump soon learn how much basal insulin is required, how often a bolus of insulin is needed, and how to set the computerized meter accordingly. To insure the availability of glucose for conversion to energy, insulin levels in the blood must be carefully regulated. Hypoglycemia in this situation always indicates an excessive blood insulin level.

If you are participating in prolonged strenuous activity such as jogging, tennis, swimming, racquetball or school athletics, decreasing insulin and/or taking a 15-20 gram carbohydrate snack every half hour to compensate for the additional caloric need can allow sports participation without undue fear or apprehension. To avoid either a hypoglycemic or a hyperglycemic reaction, diabetics are often advised to eat a meal one or two hours before beginning their work-out. Obese Type 2 diabetics generally can exercise without eating any extra food—their body's fat stores serve to meet energy needs.

Testing your blood glucose at thirty minute intervals before exercising can help you to determine whether your blood sugar is stable or falling. If you exercise for an hour or more, you may need to eat snacks during your

VIGOROUS EXERCISE

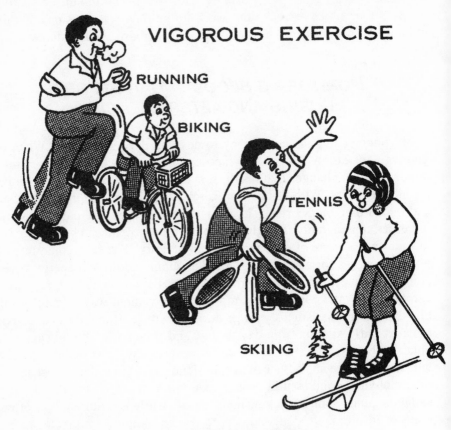

RUNNING

BIKING

TENNIS

SKIING

MODERATE EXERCISE

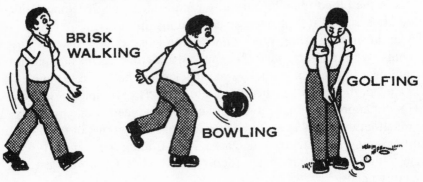

BRISK WALKING

BOWLING

GOLFING

workout. As noted, if the blood sugar is below 100mg/dl (5.55 mMol/L), a snack of 15 or 20 grams of carbohydrate should be eaten. The blood sugar should be retested in approximately twenty or thirty minutes. If it is still below 100mg/dl (5.55 mMol/L), another snack is indicated. Insulin dosage generally needs to be lowered during moderate or high intensity workouts to prevent a hypoglycemic episode. Theoretically, it would not seem to matter whether a diabetic patient reduced insulin in anticipation of prolonged physical activity or compensated with extra food in an attempt to balance energy expenditures. However, for obese diabetic patients it is more prudent to avoid the additional calories. For a growing child or teenager, however, increased food intake would probably be the better choice.

During prolonged exercise, the hormones, glucagon, epinephrine and growth hormone are secreted—all of which are insulin antagonists. Prolonged exercise may require not only additional caloric intake, but additional insulin as well. Individual variations in metabolic needs exist and diabetic patients must learn to recognize their own individual body responses. Short-burst physical activity generally requires extra short-acting carbohydrate intake at the start of the physical activity. If you feel as though you are developing hypoglycemia—feel nervous or shaky, cool and clammy, or develop a feeling of weakness—STOP exercising immediately and check your blood sugar. If there is a doubt about the status of your glucose level, eat a fast-acting sugar snack and take a 15 minute break before returning to exercise again. By carefully monitoring food and insulin needs before and after an exercise program with finger-stick blood sugars, hypoglycemia can usually be avoided.

On rare occasions, vigorous prolonged physical effort can precipitate rises in the blood sugar, making it wise to check finger-stick glucose before and after the event. This happens because the liver produces more glucose than the muscles can use immediately. This is most likely to occur when a Type 1 patient starts exercising with a high blood sugar level. If the blood sugar does not fall, ketoacidosis can develop.

If the blood sugar is 240 mg/dl or above, it is recommended that the workout period be abandoned and the urine should then be tested for ketones. Consult your physician for advice. An extra dose of insulin and increased fluid intake may be in order. Exercise may have a prolonged affect on the blood sugar, resulting in hypoglycemic episodes for up to 24 hours after exercising.

Studies have shown that hypoglycemia is even more likely to occur 4-12 hours after exercising than during the physical activity or shortly thereafter.

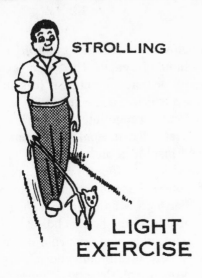

STROLLING

LIGHT EXERCISE

After you stop exercising, your body replenishes its glycogen storage depots in the muscles and liver, which exert a blood sugar lowering effect. In addition, exercise can raise the body's basal metabolic rate for hours after a work-out. This means your body continues to burn more calories than it normally does. The additional energy expenditure following a brisk walk may last for only 15 minutes. However, after a prolonged and strenuous work-out, this effect can persist for hours.

OVER EXERCISE
CAN BRING ABOUT AN INSULIN REACTION WITH SYMPTOMS OF:

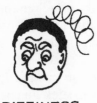

DIZZINESS

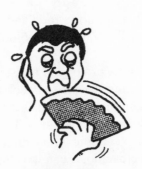

SWEATING

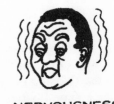

NERVOUSNESS OR SHAKINESS

COMPENSATE FOR OVER EXERCISE... EAT AN EXTRA PIECE OF FRUIT, OR SLICE OF BREAD.

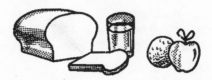

Rapid muscle movement during exercise helps to pump blood back to the heart. After exercising, if you stop abruptly, the blood supply to the heart may also drop abruptly. After strenuous exercise, no matter how tired you are, it is important to slow the pace gradually to let your body's physiological responses to aerobic exercise slowly return to normal. Spend at least three to five minutes slowing down. This means moving about at approximately 25 percent of your normal exercise rate. The cool-down phase is equally important, or perhaps more important, than the warm-up period.

SPECIAL PRECAUTIONS

Review: Exercise is very important in increasing strength and endurance, easing emotional tensions, and aiding in weight reduction. Exercise should be done regularly at a convenient time. Blood glucose levels should be monitored, and a snack should be readily available.

Even though you may have been given medical clearance to engage in an exercise program, you should be aware that persons unaccustomed to exercise are at a greater risk for a heart attack. Paradoxically, one of the best ways to avoid heart attacks is to exercise regularly. In general, the benefits of exercise outweigh the risks. To decrease your risk for serious complications stemming from exercise, you should take the following basic precautions:

1. Do not exercise outdoors during weather extremes such as hot, humid or cold weather. At such times exercise indoors.
2. Start your exercise regimen with brief non-strenuous workouts and increase gradually.
3. Never hold your breath during your work-outs.
4. After an illness or a break in your exercise schedule—even for a short time—begin slowly when you start exercising again.
5. Test your urine for ketones. If your blood sugar is elevated and ketones are present, it probably is a sign that you need more insulin. Do not begin exercising until you are ketone free.
6. Avoid alcohol before or after exercising. Alcohol is very dehydrating.
7. Drink an adequate amount of water before, during and after exercising. Older persons often lose their normal thirst signal to increase fluid intake to correct dehydration.
8. Keep your heart rate in a safe range while exercising.
9. If you take insulin, avoid hypoglycemia by eating snacks when exercising for prolonged periods.

10. When taking a shower after exercising, the water should be tepid—not hot or cold.

For an exercise program to be aerobic, the heart rate must be increased significantly for a prolonged period — 20 to 30 minutes. *Only your personal physician, who is familiar with your health status and the medications you may be taking, can advise you about the safe range in which to maintain your heart rate while exercising.*

Start your exercise routine gradually. When you become accustomed to an exercise routine, with your doctor's approval, you may increase your heart rate upward. However, even young advanced exercisers should never exceed 80 percent of their maximum rate. Listen to your body. You should feel comfortable when you exercise and be able to talk in a normal voice, even when doing aerobic activities. If you experience shortness of breath, fatigue or discomfort, adjustments in your exercise regimen are in order. You are also exercising too hard if you sweat profusely in mild heat or cold weather.

Heart attacks often give advance warning that patients ignore. Heed warning symptoms. Stop exercising immediately if you experience any shortness of breath, tightness, or chest pain radiating down the arm or into the neck or shoulders, jaw, or upper back. Other symptoms that must be respected include light-headedness, faintness, unusual fatigue, palpitations or erratic heart beat, nausea or vomiting. Any chest discomfort—pain, tightness or heavy feeling, etc.—must be considered to be cardiac in origin until proven otherwise. Contact your physician, even if the symptoms subside when you stop exercising. If the symptoms persist, and you are not allergic or have any other contra-indication to aspirin, take one tablet and call 911 or have someone take you to the nearest hospital.

C H A P T E R
• 18 •

Cardiovascular Disease and Diabetes

"Good and Bad" Cholesterol
How to Decrease Risk of Heart Disease
Drug Treatment
Diet

ATHEROSCLEROSIS AND DIABETES

More than 80 percent of diabetics die from some type of cardiovascular disease, (e.g. coronary artery disease (CAD), stroke, perpheral vacscular disease and congestive heart failure) are the leading causes of morbidity and mortality associated with diabetes. 75 percent of all hospitalizations in the diabetic population stem from a consequence of atherosclerosis. Although the mortality from cardiovascular disease has declined in the non-diabetic population during the past 25 years, during the same period it has remained steady or increased among diabetics.

Your food choices and eating habits affect not only your diabetes control, but also your general health. It is the *lipids* in your diet that play the major role in the development of cardiovascular disease (which includes various disorders of the heart and blood vessels). Lipids is the comprehensive term for a group of fat and fat-like substances that contribute to the development of atherosclerosis (hardening of the arteries). *Dyslipidemia* (pronounced dis-lip-id-eem-ee-uh) means abnormal levels of lipids in the blood. The most common type of dyslipidemia is an abnormally high blood level of **cholesterol** and **triglycerides**, a type of fat that serves as fuel storage for the body.

Everyone gets atherosclerosis as they grow older. It has long been known, however, that diabetics are prone to developing atherosclerosis and heart disease about ten to twelve years earlier than the general population. Their atherosclerosis not only develops at an earlier age than in non-diabetic persons; it also progresses more rapidly and generally is more extensive when matched for such factors as age, weight and sex. Diabetes as a primary risk factor for cardiovascular disease carries a risk equivalent to that of a non-diabetic person who already had a coronary event.

Other conditions that co-exist with diabetes that also contribute to the increased incidence of cardiovascular disease are obesity, high blood pressure, smoking, lack of exercise and decreased kidney function, which has progressed to the point where albumin (protein) is present in the urine (either microscopically or grossly). Weight control, exercise, treatment of high blood pressure, aggressive treatment of dyslipidemia and smoking cessation can go a long way towards modifying cardiovascular risks in the diabetic.

CHOLESTEROL

Although cholesterol has become a household word, much confusion remains among the public regarding this white, waxy, odorless fat-like substance. Contrary to popular belief, cholesterol is not a fat. It is a compound that belongs to the family of chemical substances called sterols. Perhaps no other element in our diet has been the source of such intense controversy. However, the jury is no longer out—a verdict has been rendered. The Framingham epidemiological study of more than 5,000 men and women over a twenty-five year period clearly demonstrated that elevated blood cholesterol levels was the chief risk factor for developing heart disease and strokes. Other risk factors identified were cigarette smoking, obesity, sedentary lifestyle, high blood pressure and diabetes.

Despite its role as the principal culprit in cardiovascular disease, cholesterol is vital for performing a number of essential biological functions. It is required for building cell membranes, transmission of nerve impulses, and the synthesis of important hormones (including the sex hormones, testosterone and estrogen, and the adrenal hormone, cortisol), as well as the bile acids. Bile is a greenish colored liquid manufactured by the liver and stored in the gallbladder. It is secreted into the intestinal tract following the ingestion of fatty foods, which it helps to emulsify and digest. The body also uses cholesterol to make Vitamin D, the vitamin responsible for strong bones and teeth. *The critical problem is not cholesterol per se, but rather the type of cholesterol and the blood cholesterol level.* More about this later.

The cholesterol in your blood is derived from the cholesterol ingested in your diet and from cholesterol produced by your body. Because cholesterol is so important, Mother Nature has programmed the liver to provide a constant supply. Even if there were no cholesterol in the foods you eat, your liver would manufacture adequate amounts to meet your body's needs.

Cholesterol obtained from dietary sources is found only in products of animal origin. Foods very high in cholesterol, such as liver or organ meats are not high on the list of the typical American diet. The one high cholesterol food that is regularly consumed is the chicken egg. All animal products—meat, fish, poultry, milk, cheese, and eggs—contain cholesterol. Food containing cholesterol contributes to elevated blood cholesterol levels, but it does not play nearly as important a role as the saturated fat content of the diet. *Saturated fats, whether derived from animal or vegetable products, stimulate cholesterol production when they are metabolized by the body.* Of course, many of the foods that are high in saturated fats are the same food substances that have a high cholesterol content.

"Oil and water don't mix." Body fluids—blood, serum, and lymph— are all water based. Lipids are not soluble in water. For lipids to enter the bloodstream and be transported throughout the body they must link up with proteins, forming compounds called lipoproteins. The protein wraps around the cholesterol and becomes the transport vehicle—the lipid is the cargo.

There are two significant types of lipoproteins involved in the transport of cholesterol. Low density lipoproteins (LDL) and high density lipoproteins (HDL). The LDL-cholesterol delivers the cholesterol to the body's cells. However, when there is an excessive amount of cholesterol in the blood the surplus may be deposited on the blood vessel walls forming scarred areas called plaques. Thus begins the atherosclerotic process—the hardening of the arteries—that can eventually choke and clog the arteries. For this reason LDL is sometimes called "Bad Cholesterol."

The HDL-cholesterol removes excess cholesterol from the blood and evidence now indicates that it sometimes removes it from plaque deposits as well, carrying it back to the liver where it can be re-used or broken down and excreted. HDL is therefore also known as "Good Cholesterol."

ATHEROSCLEROSIS—THE MANY FACES OF THIS SILENT BUT DEADLY DISORDER

The long road to atherosclerosis is an ongoing dynamic process. If the LDL-cholesterol level in the blood remains elevated through the years, the arteries may progressively narrow as a result of enlarging cholesterol deposits. Their capacity to deliver oxygen-rich blood gradually decreases as plaque deposits enlarge and the blood vessels become rigid and inflexible. Physiologically, this is the equivalent of sludge build-up in a rusted, partially blocked plumbing line.

The heart, like the rest of the body, needs a constant blood supply of oxygen and life sustaining nutrients in order to keep pumping. It gets its blood supply from the coronary arteries, vessels that branch off directly from the aorta, the large main artery that carries blood from the heart to the rest of the body. Five percent of the blood pumped into the aorta enters the coronary arteries to nourish the heart. When the blood supply to the heart decreases, the narrowed coronary arteries may be capable of delivering sufficient oxygen and nutrients to meet cardiac needs at rest or during light activities, but may be incapable of supplying sufficient oxygen and nutrients to the heart when it is being overworked and therefore needs more blood than usual. When this happens, the patient experiences discomfort in the middle of the chest, behind the breast bone. The pain often radiates across the chest. It may go down the left arm, or both arms, up to the neck or jaw. This condition, which is a consequence of the heart temporarily not getting enough oxygen-rich blood, is called coronary insufficiency or angina pectoris. Angina pectoris, or angina as it is commonly called, is sometimes experienced as a vice-like or crushing sensation of pressure in the chest. At times, it may be felt in the abdominal area or as back pain between the shoulder blades. When it is felt primarily in atypical remote areas, the symptoms are often mistaken for other illnesses. In some patients, angina may not give rise to any symptoms — a condition that is called "silent angina." Anginal pain is characteristically brought on by exertion and relieved by rest. Nitroglycerine, a coronary artery dilating medicine that is rapidly absorbed when taken sublinguinally (under the tongue), can usually relieve the discomfort of angina promptly.

When a coronary artery has been the site of significant atherosclerotic changes (cholesterol plaque build-up), it may become completely occluded by a blood clot at the site of the plaque deposits. When this happens, the segment of the heart muscle that was nourished by the blocked artery is starved for oxygen and fuel, and actual tissue death may occur. This major cardiovascular event is known medically as a myocardial infarction—commonly called a heart attack or coronary thrombosis (blood clot). A catastrophic heart attack is usually the culmination of atherosclerotic changes that have been proceeding asymptomatically beneath the surface for years. However, the majority of heart attack victims experience episodes of warning chest pain, particularly the type of angina known as unstable angina, an unpredictable form that can occur even at rest. Unstable angina must be regarded as a warning sign of greatly increased risk for a heart attack.

When atherosclerosis leads to a blood clot within one of the blood vessels that nourishes a part of the brain, the result is a cerebral thrombosis—an event that is commonly called a stroke. Another type of stroke occurs when a blood clot is dislodged from an artery and carried along by the bloodstream as a free-floating clot until it becomes lodged in and obstructs a cerebral vessel. This is called a cerebral embolism. A third type of stroke is caused by hemorrhage from the rupture of a cerebral artery. Only ten to fifteen percent of strokes are caused by hemorrhages. Hemorrhagic strokes are more likely to be fatal than thrombotic strokes.

Blood vessel walls contain smooth muscle which can narrow their diameter when they contract. Blood vessel spasm, particularly when superimposed on an already artherosclerotic coronary vessel, can cause angina. When the spasm occurs in an atherosclerotic cerebral blood vessel, it can cause neurological symptoms such as dizziness, temporary paralysis to a portion of the body, and difficulty thinking clearly. When the spasm dissipates, the paralysis and other symptoms usually subside. These temporary episodes of abnormal cerebral functioning are called transient ischemic attacks or TIAs for short.

Atherosclerosis in cerebral vessels can diminish the blood supply to the brain and give rise to a range of neurological symptoms including difficulty thinking and forgetfulness, which may progress to a permanent, gradual decline in mental acuity.

When atherosclerosis involves the aorta (the body's main artery), a portion of the wall of this large blood vessel may become weakened. The blood within the arterial system normally exerts pressure against the artery walls. It is this lateral pressure that is measured when a blood pressure reading is taken.

When a portion of the aorta is damaged by cholesterol plaque buildup, it is sometimes so weakened that the pressure exerted by the blood is sufficient to cause a portion of the weakened arterial wall to balloon out. This ballooning out of a blood vessel wall is called an aneurysm. Like an over-inflated balloon in danger of popping, an aneurysm is a grave health threat. Emergency treatment is required if a catastrophe is to be avoided.

When the atherosclerotic process involves the circulation to the lower extremities, it can decrease the blood supply to the legs and give rise to the condition known as peripheral vascular disease (PVD). PVD causes pain in the area of the calf muscles brought on by walking and relieved by rest—a symptom called intermittent claudication. When PVD progresses to an advanced state, it can impair the circulation to portions of the extremity sufficiently to cause (dry) gangrene—infarction of the tissues—of the toes, feet, or even the leg. Life-saving amputation then becomes necessary. *PVD associated with diabetes is the leading cause of non-traumatic extremity amputations in America today.*

Sigmund Freud believed that more than 90 percent of cases of impotency were caused by psychological problems. Dr. Freud was wrong. Most cases of impotency are due to organic causes, the chief of which are atherosclerosis and nerve damage. When atherosclerosis impairs the blood supply to the male sexual organ, the vascular chambers, which must fill with blood to expand and become rigid, are deprived of an adequate blood supply and lose the ability to produce and/or maintain an erection. Excluding the small percentage of men who develop impotency from psychological disorders, normal males should be able to function sexually throughout most of their life—even well into their eighties.

As if the foregoing disorders that stem from atherosclerosis of the large blood vessels (macrovascular disease) were not enough, degenerative changes in the small blood vessels (microvascular disease) give rise to eye damage, nerve damage and kidney damage. The microvascular complications are discussed in Chapter 19, *Long-Term Complications of Diabetes*. The severity of microvascular disease is related to blood sugar control and its development and progression is prevented or delayed with tight blood sugar regulation.

The Mechanism of Sudden Vascular Occlusion in Blood Vessels That Are Only Partially Blocked by Plaque Deposits

Severe lesions that occlude an important vessel certainly pose a major health risk. However, the vast majority of vessels that become completely occluded by a blood clot were not blocked for more than 30-50 percent of their diameter by plaques, prior to the rather abrupt—and at times sudden—blood clot blockage. To understand this phenomenon, it is necessary to review the changes that give rise to plaque formation and rupture.

For years, the inner lining of the blood vessels—the endothelium—was considered to be a simple semipermeable membrane. It is now known that endothelial cells produce vital substances that play key physiological roles in normal vascular function, including maintenance of the normal dilatation of the blood vessels.

The same oxygen atoms that are necessary to sustain life are sometimes transformed into a highly toxic form called free radicals. LDL-cholesterol is injurious to the endothelium when it interacts with free radical oxygen atoms and becomes oxidized. The oxygenated molecules of cholesterol can cause significant endothelial damage even when present in very small concentrations. Endothelial damage is the first step in plaque formation. The body attempts to rid itself of the toxic oxidized LDL-cholesterol by having its immune system's amoeba-like scavenger cells, called macrophages, ingest the LDL-cholesterol. The cholesterol-laden macrophages, with their ingested oxidized LDL, are transformed into what are known as foam cells. The foam cells swell and eventually rupture, discharging their lipid contents into the wall of the blood vessels forming the scarred areas called plaques. With each subsequent cholesterol deposit the plaque enlarges and the passageway through the vessel becomes narrower. The ever-enlarging plaque is covered by the endothelium, which forms a thin, unstable cap over the plaque.

The lipid-rich plaque pool is like a time-bomb waiting to go off. When the weak endothelial cap of the plaque ruptures, its lipid core comes into contact with blood. Because this material is highly thrombogenic (prone to clotting) the vessel rapidly becomes clogged with a blood clot. As we have seen, when this happens in one of the arteries that supply the heart muscle itself—a coronary artery—the blocked artery can no longer deliver oxygen and nutrients to a segment of the heart. The result is a heart attack or coronary thrombosis. This chain of events explains the not infrequent heart attacks in those with minor plaque formation (less than 30 percent blockage of a coronary artery), as well as the sudden deaths in asymptomatic individuals who have had an apparently normal electrocardiogram without clinical evidence of cardiovascular disease. Small asymptomatic plaque lesions are responsible for more than 80 percent of acute coronary events. When this process occurs in one of the blood vessels that nourish a part of the brain, the result is a cerebral thrombosis or stroke.

Dyslipidemia, high blood pressure, and tobacco use, major risk factors for heart disease, are all associated with impairment of endothelial function. Modification of these factors, particularly lowering of the LDL-cholesterol, can improve endothelial function significantly and reduce the risk of heart disease.

RISK FACTORS FOR CORONARY
ARTERY DISEASE (CAD)

Risk factors for CAD are traits or habits that make a person more likely to develop CAD. The more risk factors a person has, the greater his vulnerability for contracting the disease. Risk factors are not additive; rather they have a multiplying affect on each other. For example, a person who has three independent risk factors for CAD would not be three times as likely to get the disease, but would be 8-10 times more likely to get CAD than a person who had no risk factors. Of course, all risk factors are not equal in their propensity to cause CAD—some carry more weight than others. The four key risk factors over which you have some control are high blood pressure, dyslipidemia, smoking and diabetes.

Factors You Can Do Something About
- Current cigarette smoking
- Dyslipidemia — high blood cholesterol (high total cholesterol and LDL-cholesterol, and low HDL-cholesterol)
- High blood pressure
- Uncontrolled diabetes
- Obesity (significant — 20 percent overweight)
- Physical inactivity

Factors You Cannot Control
- Progressive age increase
      45 years or older for men
      55 years or older for women or premature menopause without estrogen replacement therapy
- Family history of premature heart disease (heart attack or sudden death)
      Father or brother — stricken before the age of 55
      Mother or sister — stricken before the age of 65

C-REACTIVE PROTEIN

When arteriosclerotic plaques are examined they show definite signs of inflammation. Recent studies have shown that our liver makes a protein called C-reactive protein (CRP). This protein is elevated by any infectious process. However, if we see an elevated CRP in persons who have no obvious focus of infection, atherosclerosis should be suspected as the cause. In fact, studies have shown CRP levels to be a better risk indicator for cardiovascular disease than cholesterol.

CRP levels can be reduced by exercise, smoking cessation and lowering cholesterol levels. Elevated CRP that is caused by atherosclerosis is responsive to aspirin therapy and the statin drugs. Diabetics show an even greater improvement in the CRP levels when treated with a statin drug than non-diabetics. A recently published study in *Lancet* (The British medical journal) showed that those with relatively normal cholesterol levels also benefited when their CRP was lowered with a statin drug. The benefits observed were decreased cardiovascular morbidity and mortality.

CHOLESTEROL LEVEL GUIDELINES

The level of cholesterol in the blood is expressed in milligrams per deciliter of blood (mg/dl). The medical guidelines for classifying blood cholesterol levels advise that a total cholesterol level of less than 200mg/dl (5.18mMol/L) is "desirable" for adults. There are three categories of total cholesterol:

Total Cholesterol Categories :

Desirable Blood Cholesterol —
less than 200mg/dl (11.1mMol/dl)

Borderline-High Blood Cholesterol —
200-239mg/dl (11.1-13.2mMol/dl)

High Blood Cholesterol —
240mg/dl (13.38mMol/dl) and above

Cholesterol levels less than 200mg/dl (11.1 mMol/dl) are considered desirable, while levels of 240mg/dl (13.3 mMol/dl) or above are high and require more specific attention. Levels from 200-239mg/dl (11.1-13.3 mMol/dl) also require attention, especially if the HDL-cholesterol is low or LDL-cholesterol level is high, or if there are other risk factors for heart disease, such as diabetes. Even borderline high blood cholesterol levels raise the risk for heart disease.

In countries where plant based foods make up the bulk of the diet, the populations have cholesterol levels of 150mg/dl (8.3 mMol/dl) or lower, and coronary artery disease (CAD) is rare. In the United States, for many years, cholesterol levels of up to 240mg/dl (13.2 mMol/dl) were considered to be normal. The fact that the average American had cholesterol levels much higher than many other areas of the world where CAD was uncommon, did not make our high average "normal," particularly in the light of the rampant rate of CAD in America. Although the current goal is to achieve total cholesterol levels below 200mg/dl (11.1 mMol/dl), any improvement is worthwhile. Research has shown that when cholesterol levels are lowered 20-25 percent, even though they may not fall within the normal range, there is a substantial decrease in CAD risk.

LDL-Cholesterol

Desirable — less than 130mg/dl (7.2 mMol/dl)
Borderline-High Risk — 130-159mg/dl (7.2 - 8.9 mMol/dl)
High Risk — above 160mg/dl (8.9 mMol/dl)

The LDL level serves as a better guide to the risk for heart disease than the total cholesterol level. Accordingly, **most physicians consider lowering LDL as the main treatment goal for a cholesterol problem.** If your LDL level puts you at high risk and you have fewer than two other risk factors for heart disease, your target goal should be an LDL level of less than 160mg/dl (8.9mMol/dl). However, if you have two or more other risk factors for heart disease, your LDL goal should be less than 130mg/dl (7.2mMol/dl). If you already have heart disease, your LDL target should be even lower — 100mg/dl (5.5mMol/dl) or less. These target goals suggested by The National Cholesterol Educational Program (NCEP) may be summarized as follows:

THE NCEP RECOMMENDATIONS

For individuals with:	Initiate drug therapy* if LDL cholesterol is:	LDL cholesterol goal is:
No coronary heart disease (CHD) and fewer than two other CHD risk factors	$\geq$190 mg/dL after $\geq$6 months of diet 10.55mMol/dl	<160 mg/dL 8.89mMol/dl
No CHD but with two or more other CHD risk factors	$\geq$160 mg/dL after $\geq$6 months 8.89mMol/dl of diet	<130 mg/dL 7.78mMol/dl
Definite CHD or other atherosclerotic disease	$\geq$130 mg/dL after 6-12 weeks of Step II diet	$\leq$100 mg/dL 5.55mMol/dl

*Following an adequate trial of diet.

National Cholesterol Education Program: Second report of the Expert Panel on Detection, Evaluation, and Treatment of High Blood Cholesterol in Adults (Adult Treatment Panel II), NIH Publication No. 93-3095, Bethesda, MD, National Heart, Lung, and Blood Institute, September 1993.

Note : There is strong evidence that diabetics should be held to the same stringent goals that the NCEP recommends for those with known cardiac disease. These goals are thought to be in order because of the accelerated atherosclerotic process and the high incidence of premature cardiovascular disease that is seen with diabetes.

The most effective way to lower LDL-cholesterol is with cholesterol lowering medications and dietary restriction of saturated fats.

HDL-Cholesterol

Normal HDL — more than 40mg/dl (2.2mMol/dl)
Low HDL — less than 40mg/dl (2.2mMol/dl)
High HDL — above 60mg/dl (3.3mMol/dl)

Unlike total cholesterol and LDL-cholesterol, the lower your HDL, the higher your risk for heart disease. An HDL level less than 35mg/dl (2.2mMol/dl) is considered low and increases your risk. *The higher your HDL, the better.* An HDL level of 60mg/dl (3.3mMol/dl)) or above is high and is associated with longevity. Alcohol raises the HDL. The benefits of alcohol are optimized with an intake of two drinks daily. For diabetics, the ingestion of alcohol poses special hazards and should not be done without their physician's approval. Although larger amounts of alcohol—more than two drinks—may raise the HDL even higher, it is still unclear whether the segment of HDL that is elevated is the protective segment. Furthermore, there is no doubt that larger amounts of alcohol are associated with an increased incidence of coronary artery disease as well as other health problems.

An HDL level below 40mg/dl (2.2mMol/dl) is considered a risk factor. An HDL over 60 (3.3mMol/dl) usually is protective—a negative risk factor.

Low HDL levels are not always associated with increased cardiovascular risk. Surprisingly, those who follow a relatively strict low fat vegetarian diet, may have low HDL levels and a decreased risk for cardiovascular disease, in contrast to most patients with low HDL levels.

Note: HDL-cholesterol can be increased by regular exercise, weight control, smoking cessation and cholesterol lowering medications.

Cholesterol/HDL Ratio

The significance of the level of total cholesterol can be determined only after evaluation of the types of cholesterol that contribute to the total reading. A frequently simplified formula that yields practical information is the ratio of total cholesterol to HDL-cholesterol.

A total cholesterol level of 260mg/dl (11.1mMol/dl) may have entirely different significance for two individuals with different lipid profiles. If the

HDL level is high, the ratio may be within normal limits and not represent a health threat despite the high total cholesterol level. If the HDL is low, the elevated cholesterol would represent a significant hazard and require management. People with normal total cholesterol, who have low HDL levels, are at a two-to-three-fold increased risk for coronary artery disease.

Even though the general guidelines state that a cholesterol level below 200mg/dl (5.18mMol/L) is desirable, if an individual with a low total cholesterol reading has a low HDL level, the ratio would be high and indicate vulnerability to cardiovascular disease. Conversely, as noted, an individual with a high total cholesterol, with a high HDL-cholesterol, might well have a satisfactory total cholesterol/HDL ratio and not be at increased risk for cardiovascular disease. The following reference values can serve as a general guide:

Coronary Heart Disease Risk*	Total Cholesterol/HDL Ratio	
	Male	Female
1/2 Average	3.4	3.3
Average (normal)	5.0	4.4
Twice Average (moderate)	9.6	7.0
Three Times Average (high)	13.4	11.0

* Data based on Framingham Study (see table to determine your risk of coronary disease)

Triglycerides

Triglycerides are fats that circulate in the blood and serve as energy sources. Based on your age, your triglyceride levels should not rise above the following:

AGE	INCREASED RISK
19-29	> 140mg/dl (7.78mMol/dl)
30-39	> 150mg/dl (8.33mMol/dl)
40-49	> 160mg/dl (8.89mMol/dl)
> 49	> 190mg/dl (10.55mMol/dl)

Triglyceride levels must be done on blood obtained after an overnight fast of at least 14 hours, otherwise erroneously high test levels could result. HDL-cholesterol levels must also be done on fasting specimens for accurate results. However, total cholesterol levels may be performed on non-fasting blood.

WHAT AFFECTS YOUR BLOOD CHOLESTEROL LEVEL?

Your blood cholesterol levels are affected by:

What you eat — The saturated fat and cholesterol in the food you eat raise total and LDL-cholesterol levels.

Obesity — Being overweight can make LDL-cholesterol levels go up and HDL levels go down.

Physical activity/Exercise — Increased physical activity helps to lower LDL-cholesterol and raise HDL-cholesterol levels.

Heredity — Your body makes all the cholesterol it needs, and your genes influence how your body makes and handles cholesterol.

Age and sex — Blood cholesterol levels in both men and women begin to go up at about age 20. Women before menopause have levels that are lower than men of the same age. After menopause, a woman's LDL-cholesterol goes up as does her risk for heart disease. The risk of CAD is increased in post-menopausal women, whether the menopause is natural, surgical, or premature.

HORMONE REPLACEMENT THERAPY (HRT)

The increased incidence of cardiovascular disease in women after the menopause was formerly thought to result from the decline of estrogen levels post-menopausally. However, we now know that HRT actually increased the risk for cardiovascular disease. Additionally, recent studies have shown that HRT also increases the risk for breast cancer. 100,000 cases of breast cancer per year in the United States are said to have been attributable to HRT. The estrogen progesterone* combination showed an even greater incidence of breast cancer than when estrogen was used alone. A recently widely publicized study appeared to show that the risk was greatest during the first years of therapy. Prior studies had indicated that the first few years of HRT did not show a dramatic rise in breast cancer. The recent study, however, clearly included women who had already developed breast cancer prior to the study, thus giving a false bias to the first year statistics.

Post-menopausal symptoms can be completely disabling. Debilitating symptoms force some women to demand HRT despite the risks. These patients should be given as little estrogen as possible to control their disabling symptoms. Progesterone, which formerly was given every day as with the popular drug combination Prem/Pro are now given every 3, 4 or sometimes 5 months. Transvaginal ultrasound, a simple non-invasive procedure, can be performed on women receiving progesterone to detect uterine cancer in its earliest stage.

*Progesterone is given to protect the uterus from cancer. Women who have had a hysterectomy do not require progesterone.

BLOOD CHOLESTEROL

Health concerned organizations such as the American Diabetes Association, the American Dietetic Association and the United States Department of Agriculture, as well as dietary advice given in popular health publications, has led to some changes in eating habits in the United States. However, despite the fact that they know better, most Americans continue to consume a diet that is outrageously high in saturated fats. Dairy products, fried foods, luncheon meats, cakes, hot dogs, hamburgers, and pizzas are but a few popular examples of foods rich in cholesterol and saturated fats. Even a lean filet mignon with no visible white streaking derives at least 30 percent of its calories from its fat content! It should come as no surprise that heart disease has reached epidemic proportions in this country.

In pre-World War II Japan, the typical Japanese diet consisted of fruits and vegetables, rice, and fish. Heart disease at that time was extremely rare among the general population. With the post-war westernization of the Japanese diet, the incidence of heart disease has steadily risen. Hyperlipidemia, high lipid levels in the blood, is the key factor in the development of hardening of the arteries.

Everyone, regardless of their blood cholesterol level, should eat in a heart-healthy way. This is true beginning with children above age five on up to their parents, grandparents, and even great-grandparents. The whole family should also be physically active. And if you have a high blood cholesterol level—whether due to what you eat, your heredity, or diabetes—it is even more important to eat healthfully and to be physically active. Adopting these behaviors can also help control high blood pressure as well as blood sugar levels.

GENERAL RULES TO LOWER BLOOD CHOLESTEROL

Choose foods low in saturated fat

All foods that contain fat are made up of a mixture of saturated and unsaturated fats. Saturated fat raises your blood cholesterol level more than anything else that you eat. It is found in greatest amounts in foods from animals, such as fatty cuts of meat, poultry with the skin, whole-milk dairy products, lard, and in some vegetable oils like coconut, palm kernel, palm oils, and hydrogenated vegetable oils. The best way to reduce your blood cholesterol level is to choose foods low in saturated fat. One way to do this is by choosing foods such as fruit, vegetables, whole grain foods, breads and cereals naturally low in fat, and high in starch and fiber.

Choose foods low in total fat

Since many foods high in total fat are also high in saturated fat, eating foods low in total fat will help you eat less saturated fat. When you do eat fat, you should substitute unsaturated fat for saturated fat. Unsaturated fat is usually liquid at room temperature and can be either monosaturated or polyunsaturated. Examples of foods high in monosaturated fat are olive and canola oils. Monosaturated fats are believed to have a more favorable affect on the lipid profile than any other type of fat. Those high in polyunsaturated fat, include safflower, sunflower, corn, and soybean oils. Any type of fat is a rich source of calories, so eating foods low in fat will also help you keep your weight under control.

Choose foods high in starch and fiber

Foods high in starch and fiber are excellent substitutes for foods high in saturated fat. These foods—breads, cereals, pasta, grains, fruits, and vegetables—are low in saturated fat and contain no cholesterol. They are also usually lower in calories than foods that are high in fat. Foods high in starch and fiber are also good sources of vitamins and minerals.

Diets low in saturated fat and cholesterol, and high in fruits, vegetables, and grain products, like oat and barley bran, and dry peas and beans, contain soluble fiber which may help to lower blood cholesterol.

Choose foods low in cholesterol

Dietary cholesterol can also raise blood cholesterol levels, although not nearly as much as saturated fat. It is important to choose foods low in dietary cholesterol. Dietary cholesterol is found only in foods that come from animals. Many of these foods are also high in saturated fat. Foods from plant sources do not have cholesterol but can contain saturated fat. Coconut is the main source of saturated fat from the plant kingdom.

Be more physically active

Being physically active helps your blood cholesterol levels: It can raise HDL and may lower LDL. Being more active can also help you lose weight, lower your blood pressure, improve the fitness of your heart and blood vessels, and reduce stress.

Lose weight, if you are overweight

People who are overweight tend to have higher blood cholesterol levels than people of desirable weight. Overweight people with an "apple" shape—bigger (pot) belly—tend to have a higher risk of heart disease than those with a "pear" shape—bigger hips and thighs.

Whatever your body shape, when you cut the fat in your diet, you cut down on the richest source of calories. An eating pattern high in starch and fiber instead of fat is a good way to lose weight. Starchy foods have little fat and are lower in calories than high fat foods. Losing even a little weight can help to lower LDL-cholesterol and raise HDL-cholesterol. You don't need to reach your desirable weight to see a significant change in your blood cholesterol levels.

REVIEW

To Lower Your Blood Cholesterol, Remember to:
- Choose foods low in saturated fat and cholesterol
- Be more physically active
- Lose weight, if you are overweight

Sources of Saturated Fat and/or Cholesterol
- Animal fats (bacon, beef, chicken, ham, lamb, pork, turkey, etc.)
- Butter
- Cocoa butter
- Coconut
- Coconut oil
- Cream
- Egg and egg yolk solids
- Hydrogenated (hardened) vegetable oils
- Hardened fat or oil
- Lard
- Palm kernel oil
- Vegetable oil*
- Vegetable shortening
- Whole milk solids

* Could be coconut or palm oil or hydrogenated or partially hydrogenated oil

SPECIAL DIETARY ADJUNCTS TO REDUCE LDL CHOLESTEROL

Increase soy products in your diet
A number of studies credit soy products with significantly lowering LDL-cholesterol levels without decreasing HDL-cholesterol levels. Soy products are excellent substitutes for animal protein, which usually contains

a large percentage of saturated fats and cholesterol. Soy bean products such as tofu, vegetarian soy "hamburgers," soy bean milk, etc. are available in health food markets, and are beginning to appear on the shelves of many supermarkets.

Include garlic in your diet

Several large retrospective studies have shown that the daily intake of one medium-sized garlic clove or 900 -1800mg of garlic in capsule form can reduce LDL-cholesterol levels an average of 9 percent, while raising HDL-cholesterol slightly. High intake of garlic is believed to be associated with a decreased incidence of cardiac disease and mortality, and certainly not associated with any side effects, except, perhaps, bad breath. Some recent small scale studies have failed to demonstrate any favorable benefits on lipid metabolism from ingesting tablets that contained 300mg of Kwai garlic powder or 5mg of garlic oil, which is the equivalent of 4 or 5 grams of fresh garlic cloves (1 gram = 1000 mg).

Increase intake of monosaturated fats

Polyunsaturated fats—corn oil, soybean oil and most margarines—have been associated with increased rates of LDL-cholesterol oxidation, which, as we have seen, is the first step along the metabolic pathway to plaque formation. They also increase platelet agglutination, which can promote blood clotting. Monosaturated fats such as canola oil or olive oil decrease rates of LDL oxidation and are preferable to polyunsaturated oils.

A large experimental study based on a variation of the so-called mediterranean diet, which emphasizes olive oil and monosaturated fats, and omega-3* oils with multiple servings of legumes daily, showed a significant reduction in cardiovascular disease. The study demonstrated a startling overall decrease in mortality of more than 70 percent over those who followed the control, typical French diet. Both the experimental and the standard French diet derived about 30 percent of their calories from fat. The differences in mortality suggest that factors other than simply the cholesterol and saturated fat content of the diet were responsible for the differences observed. Dietary sources which may have played a role were foods rich in omega-3 oils and monosaturated fats, such as seafood and nuts, particularly almond, hazelnut, pecan, cashew and macadamia nuts.

Read food labels critically. The hype on food labels is often misleading.

NUTRITION INFORMATION

Look for the amount of saturated fat, total fat, cholesterol, and calories in a serving of a product. Compare similar products to find the one with the smallest amounts. If you have high blood pressure, do the same for sodium. The ingredient in the least amount is listed last. So, to choose foods low in saturated fat or total fat, limit your use of the products that list any fat or oil first—or that list many fat and oil ingredients. If you are watching your sodium intake, do the same for sodium or salt.

Aside from nutrition and the ingredients list, some labels make claims such as "low fat" or "light." These vague terms are applied loosely and often have little meaning. Aside from the nutrition information required by law, labels are usually designed, not to inform, but to sell a product. State and Federal statutes require that labels be truthful, but they are often misleading and fail to tell the whole story. For example:

Natural—This literally means occurring in nature. Everything existing on this planet is natural, including poisons.

Low calorie—If the caloric content per serving is less than 40 and the food has less than 0.4 calories per gram, a food may be classified as low calorie, even if all the calories are from fats and simple sugars.

Lean—If the product contains 25 percent fewer calories than the standard product of the manufacturer (which may have been extremely high in calories), it qualifies for the lean designation.

No artificial flavors—This category may ignore artificial preservatives, many of which are highly allergenic and possibly carcinogenic.

No cholesterol—May not contain cholesterol, but can be high in saturated fats that stimulate body cholesterol metabolism.

Serving size—Manufacturers often make the serving size smaller than what is usually considered to be a normal portion. This makes calorie and fat content appear to be less than they really are.

Sugar free—This designation usually refers only to the sucrose content. Honey and fructose, for example, which are also sugars, are exempted from this designation.

Non-fat—If the fat content per serving is less than 0.5 gram, the fat content can be ignored. If the serving size is small, the food may contain significant amounts of fat and yet bear a label that loudly proclaims it to be free of fat.

May contain one or more of the following fats—Always assume that it contains the worst hydrogenated fat or saturated fat listed.

Shortening—Usually indicates a saturated fat or vegetable oil that has been made solid by hydrogenation.

PRODUCT: **CHECK FOR:**

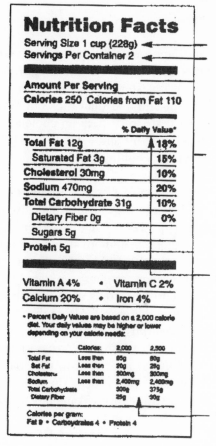

- Serving size
- Number of servings

- Calories
- Total fat in grams
- Saturated fat in grams
- Cholesterol in milligrams

Here, the label gives the amounts for the different nutrients in one serving. Use it to help you keep track of how much fat, saturated fat, cholesterol, and calories you are getting from different foods.

- The "% Daily Value" shows you how much of the recommended amounts the food provides in one serving, if you eat 2,000 calories a day. For example, one serving of this food gives you 18 percent of your total fat recommendation.

- Here you can see the recommended daily amounts for each nutrient for two calorie levels. If you eat a 2,000 calorie diet, you should be eating less than 65 grams of fat and less than 20 grams of saturated fat. Your daily amounts may vary higher or lower depending on your calorie needs.

Some foods may at first glance appear to be low fat. Two percent milk, for example, doesn't sound like a high fat food until you realize that whole milk is 3.5 - 4 percent fat. The 2 percent refers to the fat content by overall weight. Because milk is primarily water, its fat content, as a proportion of the entire weight of a serving might seem small, but the fat content is responsible for approximately 38 percent of the total calories. Skim milk has no fat and retains the vitamin and protein content. All forms of cow milk, however, contain cholesterol.

Partially Hydrogenated Vegetable Oils, and Trans Fats — Man-Made Fats that Masquerade as Heart-Healthy Foods

The type of fat you eat is even more important than the total amount consumed. As emphasized throughout this chapter, lipid control requires a reduction in the intake of saturated fats and cholesterol. Fats that are liquid at room temperature are generally more unsaturated than those that are solid. The liquid fats which have the most favorable affect on cholesterol levels are the monosaturated fats, such as olive oil and canola oil. These fats are heat stable and remain unchanged by cooking. (More about this later.)

Researchers have identified highly atherogenic* fats that are routinely found in commercial baked products and margarines. These undesirable fats, called hydrogenated fats, are derived from vegetable oils. When subjected to chemical treatments designed to make them more stable and prolong the shelf life of foods to which they are added, these fats are transformed into a new type of fat which has properties similar to saturated fats. Through a process called hydrogenation, hydrogen atoms are added to the unsaturated portion of the molecular structure, thereby changing them into a more solid form that is, for all intents and purposes, either a partially or completely saturated fat. To make matters even worse, when these transformed fats are heated, they undergo a physical alteration in the spatial arrangement of their atoms, which changes their properties. The new spatial arrangement of the molecule is called the trans form. Trans fats have a worse affect on cholesterol levels than ordinary saturated fats, not only causing LDL-cholesterol levels to rise, but also decreasing HDL levels. Additionally, they may be carcinogenic making them even more hazardous. They impersonate heart-healthy fats because they are derived from unsaturated liquid oils and are not required to be listed in the saturated fat category on food labels.

How Much Cholesterol Reduction Can Be Expected From Dietary Modification?

How effective your diet is in lowering your LDL-cholesterol level depends on your dietary habits before starting the diet, how well you follow your diet, how your body responds to your new way of eating and how rigid a dietary regimen you follow. In general, those with higher cholesterol lev-

---

*Substances that cause hardening of the artery.

els have greater reductions in LDL-cholesterol levels than those with lower starting levels. If you are overweight and lose weight, a low saturated-fat, low cholesterol diet may work even better to lower your high cholesterol.

A low saturated-fat diet can reduce total cholesterol levels in patients who are consuming an average American diet by about 8 to 14 percent. Many people who have blood cholesterol levels higher than average will often have an even bigger reduction. Every one percent reduction in cholesterol levels lowers your risk for a future heart attack by about two percent. So, an 8 to 14 percent reduction in cholesterol levels would lower the CAD risk by about 16 to 28 percent.

LIFETIME CHANGES IN DIET

For people with diabetes, advice from a registered dietician or other qualified nutritionist can help to insure success with their diet. Whoever prepares the meals in your house should also participate in these sessions. Your new diet should be maintained for life. You may want to continue diet education sessions with your dietician quarterly for the first year of long-term monitoring and once or twice yearly thereafter.

DRUG THERAPY TO TREAT DYSLIPIDEMIA

When lifestyle changes — particularly diet and exercise — are insufficient to meet target lipid profile goals, drug treatment is usually necessary.

HMG-CoA Reductase Inhibitors

The introduction of this new class of cholesterol-lowering drugs has revolutionized the treatment of dyslipidemia. The HMG-CoA reductase inhibitors, or "statins," herald a new era of treatment for hypercholesterolemia. The enzyme HMG-CoA reductase plays a key role in the synthesis of glucose by the liver. The "statins" prevent theHMG-CoA reductase enzyme from functioning and thereby inhibit cholesterol production.

There are currently six statin drugs on the market in the United States. Included in this category of drugs are Lovastatin (Mevacor®), Simvastatin (Zocor®), Atorvastatin (Lipitor®), Rosuvastatin(Crestor®), Fluvastatin (Lescol®), and Pravastatin (Pravachol®).

The statins lower LDL-cholesterol levels more effectively than any of the other types of cholesterol lowering drugs. They work by inhibiting an enzyme, HMG-CoA reductase, that controls the rate of cholesterol production in the liver. This lowers cholesterol by slowing down the production of cholesterol. They also increase the liver's ability to remove LDL-cholesterol already in the blood. Statins were initially used to lower cholesterol levels in two large studies, the Scandinavian Simvastatin Survival Study (4S) and Cholesterol and Recurrent Events (CARE). The large reductions in total and LDL-cholesterol produced by these drugs resulted in significant reductions in heart attacks and coronary heart disease (CHD) deaths. Thanks to their track record in these studies and their ability to lower LDL-cholesterol, statins have become the drugs most frequently prescribed when a person needs a cholesterol-lowering medicine.

Studies using various statins report from 20 to 60 percent lower LDL-cholesterol levels in patients on these drugs. Statins also produce a modest increase in HDL-cholesterol and reduce elevated triglyceride levels.

The statins are usually given in a single dose with the evening meal or at bedtime to take advantage of the fact that the liver makes more cholesterol at night than during the day. However, Lipitor®, which has a long half-life, may be taken any time of the day.

In November 1994, the five-year 4S Study provided a controlled scientific look at more than 4000 men who had survived a heart attack or had angina pectoris (coronary insufficiency). Cholesterol levels of the subjects averaged 260mg/dl (14.4mMol/dl). The study had a double-blind, placebo controlled format. The participants were divided into two groups. Half of them received Simvastatin and the other half were given placebo pills. The results clearly demonstrated the benefits of lowering blood cholesterol levels with medication. Those receiving the cholesterol lowering drugs had a much lower incidence of coronary bypass surgery or balloon angioplasty, treatments for advanced coronary artery disease. The overall mortality within the treated group was 30 percent less than in the control group. In other words, not only did far fewer patients require surgical intervention for advanced coronary disease, but the improved lipid profile was accompanied by an overall improvement in health and decreased mortality.

In November 1995, Dr. James Shepherd of the University of Glasgow, reported the results of the landmark Pravachol Primary Prevention Study, also known as the West of Scotland Coronary Prevention Study (WOSCOPS), in the prestigious New England Journal of Medicine. This double-blind, four-year study involved more than 6500 Scottish men, aged 45-64, with cholesterol levels of 250-300mg/dl (13.88 - 16.66mMol/dl), with no known heart disease, who were treated with Pravastatin.

The results far exceeded the anticipated benefits of even the most optimistic proponents of drug intervention. The treated group had 33 percent decrease in coronary heart disease, 22 percent fewer deaths from all causes, and 37 percent fewer bypass surgical procedures. The importance of treating a large segment of the population that has no known heart disease, but does have elevated cholesterol levels, was clearly demonstrated by the WOSCOPS.

The study showed that drug intervention should be resorted to earlier than previously believed. If diet and exercise cannot achieve satisfactory reduction in abnormal lipid levels, drug therapy is definitely indicated. Those with additional risk factors are particularly vulnerable. These are the asymptomatic hyperlipidemic individuals with silent underlying cardiovascular disease who may die without warning symptoms.

Cross Section of Blood Vessels

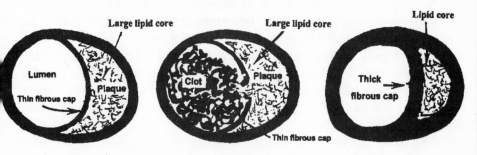

"Vulnerable" Plaque

Plaque Rupture with Clot Formation

"Stable" Plaque

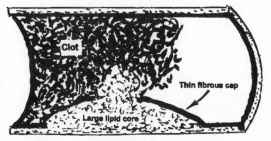

Longitudinal View
Vulnerable Plaque with Rupture and Clot Formation

coronary artery events (heart attacks and unstable angina) as early as six months to one year after instituting therapy.

CAUTION: Do not take statin drugs with grapefruit juice. Doing so reduces the effectiveness of the drug. The exception to this rule is Pravachol which is unaffected by grapefruit juice because it is metabolized by a different metabolic pathway than the other statin drugs.

It is desirable to take the over the counter antioxidant CoQ-10 when on statins. This is particularly important if you are taking any vitamin E.

As already noted, the stability of plaques and the condition of the inner lining of the blood vessel play major roles in acute coronary events.

Vulnerable plaques have a large lipid core with only a thin fibrous cap separating the highly thrombogenic core material from the circulating blood. Stable plaques have a thick fibrous cap which seals off the lipid core.

Patients on the "statins" must be monitored by their physician for adverse side effects such as elevated liver enzymes. In general, however, this class of drugs is well tolerated. Side effects are usually mild and reversible. Blood tests to monitor liver function should be done periodically. Muscle inflammation, called myopathy, is a rare and potentially serious side effect that has been seen in less than one half of one percent of those on these medications.

The incidence of myopathy is increased when these drugs are taken along with Gemfibrozil or nicotinic acid at lipid lowering doses (greater than 1 gram per day). The possible benefits of combined therapy with Gemfibrozil and a statin are not considered to be sufficient to outweigh the risk for developing myopathy. However, some physicians employ this drug combination when they are able to monitor the creatinine phosphokinase (CPK) enzyme and liver function tests periodically in reliable patients who will not get lost to medical follow-up. Patients with renal insufficiency, particularly the type associated with diabetes, are also at increased risk for developing myopathy.

If you take a statin you must familiarize yourself with the symptoms associated with myopathy: muscle aches or pains, and muscle tenderness or weakness, particularly if accompanied by malaise, fever and a brown discoloration of the urine. CPK is one of the blood enzyme tests performed periodically to monitor liver function in patients taking a statin. If the CPK level is elevated, or myopathy is suspected, the statin therapy must be discontinued.

Bile Acid Resins

Bile acid resins bind with cholesterol-containing bile acids in the intestines and are then eliminated in the stool. The major effect of bile acid resins is to lower LDL-cholesterol by about 10 to 20 percent. Small doses of resins can produce useful reductions in LDL-cholesterol. Bile acid resins are sometimes prescribed with a statin for patients with CAD to increase cholesterol reduction. When these two drugs are combined, their effects are added together to lower LDL-cholesterol by over 40 percent. Cholestyramine and colestipol are the two main bile acid resins currently available. These two drugs are available as powders or tablets. They are not absorbed from the gastrointestinal tract and 30 years of experience with the resins indicate that their long-term use is safe.

Bile acid resin powders must be mixed with water or fruit juice and taken once or twice (rarely three times) daily with meals. Tablets must be taken with large amounts of fluids to avoid gastrointestinal symptoms. Resin therapy may produce side effect symptoms including significant constipation, bloating, nausea, and gas.

The bile acid resins are not prescribed as the sole medicine to lower your cholesterol if you have high triglycerides or a history of severe constipation. Although resins are not absorbed, they may interfere with the absorption of other medicines if taken at the same time. Other medications, therefore, should be taken at least one hour before or four to six hours after the resin. If you take a resin, talk to your doctor about the best time to take this medicine, especially if you take other medications.

Nicotinic Acid (Niacin)

Nicotinic acid or niacin, the water-soluble B vitamin, improves lipoproteins when given in doses well above the vitamin requirement. However, nicotinic acid may increase insulin resistance, it worsens glucose intolerance, thereby elevating blood glucose levels (therefore it is generally not prescribed for diabetics). Nicotinic acid lowers total cholesterol, LDL-cholesterol, and triglyceride levels, while raising HDL-cholesterol levels. There are two types of nicotinic acid: immediate release and timed release. Most experts recommend starting with the immediate-release form. Nicotinic acid is inexpensive and widely accessible to patients without a prescription but must NOT be used for cholesterol lowering without the monitoring of a physician because of potential side effects. (Nicotinamide, another form of the vitamin niacin, does not lower cholesterol levels and should not be used in place of nicotinic acid).

All patients taking nicotinic acid to lower serum cholesterol should be closely monitored by their doctor to avoid complications from this medication. Self-medication with nicotinic acid should definitely be avoided because of the possibility of failing to detect a serious side effect if not under a doctor's care.

Patients on nicotinic acid are usually started on low daily doses and gradually increase to an average daily dose of 1.5 to 3 grams per day.

Nicotinic acid reduces LDL-cholesterol levels by 10 to 20 percent, reduces triglycerides by 20 to 50 percent, and raises HDL-cholesterol by 15 to 35 percent.

A common and troublesome side effect of nicotinic acid is flushing or hot flashes, which are the result of the dilatation of blood vessels. Most patients develop a tolerance to flushing, and in some patients, it can be decreased by taking the drug during or after meals. The effects of high blood pressure medicines may be increased while you are on niacin. If you are taking high blood pressure medication, it is important to set up a blood pressure monitoring system while you are getting accustomed to a new niacin regimen.

A variety of gastrointestinal symptoms, including nausea, indigestion, gas, vomiting, diarrhea, and the activation of peptic ulcers, have been seen with the use of nicotinic acid. Other major adverse effects include liver problems, gout, abnormal heart rhythms and elevation of blood sugar. Risk of the these side effects is dose related and increases as the dose of nicotinic acid is raised.

OTHER DRUGS

Fibrates (Fibric Acid Derivatives)

The cholesterol-lowering drugs called fibrates are primarily effective in lowering triglycerides and, to a lesser extent, in increasing HDL-cholesterol levels. Gemfibrozil (Lopid®), the fibrate most widely used in the United States, can be very effective for patients with high triglyceride levels. However, it is not very effective for lowering LDL-cholesterol. As a result, it is used less often than other drugs in patients for whom LDL-cholesterol lowering is the main goal of treatment.

Fibrates are usually given in two daily doses 30 minutes before the morning and evening meals. Triglyceride reductions generally are in the range of 20 to 50 percent with increases in HDL-cholesterol of 10 to 15 percent.

Fibrates are generally well tolerated by most patients. Gastrointestinal complaints are the most common side effect. Fibrates also appear to increase the likelihood of developing cholesterol gallstones. They can increase the effect of medications that thin the blood, which necessitates close monitoring by a physician.

Combination Drug Therapy

If your goal LDL level is not reached after three months with a single drug, your doctor may consider increasing the dosage of your medication or starting a second medicine to go with it. Combination therapy can increase your cholesterol lowering, reversing or slowing the advance of atherosclerosis and further decreasing the chance of a heart attack.

ASPIRIN AND CARDIOVASCULAR DISEASE

For the blood clotting mechanism to begin, certain particles that normally circulate in the blood, called platelets, are required. The blood clotting process is initiated when the platelets become sticky and adhere to one another and the blood vessel wall. Ordinary aspirin has the effect of preventing this platelet stickiness from developing. Aspirin, in low doses, has been used to reduce the risk of heart attacks by preventing platelets from sticking together. The major risk of aspirin therapy is irritation to the stomach lining causing gastrointestinal irritation or hemorrhage and stroke. These side effects are dose related and are reduced to approximately placebo levels when enteric coated 81mg aspirin tablets are used. This small dose of aspirin is just as effective as higher doses (1 adult tablet contains 325mg of aspirin). Contraindications to aspirin therapy include allergy to aspirin, bleeding tendency, liver disease or history of peptic ulcer. **Only a doctor who knows your complete medical history and current health status can judge whether the benefits you may gain from aspirin outweigh any risks.** Only a doctor who knows your complete medical history and current health status can judge whether the benefits you may gain from aspirin outweigh the risks.

HOMOCYSTEINE: AN INDEPENDENT RISK FACTOR FOR HARDENING OF THE ARTERIES

High blood cholesterol levels and the other generally recognized risk factors for atherosclerosis do not explain all cases of premature heart disease. Some coronary artery disease (CAD) patients do not have abnormalities in their lipid profile and are unresponsive to cholesterol-lowering drugs. Many of these cases may be due to abnormalities in the way their body metabolizes homocysteine, a little known amino acid.

Homocysteine is produced by the body's cells in the normal course of their metabolism. Under usual conditions the body can rapidly dispose of any excess amounts of homocysteine produced. Some people, however, are born with defective metabolic pathways for handling homocysteine, which results in marked elevations of homocysteine levels. These individuals develop premature atherosclerosis. Their bodies undergo an accelerated aging process and they may experience strokes and heart attacks at an early age, even before they attain adulthood. Physiologically their young bodies are those of elderly persons.

Although these congenital forms of marked elevation of homocysteine levels are rare, it has been theorized that milder but prolonged elevations of homocysteine levels in the blood of otherwise normal people can slowly and asymptomatically take their toll on the body's vascular system. Homocysteine levels in the blood can be measured by a laboratory test. In general, plasma homocysteine levels of 12mM/l or less are considered normal. Concentrations between 12-15 mM/l are considered borderline, and concentrations greater than 15mM/l are believed to be associated with a high risk for cardiovascular disease. Studies indicate that risk for cardiovascular disease correlates directly with homocysteine levels, and declines in risk are proportional to decreases in homocysteine levels. Elevated homocysteine levels are often encountered in those with a family history of premature heart disease, particularly occurring in the absence of the usual risk factors.

It is believed that many cases of homocysteine elevation result from dietary deficiencies. A diet low in plant foods and, therefore, deficient in folic acid (or folate) as well as vitamins B-6 and B-12, may predispose to abnormally high levels of homocysteine. Many patients with elevated homocysteine levels respond to supplements of folic acid. The optimal dosage is believed to be between 650 to 1000 micrograms daily. The typical American diet supplies approximately 200mcg/day. Many multiple vitamin and mineral supplements supply an additional 400 micrograms. Furthermore, in January 1998, the Food and Drug Administration mandated that all grains and cereals be fortified with folic acid. Generally, the simple measure of taking a daily dietary supplement of folic acid and Vitamin B-6 suffices to prevent homocysteine levels from rising too high. Although citrus fruits, vegetables and beans are good sources of folate, large quantities must be consumed to insure an adequate protective intake. Folic acid supplements are safe, except for the possibility that they may mask Vitamin B-12 deficiency. But, this does not pose a problem because Vitamin B-12 is usually included in most multiple vitamin supplements containing folic acids. Despite the compelling evidence for the relationship between homocysteine and atherosclerosis, the definitive studies to determine if reducing homocysteine levels prevents atherosclerosis have not yet been completed. However, abnormally high homocysteine levels in the blood must be considered a major risk factor for cardio-vascular disease. Everyone should protect himself against this threat. Prevention or treatment of elevated homocysteine levels is straightforward and risk free. The disorder is usually corrected by simply taking vitamin supplements containing folic acid, B-6 and B-12.

Both Type 1 and Type 2 diabetic patients have been shown to have elevated homocysteine levels. However, to date no studies have showed a reduction of CAD with reduction of homocysteine levels. Studies in non-diabetics with homocysteine levels greater than 15Mmol/L have shown benefit with treatment of folic acid.

SYNDROME X: THE METABOLIC CARDIOVASCULAR SYNDROME

A syndrome is a group of signs and symptoms that occur together in a particular disease process or abnormal condition. Syndrome X is the name given to the association and complex interrelationship between dyslipidemia (especially elevated triglycerides), glucose intolerance, high blood pressure, excessive abdominal fat (central obesity), insulin resistance (the inability of the body to respond normally to insulin resulting in high blood insulin levels), and Coronary Artery Disease (CAD).

Aside from putting an individual at risk for developing diabetes, Syndrome X also predisposes to atherosclerosis. Many studies have shown Syndrome X to pose as great a risk for cardiovascular disease as does elevated blood cholesterol levels. Syndrome X may be responsible for many heart attacks despite the fact that those with this condition usually have total cholesterol levels within the normal range.

Once the cluster of symptoms that constitute Syndrome X is recognized, measures can be taken to control and eliminate this health threat. Syndrome X is not difficult to recognize when one is alert to the three main elements that make up the syndrome.

1. Excessive abdominal fat. A waistline measurement greater than 39 inches in either men or women suggests Syndrome X.
2. A ratio of total cholesterol to HDL-cholesterol greater than 5 may indicate Syndrome X.
3. Elevated triglyceride levels—usually above 150mg/dl (3.89mMol/L)—associated with normal total cholesterol and high LDL-cholesterol levels—along with low HDL-cholesterol point to Syndrome X.

How to Prevent or Reverse Syndrome X

Once the cluster of symptoms that constitute Syndrome X are recognized, measures can be taken to lower or even normalize the risks of this health threat. The key to preventing or reversing the syndrome is diet and exercise. With weight loss and a decrease in abdominal fat, there is improvement in insulin sensitivity, the main factor responsible for Syndrome X. Exercise not only helps to restore muscle tone, but also promotes improvement in insulin sensitivity. Certain high blood pressure medications, Beta blockers and diuretics, tobacco use, and a diet high in saturated fats may increase the risk of developing syndrome X.

Order of Priorities for Treatment of Dyslipidemia in Adults with Type 2 Diabetes

Lower LDL-cholesterol
1. Control of blood sugar with lifestyle modification. Low saturated fat, low cholesterol diet, aerobic exercise regimen.
2. If unresponsive to lifestyle measures alone start HMG CoA reductase inhibitor (statin).
3. If still unable to reach target goal, add bile acid binding resin to medication regimen.

(Lifestyle modification + statin + resin)

Raise HDL-cholesterol
Weight loss, increased aerobic physical activity and smoking cessation may help. Nicotinic acid raises HDL-cholesterol, but worsens glucose control. It is therefore relatively contraindicated in diabetes and generally not used.

Lower Triglyceride Levels
1. Control of blood sugar first priority with dietary restriction of simple sugars and avoidance of alcohol.
2. Fibric acid derivative—gemfibrozil (Lopid®).

Note: Statins are effective at high doses in patients with elevated triglycerides who also have high LDL-cholesterol levels. There is a relative contraindication to their use with gemfibrozil.

Treat Combined Hyperlipidemia Aggressively
1. Improve blood sugar regulation with diet plus high dose of a statin.
2. Alternative treatment improved diet for blood sugar control plus resin plus gemfibrozil.
3. If not controlled: stringent dietary control + statin + gemfibrozil.* Evaluate benefits vs. risks.

* CAUTION: The incidence of myopathy, a serious side effect that is rarely seen with statin therapy, is increased when gemfibrozil is taken along with a statin. Monitoring of liver enzyme levels such as the CPK must be done when this combination of medications is used. Many physicians believe the benefits offered by this combination of medications do not outweigh the risks entailed by their use. Nicotinic acid along with a statin drug is also associated with increased myopathy risk, although to a lesser degree. Patients with kidney disease (nephropathy) are at a high risk for side effects when combinations of these drugs are used.

Treatment of Dyslipidemia in Type 1 Diabetic Patients

Type 1 patients who maintain good blood sugar control generally have lipid levels that are within the normal range. The composition of their lipids, however, is abnormal. The effect of these abnormalities on cardiovascular disease are not completely known. The ADA recommends aggressive treatment of all Type 1 patients who have LDL-cholesterol levels above 130mg/dl (3.37mMol/L) or above 100mg/dl (2.59mMol/L) in patients with known CAD. Optimal blood sugar control is the key to prevention and treatment of dyslipidemia in Type 1 patients.

ALCOHOL AND HEART DISEASE —THE FRENCH PARADOX

As long ago as 1819, Samuel Black, an Irish physician, noted that coronary artery disease was not an uncommon post-mortem finding in his country, and relatively rare in France and the Mediterranean countries. He ascribed the discrepancy to some unknown differences in lifestyle and/or diet.

Despite the fact that the French eat three times as much saturated fat as their American counterparts, the incidence of coronary artery disease in France is only one-third of that in the United States. In 1991, this was the subject of a report on the CBS television show 60 Minutes. The phenomenon became known popularly as the "French Paradox."

There are significant dietary differences between the eating habits in the two countries. The French drink less milk than Americans, and eat more fresh vegetables, fruit, garlic and cheese. They also consume considerably more wine.

Many epidemiological studies have demonstrated that alcohol exerts some sort of protective effect against heart disease. The equivalent of two drinks per day has been shown to cause a significant decrease in heart disease. Higher doses of alcohol, however, can raise blood pressure and are associated with an increased incidence of heart attacks and strokes. The protective affect of alcohol is to some degree associated with the ability of alcohol to raise the HDL-cholesterol. Red wine seems to have a particularly beneficial effect. The unique protective quality of red wine is believed to reside in its high content of polyphenols—powerful anti-oxidants— which are not present in white wine (except champagne) and are absent from beer, with the exception of dark beers. Grape juice has about one third to one half the amount of flavinoids as red wine.

Alcoholic Beverages and Diabetes

Only your personal physician can tell you whether it's safe for you to drink alcoholic beverages occasionally. Most people with diabetes—with their doctor's approval—can drink alcohol safely if they drink in moderation (one or two drinks occasionally). Higher quantities of alcohol can cause health problems. Naturally, diabetics must observe the same precautions regarding the use of alcohol as the general public.

Alcohol has empty calories without the vitamins, mineral, and other nutrients that are essential for maintaining good health. People who are trying to lose weight need to account for the calories in their alcoholic drinks. One alcoholic beverage=12ozs. of beer, 5ozs. of wine, or 1-1/2ozs. of distilled spirits. Ordinarily, to avoid alcohol-induced hypoglycemia, diabetics should never drink alcohol on an empty stomach. When calories from alcohol need to be calculated as part of the overall caloric intake, it probably is best to substitute alcohol for fat exchanges (1 alcohol beverage =2 fat exchanges). Alcohol abstention is necessary during pregnancy and in those with a history of alcohol abuse, liver disease or other medical contraindication to its use.

FREE RADICALS AND ANTI-OXIDANTS

Free radical oxidation of LDL-cholesterol is the initial step in plaque formation. Free-radicals are highly reactive atoms or molecules that form in our body as by-products of normal cell metabolism. Oxygen's unique chemical structure makes it particularly vulnerable to free-radical conversion. Oxygen is essential for all life processes. However, when an oxygen atom is converted into a free-radical it becomes extraordinarily toxic, capable of causing cell damage. There is a constant tug of war between free-radicals and anti-oxidant molecules to maintain equilibrium. Anti-oxidants are certain nutrients found in fruits and vegetables that protect against the oxygen-induced damage which free-radicals cause. Free-radicals generally exist for only extremely short periods of time before they are neutralized by an anti-oxidant. Exposure to a large quantity of anti-oxidants poses a threat that the anti-oxidant defense system could be overwhelmed. Aside from being generated by the body's own metabolism, free-radical molecules abound in our environment. They are formed by solar radiation, x-rays, insecticides, auto exhaust fumes, cigarette smoke and other pollutants. We are currently exposed to more environmental pollutants that generate free-radicals than at any time in the past. Our need for an adequate supply of dietary anti-oxidants to combat this threat is greater than ever.

It is important to include adequate amounts of anti-oxidants in the diabetic diet because of their role in preventing some of the long-term complications of diabetes. The destructive effects of smoking includes an increased rate of free radical formation. We know that smoking also causes the formation of Accelerated Glycosylated End products (AGE's) that play a major role in the tissue damage that gives rise to long-term diabetic complications (see Chapter 27, *Diabetes: The Cure*). One more reason that it is imperative for diabetics to stop smoking: Anti-oxidants provide some benefit against the accelerated cardiovascular and renal disease that frequently accompany diabetes, as well as the other long-term end organ tissue damage that is probably related to AGEs formation.

Potent anti-oxidants that can mop up free-radicals before they do harm include selenium, vitamin C, vitamin E, the carotenoids—precursors to vitamin A, and phytochemicals. Tea leaves, particularly green tea, are high in anti-oxidants called polyphenols.

Epidemiologic studies have shown that diets rich in fruits and vegetables were associated with a decreased incidence of coronary artery disease (CAD). It is believed that the high anti-oxidant content of these foods decreases LDL oxidation, thereby reducing plaque formation. Many cardiologists recommend including foods high in Vitamin C, a potent anti-oxidant, for their patients. It is most desirable to get your Vitamin C from natural sources. A glass of freshly squeezed orange juice, for example, contains approximately 150mg of Vitamin C. Vitamin E, another potent anti-oxidant with cardio-protective qualities is found in whole grains, vegetables, particularly leafy vegetables and nuts. Some studies point to the cardio-protective benefits of taking Vitamin E supplements at a dosage of 400 I.U. daily. The typical American diet falls woefully short of supplying this amount of the vitamin.

Vitamin E

Vitamin E decreases the oxidation of LDL-cholesterol, which as we have seen is the first step in plaque formation. Vitamin E also helps to prevent platelet agglutination, the initial step in blood clot formation.

At times, Vitamin E, when outdated or stored improperly, can have a pro-oxidant effect, characteristics which are the opposite of an anti-oxidant. This rare exceptional reaction is avoided when Vitamin C is taken along with Vitamin E.

The daily allowance (RDA for vitamin E set by the FDA is 15 IU. Most people get less than 11 IU of Vitamin E from their diet. The only active form of Vitamin E is the d-Alpha Tocopherol. A mirror image chemical form, l-Alpha Tocopherol is inert.* Vitamin E in mega doses (beyond 1000 I.U.) is to be avoided because it may cause side effects in some persons, including fatigue. Excellent natural sources of Vitamin E are whole grains, nuts, seeds and vegetables.

Vitamin C

Vitamin C is a less potent anti-oxidant than Vitamin E. Vitamin C is a water soluble vitamin that is present in many fruits and vegetables. An average glass of orange juice contains about 150mg of Vitamin C. Despite the claims of benefit for megadoses of Vitamin C for illness and general health, supporting evidence for such benefits is not only lacking, but some studies indicate toxic side effects at doses beyond 500mg/day. Ascorbic acid levels are 20 percent lower in diabetics than in non-diabetics. They are also low in smokers. Diabetics should include foods high in Vitamin C routinely in their diet. An additional benefit of Vitamin C was documented in patients undergoing angioplasty for coronary disease. Those who took

---

*When purchasing Vitamin E, always read the fine print on the label. The d-L Alpha Tacopherol Vitamin E contains only one half of the active form. Therefore, 800 IU of the d-L form is equal to 400 units of the d form. Natural Vitamin E is all d-Alpha Tocopherol.

60mg of Vitamin C daily had only half the failure rate of those not taking any supplemental Vitamin C.

Get your vitamin C from fresh citrus or other Vitamin C containing fruits and vegetables such as tomatoes, peppers, and strawberries.

The Carotenoids

Betacarotene and other carotenoids are derived from plants. The carotenoids are the colored pigments in many yellow or orange fruits, as well as green leafy vegetables. Protective benefits of the carotenoids, when taken in pill form, has not been consistently demonstrated. Studies, however, did show benefit from carotenoids obtained from natural dietary sources.

Selenium

This mineral is a potent anti-oxidant. However, in large doses selenium is toxic. Daily doses of 200mcg are adequate. Dietary sources of selenium vary considerably in different areas of the country, depending on such factors as the selenium content of the soil where foods are grown.

Green Tea

Green tea is rich in anti-oxidants that have a favorable affect on lipid metabolism. The active ingredient is a catechin, a compound that belongs to the chemical group called polyphenols. The catechins present in green tea, along with other polyphenols may be effective in preventing LDL-cholesterol from undergoing oxidation, one of the initial steps in plaque formation.

Green tea has other beneficial affects on lipid metabolism. One recent study demonstrated a nine point decrease in total cholesterol level in men who drank green tea daily. The catechins present in green tea are also purported to help prevent lung cancer and certain skin cancers. Although massive doses of catechins are toxic, drinking several cups of green tea daily is safe and appears to offer health benefits.

Note: As with all vitamins and supplements, it is most desirable to get these nutrients from their natural food sources. Taking a supplement in pill form may not be adequate because other, sometimes poorly understood, additional nutrients in the natural food may be lacking in the supplement.

THE PRITIKIN PROGRAM , DIABETES
AND ATHEROSCLEROSIS

In 1957, Nathan Pritikin was diagnosed with life-threatening heart disease and a high blood-cholesterol level. In defiance of what was then medical convention, Pritikin decided he would treat himself—with a low-fat, high-fiber diet and regular aerobic exercise. Twelve months later, his blood cholesterol had dropped 140 points. By 1966, his cardiovascular endurance had so improved that he was able to run seven miles a day. His stress tests no longer showed evidence of coronary insufficiency. Pritikin had turned his life around. And, he felt wonderful.

The backbone of the Pritikin food plan is carbohydrates. Seventy-five to eighty percent of your daily calories will be in the form of unrefined carbohydrates (vegetables, fruits, grains, pastas, legumes, breads). These are great energy sources, so you'll have plenty of pep on this plan. And since unrefined carbohydrates (whole-grain bread, brown rice) are emphasized here, your vitamin, mineral, and fiber requirements will be easily satisfied.

The Pritikin program can improve your health. Stress, exercise, and smoking do influence health, but nutrition is the key to preventing, halting, and even reversing atherosclerosis.

The Pritikin Program is high in fiber, the indigestible part of plant cells. It adds bulk to waste products passing through your digestive system. Researchers believe a high-fiber diet keeps blood sugar levels in balance and may therefore help control diabetes. Soluble fiber—the type found in oat bran, legumes (navy, lima and kidney beans), vegetables (corn), fruits (apples and oranges) and brown rice—actually *lowers* cholesterol.

You would probably have to triple the amount of fiber you're currently getting in order to meet the 25 to 35 grams per day standard set by the American Dietetic Association. On the Pritikin Program, you will be assured of at least 40 grams daily. The amount of protein you'll get on the Pritikin Program is the same amount most Americans currently consume— 10 to 15 percent of daily calories. The difference is in the *source* of protein. On the Pritikin Program, most of the protein comes from vegetables, grains, and legumes rather than from animal products. These foods are good sources of protein and don't carry the dietary fat and cholesterol of animal products. Protein, which aids tissue repair, is only needed in small amounts. Instead of eating meat as a main course, you'll be eating mostly vegetable and grain entrees, with fish, poultry, and lean meats functioning either as a side dish or condiment in a main dish. To ensure daily cholesterol intake does not exceed 100 milligrams, an amount most people can handle, the Pritikin Program recommends that meat intake be kept to 3.5 ounces daily.

Even if you already have evidence of atherosclerosis, it is never too late to lower your cholesterol. By lowering it, you may prevent further development of disease, and in some cases, even reverse the process.

The recommended level for blood cholesterol on the Pritikin Program is 160 milligrams per deciliter of blood, or 100 plus your age, whichever is lower. This figure is based on population studies in nations with a low incidence of cardiovascular disease. Research shows that there is almost no risk for heart disease associated with a cholesterol level below 150.

On the Pritikin program you will be getting 100 milligrams (or less) of cholesterol daily. Compare this with the 400 to 500 milligrams most Americans consume daily.

Diet is one of the most important keys to controlling diabetes. Most diabetics quickly master the art of avoiding too many simple sugars and many of the fatty foods they had previously found difficult to resist. The standard diabetic diet is based upon food exchanges, total calories, and proportions of carbohydrates, proteins, and fats as described in Chapter 7, *Guidelines for Healthier Eating With Diabetes*. These diets are excellent for most people, particularly young persons. However, there is no emphasis on preventive measures against the long-term degenerative complications of diabetes. The Pritikin approach seeks to combat the "Deadly Quartet"—a constellation of the disorders that are associated with insulin resistance and lead to the long-term complications.

Included in the "quartet" are obesity—particularly abdominal fat deposits—high blood pressure, and elevated levels of cholesterol and triglycerides in the blood. The "Deadly Quartet" increases the risk of microvascular disease—changes in the small blood vessels (capillaries)—that develop when the blood sugar is chronically uncontrolled. The Pritikin approach to diabetes emphasizes the importance of preventing and treating obesity associated with Type 2 diabetes and stresses the importance of diet, exercise, and behavioral changes.

The Pritikin diet emphasizes complex carbohydrates, taking into account the preparation, refining, milling, and breakdown of carbohydrates. The dietary program taught at the Pritikin Longevity Center influences the rapidity of digestion and absorption of nutrients and therefore, the effect on blood sugar levels. Unrefined carbohydrates make the body work harder to refuel itself by requiring physiological processes to gradually convert the complex carbohydrates to simple sugars, a process that maintains a more stable blood glucose pattern.

Researchers refer to a food's immediate, post-meal effect on blood sugar as "glycemic-index." In one study, low glycemic-index wheat flour and potatoes had the same percentage of fat and fiber, but the low glycemic-index foods reduced blood sugar more efficiently by 11-20 percent.

The ingestion of unrefined carbohydrates makes it easier to lose weight by prolonging the feeling of satiety (fullness) and they are more slowly absorbed, adding to the benefit for stabilizing the blood glucose levels in diabetics.

A high soluble fiber diet content also has the important added benefit of slowing the digestive process, improving insulin sensitivity, and lowering the levels of cholesterol and triglycerides — effects that lower the risk for developing vascular disease.

Whole grain hot cereal is better for you than whole wheat bread. Corn on the cob is better than cornmeal. A fresh apple is better than a dried apple.

Vegetarian chili, split pea, and barley soup, as well as corn chowder and lentil soup, all contain the right foods; the unrefined carbohydrates and the high soluble fiber meet the criteria for aiding in controlling blood sugar levels. In short, the Pritikin program may offer protection against the rate of development of many of the long-term complications of diabetes. The Pritikin program recommends eating five to eight small meals every day rather than two or three large meals. This helps to avoid spikes in blood sugar and seems to control appetite and hunger to a greater degree.

Another mainstay in the Pritikin approach is exercise. Exercise lowers and stabilizes blood sugar, improves glucose tolerance, and reduces insulin resistance. Exercise also facilitates the lowering of cholesterol and triglycerides, and raises the "good" cholesterol, HDL, all of significant benefit to the diabetic. The exercise should be regular and sustained. Along with the prescribed diet, it will assist in weight loss in the obese diabetic. Most exercise derives 50 percent of calories from fat and 50 percent from carbohydrate. Sustained physical activity will use up fat stores leading to weight loss.

Moderate activities are preferable because high intensity exercise may release hormones which can raise blood sugar levels. Your physician, knowing your status regarding possible retinopathy, hypertension, and circulatory problems, can prescribe the best type of exercise for you.

The Pritikin program is *not for everyone*. It requires dedication and dietary sacrifices that many people are unwilling to make. Of course, varying degrees of modification can be incorporated into your diabetes control regimen in consultation with your dietitian and physician. This plan is particularly suitable for obese Type 2 diabetics who may be able to discontinue their medications after following the program. Everyone presents his own unique requirements. Therefore, before undertaking any radical change in your diet, consult your diabetologist for approval and recommendations.

CHAPTER
• 19 •

Long-Term Complications of Diabetes

Neuropathy
Cardiovascular Disease
Retinopathy
Nephropathy

Diabetes can affect many parts of the body. It can damage the kidneys, eyes, nervous system, blood vessels and heart causing kidney failure, vision loss, nerve damage, heart attacks, and strokes. These complications develop slowly over the years as a consequence of the chronically elevated blood sugar.

DIABETIC NEUROPATHY

What is Diabetic Neuropathy?

Diabetic neuropathy is a nerve disorder caused by diabetes. Symptoms of neuropathy include numbness and sometimes pain in the hands, feet, or legs. Nerve damage caused by diabetes can also lead to problems with internal organs such as the heart, sexual organs and digestive tract, causing indigestion, diarrhea or constipation, dizziness, bladder infections, and impotence. In some cases, neuropathy can flare up suddenly, causing weakness and weight loss. Depression may follow. While some treatments are available, a great deal of research is still needed to understand how diabetes affects the nerves and to find more effective treatments for this complication.

What Causes Diabetic Neuropathy?

Scientists do not know the precise biochemistry of what causes diabetic neuropathy, but several factors are likely to contribute to the disorder. High blood glucose causes chemical changes in nerves. These changes impair the nerves' ability to transmit signals. High blood glucose also damages blood vessels that carry oxygen and nutrients to the nerves. In addition, inherited factors probably unrelated to diabetes may make some people more susceptible to nerve disease than others.

How high blood glucose leads to nerve damage is a subject of intense research. Normally, glucose is metabolized (broken down for energy) to carbon dioxide and water. When blood sugar levels are high, some glucose is metabolized using an alternative pathway that produces a substance called sorbitol and depletes a substance called myoinositol that may cause nerve damage.

How Common is Diabetic Neuropathy?

People with diabetes can develop nerve problems at any time. Significant clinical neuropathy can develop within the first 10 years after diagnosis of diabetes and the risk of developing neuropathy increases the longer a person has diabetes. The various neuropathies are one of the most common long-term complications of diabetes, eventually affecting up to 70 percent of diabetics.

Diabetic neuropathy appears to be more common in smokers, people over 40 years of age and—as would be expected—among those who have had problems controlling their blood glucose levels.

Recently, researchers have focused on the effects of excessive glucose metabolism on the amount of nitrous oxide in nerves. Nitrous oxide dilates blood vessels. In a person with diabetes, low levels of nitrous oxide may lead to constriction of blood vessels supplying the nerve, contributing to nerve damage. Another promising area of research centers on the effect of glucose attaching to proteins when blood sugar is elevated, altering the structure and function of the proteins and affecting vascular function.

Scientists are studying how these changes occur, how they are connected, how they cause nerve damage, and how to prevent and treat damage.

What Are the Symptoms of Diabetic Neuropathy?

The symptoms of diabetic neuropathy vary. Numbness and tingling in feet are often the first sign. Some people notice no symptoms, while others are severely disabled. Neuropathy may cause both pain and insensitivity to pain in the same person. In some people, mainly those afflicted by focal neuropathy, the onset of pain may be sudden and severe. Unfortunately, because symptoms are slight at first, and because most nerve damage occurs over a period of years, mild cases may go unnoticed for a long time before measures are instituted to prevent permanent damage.

WHAT ARE THE MAJOR TYPES OF NEUROPATHY?

The symptoms of neuropathy also depend on which nerves and what part of the body is affected. Neuropathy may be **diffuse**, affecting many parts of the body, or **focal**, affecting a single, specific nerve and part of the body.

Diffuse Neuropathy

The two categories of diffuse neuropathy are peripheral neuropathy, affecting the feet and hands, and autonomic neuropathy, affecting the internal organs.

Peripheral Neuropathy

The most common type of peripheral neuropathy damages the nerves of the limbs, especially the feet. Nerves on both sides of the body are affected. Common symptoms are:
— Numbness or insensitivity to pain or temperature
— Tingling, burning or prickling
— Extreme sensitivity to touch, even light touch
— Loss of balance and coordination

These symptoms are often worse at night. The damage to nerves often results in loss of reflexes and muscle weakness. The foot often becomes wider and shorter, the gait changes, and foot ulcers appear as pressure is put on parts of the foot that are less protected. Because of the loss of sensation, injuries may go unnoticed and often become infected. If ulcers or foot injuries are not treated in time, the infection may involve the bone and require amputation. However, problems caused by minor injuries can usually be controlled if they are caught in time. Avoiding foot injury by wearing well-fitted shoes and examining the feet daily can help prevent amputations.

Autonomic Neuropathy
(*also called visceral neuropathy*)

Autonomic neuropathy is another form of diffuse neuropathy. It affects the nerves that serve the heart and internal organs and produces changes in many processes and systems.

Autonomic neuropathy most often affects the organs that control urination and sexual function. Nerve damage can prevent the bladder from emptying completely, promoting bacterial growth more easily in the urinary tract (bladder, ureter and kidneys). When the nerves of the bladder are damaged, a person may have difficulty knowing when the bladder is full, resulting in urinary incontinence.

The nerve damage and circulatory problems of diabetes can also lead to a gradual loss of sexual response in both men and women, although sex drive is unchanged. A man may be unable to have erections or may reach sexual climax without ejaculating normally.

Autonomic neuropathy can affect digestion. Nerve damage can cause the stomach to empty too slowly, a disorder called gastric stasis. When the condition is severe (gastroparesis), a person can have persistent nausea and vomiting, bloating, and loss of appetite. Blood glucose levels tend to fluctuate greatly with this condition. Therefore, gastroparesis should be considered as a possible cause of unexplained poor glycemic control in a previously stable patient, even in the absence of GI symptoms.

If nerves in the esophagus are involved, swallowing may be difficult. Nerve damage to the bowels can cause constipation or frequent diarrhea, especially at night. Problems with the digestive system often lead to weight loss.

Autonomic neuropathy can affect the cardiovascular system, which controls the circulation of blood throughout the body. Damage to this system interferes with the nerve impulses from various parts of the body that signal the need for blood and regulate blood pressure and heart rate. As a result, blood pressure may drop sharply after rising to a standing position following prolonged sitting, causing a person to feel dizzy or light-headed, or even to faint (orthostatic hypotension).

Neuropathy that affects the cardiovascular system may also affect the perception of pain from heart disease. For example, those with coronary artery disease may not experience anginal pain as a warning sign of heart disease or they may suffer painless heart attacks. It may also raise the risk of a heart attack during general anesthesia.

Autonomic neuropathy can hinder the body's normal response to low blood sugar or hypoglycemia, which makes it difficult to recognize and treat an insulin reaction. Autonomic neuropathy can also affect the nerves that control sweating. Sometimes nerve damage interferes with the activity of the sweat glands, making it difficult for the body to regulate its temperature. Other times, the result can be profuse sweating at night or while eating (gustatory sweating).

Focal Neuropathy *(including multiplex neuropathy)*

Occasionally, diabetic neuropathy appears suddenly and affects specific nerves, most often in the torso, leg, or head. Focal neuropathy may cause:

— Pain in the front of a thigh
— Severe pain in the lower back or pelvis
— Pain in the chest, stomach, or flank
— Chest or abdominal pain sometimes mistaken for angina, heart attack, or appendicitis
— Aching behind an eye
— Inability to focus the eye
— Double vision
— Paralysis on one side of the face (Bell's palsy)
— Problems with hearing

This kind of neuropathy is unpredictable and occurs most often in older people who have mild diabetes. Although focal neuropathy can be painful, it tends to improve by itself after a period of weeks or months without causing long-term damage.

People with diabetes are also prone to developing compression neuropathies. The most common form of compression neuropathy is carpal tunnel syndrome. Asymptomatic carpal tunnel syndrome occurs in 20 to 30 percent of people with diabetes, and symptomatic carpal tunnel syndrome occurs in 6 to 11 percent. Numbness and tingling of the hand are the most common symptoms. Muscle weakness may also develop.

How do Doctors Diagnose Diabetic Neuropathy?

A doctor diagnoses neuropathy based on symptoms and a physical exam. During the exam, the doctor may check muscle strength, reflexes, and sensitivity to position, vibration, temperature, and light touch. Sometimes special tests are also used to help determine the cause of symptoms and to suggest treatment.

A simple *screening test* to check point sensation in the feet can be done in the doctor's office. The test uses a nylon filament mounted on a small wand. The filament delivers a standardized 10-gram force when touched to areas of the foot. Patients who cannot sense pressure from the filament have lost protective sensation and are at risk for developing neuropathic foot ulcers.

Nerve conduction studies check the flow of electrical current through a nerve. With this test, an image of the nerve impulse is projected on a screen as it transmits an electrical signal. Impulses that seem slower or weaker than usual indicate possible damage to the nerve. This test allows the doctor to assess the condition of the nerves in the arms and legs.

Electromyography (EMG) is used to see how well muscles respond to electrical impulses transmitted by nearby nerves. The electrical activity of the muscle is displayed on a screen. A response that is slower or weaker than usual suggests damage to the nerve or muscle. This test is often done at the same time as nerve conduction studies.

Ultrasound employs sound waves. The sound waves are too high to hear, but they produce an image showing how well the bladder and other parts of the urinary tract are functioning.

Nerve biopsy involves removing a sample of nerve tissue for examination. This test is most often used in research settings.

If your doctor suspects autonomic neuropathy, you may also be referred to a physician who specializes in digestive disorders (gastroenterologist) for additional tests.

How is Diabetic Neuropathy Usually Treated?

Treatment aims to relieve discomfort and prevent further tissue damage. The first step is to bring blood sugar under control by diet and oral drugs or insulin injections, if needed, and by careful monitoring of blood sugar levels. Although symptoms can sometimes worsen at first as blood sugar is brought under control, maintaining lower blood sugar levels helps reverse the pain or loss of sensation that neuropathy can cause. Good control of blood sugar may also help prevent or delay the onset of further problems.

Relief of Pain

For relief of pain, burning, tingling, or numbness, the doctor may suggest Gabapentin, a drug manufactured by the Parke-Davis Co. under the trade name Neurontin, which has been quite effective in relieving the pain of diabetic neuropathy side effects including fatigue and sleepiness, and analgesics such as aspirin or acetaminophen or anti-inflammatory drugs containing ibuprofen. Nonsteroidal anti-inflammatory drugs should be used with caution in people with renal disease. Antidepressant medications such as amitriptyline or nerve medications such as carbamazepine or phenytoin sodium may be helpful. Codeine is sometimes prescribed for short-term use to relieve severe pain. In addition, a topical cream, capsaicin, is available over-the-counter to help relieve the pain of neuropathy.

Other treatments include hypnosis, relaxation training, biofeedback, and acupuncture. Some people find that walking regularly or using elastic stockings helps relieve leg pain. Warm (not hot) baths, massage, or an analgesic ointment may also help. After age forty, **never** massage your legs. Many adults have asymptomatic blood clots in their deep veins that will never cause a problem unless they are dislodged by vigorous manipulation such as massage therapy.

Gastrointestinal Problems

Indigestion, belching, nausea, or vomiting are symptoms of gastroparesis. For patients with mild symptoms of slow stomach emptying, doctors suggest eating small, frequent meals and avoiding fats. Eating less fiber may also relieve symptoms. For patients with severe gastroparesis, the doctor may prescribe metoclopramide, which speeds digestion and helps relieve nausea. Other drugs that help regulate digestion or reduce stomach acid secretion may also be used. In each case, the potential benefits of these drugs need to be weighed against their side effects.

A wheat-free diet may also bring relief since the gluten in flour sometimes causes diarrhea.

Neurological problems affecting the urinary tract can result in infections or incontinence. The doctor may prescribe an antibiotic to clear up an infection and suggest drinking more fluids to prevent further infections. If incontinence is a problem, patients may be advised to urinate at regular times (every 3 hours, for example) since they may not be able to tell when the bladder is full.

Dizziness, Weakness

Sitting or standing up slowly may help prevent light-headedness, dizziness, or fainting, which are symptoms that may be associated with some forms of autonomic neuropathy. Raising the head of the bed and wearing elastic stockings which aid the venous blood may also help.

Muscle weakness or loss of coordination caused by diabetic neuropathy can often be helped by physical therapy.

Urinary and Sexual Problems

Nerve and circulatory problems of diabetes can disrupt normal male sexual function, resulting in impotence. After ruling out a hormonal cause of impotence, the doctor can provide information about methods available to treat impotence caused by neuropathy. (See Chapter 23, *Diabetes and Impotence.*)

In women who feel their sexual life is not satisfactory, the role of diabetic neuropathy is less clear. Illness, vaginal or urinary tract infections, and anxiety about pregnancy complicated by diabetes can interfere with a woman's ability to enjoy intimacy. Infections can be reduced by good blood glucose control. Counseling may also help a woman identify and cope with sexual concerns.

**Why is Good Foot Care Important for
People With Diabetic Neuropathy?**

People with diabetes need to take special care of their feet. Neuropathy and blood vessel disease both increase the risk of foot ulcers. The nerves to the feet are the longest in the body, and are most often affected by neuropathy. Because of the loss of sensation caused by neuropathy, sores or injuries to the feet may not be noticed and complications may progress asymptomatically.

At least 15 percent of all people with diabetes eventually have a foot ulcer, and 6 of every 1,000 people with diabetes experience dry gangrene of the foot requiring amputation. However, doctors estimate that nearly three quarters of all amputations caused by neuropathy and poor circulation could be prevented with careful foot care. Read the rules for foot care spelled out in Chapter 22, *Care of the Feet.*

DIABETIC RETINOPATHY

Blindness is one of the most feared complications of long standing diabetes. It is true that diabetes mellitus is the leading cause of blindness in the United States and is one of the most feared complications. The incidence of blindness from diabetic retinopathy is 0.2 percent per year in all diabetics, but this fact may be somewhat misleading. "Legal" blindness is defined as vision 20/200 or less, and does not necessarily mean "total blindness." A person may be legally blind and still be able to perform most of his daily chores with the exception of driving and tasks that obviously require more acute vision. In fact, not more than 5 percent of the diabetic population is completely blind. This low figure is a result of new and modern scientific treatments available for diabetic eye problems.

The eye is actually a small sphere filled with a clear gel called the vitreous. The retina is a delicate membrane of nerve tissue that lines the inside of the eye chamber. It acts like a photographic film that receives visual stimuli and transmits the "picture" to the brain for interpretation. This visual impulse passes along the optic nerve and goes directly to the visual center located in the back of the brain. Indeed, the optic nerve itself is a direct extension of the brain.

Your doctor can visualize the inside of the eye and the optic nerve with an instrument called an ophthalmoscope. The tiny blood vessels that provide nourishment to the eye can be seen radiating out from this "optic disc." With long-standing diabetes, these "retinal" vessels can weaken and subsequently develop tiny "blow outs" called microaneurysms that can leak plasma out of the confines of the tiny capillary. In some, this is followed by the formation of new blood vessels associated with scar formation of the damaged tissues, resulting in visual loss.

The above sequence of events is given the generic name, Diabetic Retinopathy. Retinopathy can be divided into two major categories: *non-proliferative* (background retinopathy) and *proliferative* retinopathy. The former includes venous abnormalities, microaneurysms, retinal bleeding and accumulations of lipid or protein containing fluid called exudates. The abnormality in non-proliferative retinopathy can be seen with a procedure known as fluorescein angiography and often can be reversed with excellent glucose control. Edema of the retina is due to abnormal capillary permeability and poor blood supply (ischemia). "Macular" edema is a serious complication and must be treated early by photocoagulation. This treatment will be discussed later.

The hallmark of *proliferative* retinopathy is new blood vessel formation (neo-vascularization). These tiny vascular loops grow on the surface of the retina or extend into the vitreous. Traction may develop between the vitreous and the neovascular elements leading to another serious complication, retinal detachment. A table showing the types of diabetic retinopathy follows:

A. Background retinopathy or non-proliferative retinopathy
1. Microaneurysms with or without tiny hemorrhages.
2. Exudates (hard)
3. Venous and arteriolar abnormalities
5. Retinal edema

B. Preproliferative retinopathy
1. Soft exudates or "cotton wool" spots
2. Intra-retinal vascular abnormalities

   3. Areas of "non perfusion"
   4. Macular edema

C. Proliferative Retinopathy
   1. New vessels on the optic disc
   2. New vessels in other areas
   3. Growth of fibrous tissue
   4. Contraction of fibrous tissue with retinal hemorrhage
      or retinal detachment.

Don't let these terms scare you. Actually, non-proliferative, or background retinopathy, usually does NOT interfere with vision except when there is an accumulation of fluid in the macular area, and this complication can now be treated quite successfully when treatment is started early. Remember, most of these conditions can be adequately treated and only 5 percent of diabetics go on to complete loss of vision.

Type 1 diabetics usually develop mild reversible changes such as some leakage of retinal vessels within a few years of onset of abnormally high glucose levels. In approximately ten years, they will usually have microaneurysms and some exudate on the retina that can be visualized with the ophthalmoscope by the attending physician. With poor control of blood sugars, hemorrhages, fibrous tissue, and some dimming of vision may occur because of changes in the retina.

The retinal changes in Type 2 diabetes have an unpredictable course and may go unnoticed for years. Careful examination of the eyes on each medical visit enables the treating physician to document any progressive changes and to note the development of tiny hemorrhages or exudate on the retina.

Diabetics may experience temporary blurring of vision and changes in refraction most likely due to osmotic changes in the shape of the lens as a result of fluctuations in blood sugars. While uncomfortable, new refractions and glasses for the eyes should NOT be obtained until a steady period of glucose control occurs. It may take 6-8 weeks before the changes in visual acuity become stabilized.

Remember, every visual defect in the diabetic is not necessarily a consequence of retinopathy. Eye disorders that occur in the general population, *i.e.,* glaucoma, cataracts, conjunctivitis, etc., occur with increased frequency in diabetics. Glaucoma (increased pressure in the interior of the eye) is particularly common in older diabetic patients.

Treatment of Diabetic Retinopathy

Studies have shown that rigid control of blood sugars can improve the optic nerve and vascular changes seen in diabetes. Animal research seems to indicate that good control of glucose can slow or even stop the progression of retinopathy.

Photocoagulation is a method of focusing a light beam on the retina to produce a burn or coagulation in a precisely defined area. This allows the ophthalmologist to destroy microaneurysms, leaky vessels, neovascular areas, and areas of edema to prevent further deterioration. It has been shown by trials carried out by the Diabetic Retinopathy Study Research Group that photocoagulation decreases the incidence of retinal detachment, hemorrhage and loss of visions. While the Argon Laser has proved to be a valuable tool for photocoagulation, newer and better instruments are presently in use in many centers specializing in retinal diseases. A procedure called vitrectomy can be performed when necessary in severe cases to remove hemorrhagic and fibrous tissue blocking vision. This procedure involves introducing a hollow needle with a cutting device attached into the vitreous and removing the material affecting vision. The vitreous gel is replaced with a saline solution. This operation has proven very helpful in patients who have an accumulation of material interfering with vision. Only highly trained ophthalmologists are qualified to perform this delicate operation.

The Diabetes Control and Complications Trial (DCCT) showed that with "intensive control," patients had a 76 percent reduction in the risk of retinopathy. This finding stands as a motivating factor to all diabetic patients who want to avoid future visual problems. Careful examination and evaluation of your eyes by your diabetologist and opthalmologist can initiate early treatment if necessary and prevent many of the major visual complications of diabetes.

NOTE: Opticians are called "doctor," but they are not physicians and do not have the medical training to evaluate and treat medical problems of the eyes. Even family practitioners and diabetologists are limited in their ability to visualize the retina. Only opthamalogists, physicians who specialize in eye care, have the equipment and expertise to visualize more than 95 percent of the retina and render treatment early enough to prevent or reverse eye damage. Diabetics should be monitored on a regular basis by their opthamologist.

DIABETIC NEPHROPATHY

The kidneys filter waste products from the blood while preserving the important elements the body requires for future use. When protein is metabolized, nitrogenous waste products are produced that are eliminated by the kidneys. Nephropathy refers to changes in the kidneys due to infection or hardening of the small arteries that nourish the kidneys, and damage to the filtering systems within the kidney tissue. With progressive diabetic damage, protein, which is usually conserved by the kidney, begins to appear in tiny amounts in the urine. The excretion of the microscopic protein (albumin) is an important measurement that can serve as an early indicator in detecting beginning pathologic changes in the kidney. It can also be used as a guide to monitor the rate of progression of renal disease.

Persistent microalbumin levels of 20-200 micrograms or more over a six-month period indicate a diagnosis of early diabetic nephropathy. The thickening of the basement membrane, described earlier as a part of vascular disease, also takes place in the renal vessels and accounts for much of the gradual deterioration of kidney function, leading to end-stage renal disease. Experimental evidence strongly suggests that persistently elevated blood sugars play a major role in causing diabetic nephropathy. Islet cell transplant experiments done in rodents have resulted in marked reduction in the pathologic changes seen in diabetic nephropathy.

The key to treating nephropathy is to control the blood pressure, to provide strict management of blood sugar, and to decrease the work load of the kidneys by placing the patient on a moderately low-protein diet along with "tight" management of blood glucose. Some studies clearly indicate that vegetable protein is not toxic to the kidneys as is animal protein. The substitution of soy protein—a vegetable protein—is an excellent alternative to animal protein sources. Anti-hypertensive drugs of the angiotensin converting enzyme (ACE inhibitor) class, have been shown to help preserve renal function, even in patients who do not have high blood pressure. When taken by patients who exhibit micro-albuminuria (an early indicator of kidney disease), ACE inhibitors can exert a protective role in slowing or halting kidney damage.

When end-stage nephropathy reaches the point of threatening the way of life and even possibly proving fatal to the diabetic patient if untreated, renal dialysis or kidney transplant can compensate for, or take the place of, the patient's own failing kidneys. Thus, there are treatment modalities available now that will extend longevity to diabetics with advanced nephropathy and allow a return to near normal existence.

HYPERTENSION (HIGH BLOOD PRESSURE) AND DIABETES

Hypertension associated with diabetes is a different disorder than that in the non-diabetic population. Hypertension is well documented as a major risk factor of the microvascular complications that damage the retina and kidneys leading to blindness and end stage renal disease. Successful treatment requires achieving target BP levels. A blood pressure of 129/139 in a diabetic is physiologically equivalent to a reading of 150/160 in a non-diabetic. The systolic, the upper number of the blood pressure reading is the most significant. The bottom number, or diastolic pressure, naturally declines with age and does not correlate with any of the complications of hypertension that we seek to prevent with treatment. For years a BP of less than 140 systolic and less than 90 diastolic was considered acceptable. At these levels hypertension silently takes its toll over time. About eight years ago the accepted normal level was lowered to 130/80. We now know that 120/70 is preferable. Treatment of high blood pressure helps to prevent kidney disease (nephropathy) and cardiovascular disease (heart attacks and strokes) two of the major complications associated with diabetes. Diabetic patients should be given three, four or even five drugs, whatever is required, to achieve target BP levels. Two classes of drugs seem to be particularly beneficial in offering protection to the kidneys. These are the angiotensin converting enzymes, better known as ace inhibitors (ACE) and the angiotensin receptor blocker (ARBs) drugs. Both seem to have a favorable effect on kidney function and decrease or eliminate albumin excretion by the diabetic kidney as they preserve kidney function. There is a lineal relationship between rising blood pressure and kidney disease as well as cardiovascular disease.

An interesting five year study of two groups of diabetics, one with an average systolic BP of 140 and the other with a systolic BP of 126 was conducted. At the completion of the study those in the 126 group preserved their kidney function. The 140 group showed progressive kidney damage necessitating dialysis in many cases if they hadn't already succumbed to a heart attack or stroke as did many members of their group. *All over a 14 point difference in systolic BP!* Kidney artery disease is as common as coronary artery disease in the diabetic population.

A two year study of ACE inhibitors in normotensive (average BP 122/74) diabetics showed no change in kidney function and a decrease in urinary albumin excretion. The proven prevention of kidney disease with early treatment makes diligent screening and treatment mandatory.

Hypertension occurs with greater frequency in both Type 1 and Type 2 diabetes than in the population at large. Uncontrolled diabetes not only contributes to the accelerated atherosclerotic process that often accompanies diabetes, but also plays a prominent role in the frequently associated high blood pressure. However, atherosclerosis alone does not explain the high rate of hypertension found in diabetics except in those instances when there is moderate to severe involvement of the blood supply to the kidneys because of changes caused by fatty deposits in the arteries.

It has been theorized that the hypertension may, in some way, be related to the insulin resistance that is found not only in diabetes but also in obesity. A recent study has indicated that elevated systolic blood pressure may increase the death rate from diabetic complications more than any other single risk factor.

The diabetes must be kept under control by utilizing glucose monitoring as well as laboratory determinations. Diet and weight control play important roles in the management of the hypertensive diabetic patient. Obesity makes control of high blood pressure more difficult. Quitting smoking is of extreme importance as well as maintaining a low-salt, low-saturated fat diet. If blood lipids are high, additional medications to lower total cholesterol, low-density cholesterol (LDL), and raise high-density cholesterol (HDL) may be in order if lifestyle changes are unable to correct the dyslipidemia (elevated blood lipids). (See Chapter 18, *Cardiovascular Disease and Diabetes.*)

In summary, the problem of hypertension and concomitant cardiovascular problems are more prevalent in the diabetic than in the general population. The patient and his doctor must work together to control the blood sugar, keep the blood pressure within normal range, treat hyperlipidemia if present, and attempt to keep weight within normal limits. While these endeavors may require constant vigil, the long-term bebeficial results will make the effort worthwhile.

C H A P T E R
• 20 •

Travel and the Diabetic

Planning a Trip
Equipment to Take When Traveling
Necessary Precautions

Diabetes should not interfere with travel. By taking simple precautions, you can enjoy the mountains, museums, camping, athletic events, and cruises. You can participate with others on exciting tours and visits to foreign lands and meet people of many cultures.

All travelers have the opportunity and pleasure of planning their vacation as well as preparing for glitches or emergencies that may arise. Diabetic patients have an even greater obligation to plan ahead, check the areas they will be visiting, obtain knowledge in advance of the medical facilities available, and make certain to bring adequate supplies of medications, including insulin, syringes, and any other items their doctor recommends for the trip. When asked, physicians usually will provide their patients with a medical report of their history, a list of medications, and significant information for other medical personnel, should the need for treatment arise. The report will also help to avoid problems with police or customs officials who may wish to know why there are drugs and/or syringes in your luggage.

Your doctor can prescribe medications in advance for treatment of minor common ailments such as diarrhea, mild gastrointestinal symptoms or colds. All travelers arriving in new surroundings and cultures should avoid eating unpeeled fruits, leafy vegetables, undercooked meats, cheeses or cream sauces. It is wise to avoid local drinking water and ice cubes unless you are certain it is safe. Montezuma's Revenge (prolonged diarrhea) has been experienced by many U.S. visitors to Mexico. It is interesting to note that Mexican visitors to the U.S. also often experience bouts of diarrhea from local water supplies that meet strict public health standards. This occurs because each country has its own unique strains of bacteria which cause problems in those who are not accustomed to them. It is also prudent to avoid milk products such as cheese, ice cream and cream sauces.

The names and addresses of competent medical providers can be obtained, before starting your trip. The International Association for Assistance to Medical Travelers is a non-profit organization located at 417 Center Street, Lewiston, NY 14092. They publish a directory that lists addresses and phone numbers of English-speaking physicians throughout the world, whose qualifications and standards are deemed satisfactory. The Public Health Service in most communities can also give free advice about the need for required immunization procedures as well as information regarding endemic diseases in various parts of the world. Make certain you receive any necessary immunizations well in advance of your departure. This will allow adequate time to deal with any side effects, including interference with your diabetes control. If you are prone to motion sickness be sure to take along preventative medications.

Health Information for International Travelers, a publication by the Centers for Disease Control, can be obtained from the U.S. Government Printing Office, Superintendent of Documents, P.O. Box 371954, Pittsburgh, PA., 15250-7954, phone 202-512-7954.

In an urgent situation, American embassies often are of great help in obtaining prompt and qualified medical attention. Check with your insurance carrier before your trip to ascertain coverage should the need for emergency medical or surgical care arise.

If you are unfamiliar with the local language, carry a phrase book or pocket computer-translator. Most countries measure blood sugar levels in milligrams per deciliter (mg/dl) as is done in the United States. However, in the United Kingdom, and some other countries, the Système Internationale is used. Blood sugars are reported in millimols/liter (mM/l). To convert mg/dl to mM/l, divide by 18. Conversely, to change mM/l to mg/dl, multiply by 18.

When buying your boat or plane ticket, always request a diabetic diet. If this service is not provided, you may order a regular diet and use your own knowledge and judgment in deciding which foods would have the least impact on your blood sugar levels.

Wearing a medic-alert medallion and identification bracelet is always desirable, but even more so when traveling in strange and exotic places. Medic-Alert, 2323 Colorado Avenue, Turlock, CA 95382, is a non-profit organization that can help you to obtain materials to communicate vital medical information. For membership information, call 800-432-5378, or visit their web site at www.medicalert.org.

It is prudent to take extra supplies of all items related to your diabetes when traveling. This includes your testing devices for blood sugar, extra batteries for glucose monitoring meters, lancets, test strips, alcohol, cotton, band-aids, syringes, vials of insulin and soap for washing hands and cleansing the skin.

If you take insulin, be sure to take into account changes in time zones when traveling long distances. Discussion with your doctor or diabetic educator regarding changes in the timing and dosage of insulin is in order for trips that will cross several time zones. Upon arrival, you can adjust your meal and insulin schedule based on local time. Do not take your mealtime insulin unless you are sure that the anticipated food will follow. Having your glucose test meter along will make it easier to regulate your blood sugar levels regardless of the changes in local time, climate, and diverse food availability.

A good tip to remember is that traveling west lengthens the day and increases the need for insulin and snacks. If the time difference is less than three hours no adjustment is necessary.

Luggage can be misplaced or lost. It is vitally important that your diabetic supplies, along with your wallet, passport, hotel and train reservations, and money are kept in a carry-on bag, not in checked luggage. Stored baggage cannot only be lost, but the cargo area of the plane—particularly at high altitudes—may be subject to freezing. Your carry-on tote bag should be secure and always under close observation. Crime exists all over the world. It is better to be safe than sorry. Take twice as much insulin, syringes, test equipment and other supplies than you think you will need. Divide your insulin and other diabetes supplies between two different bags. Then, if a bag is misplaced, you won't have lost all of your supplies. Your type, brand, species, and concentration of insulin(s) may not be available in other countries. Having to switch insulins in the middle of your trip could affect control. Be sure to bring along sufficient supplies to last the entire trip.

Whenever possible, keep insulin refrigerated between use. However, insulin that is not refrigerated remains stable for one month provided it is kept in a cool place (below 86 degrees F). Make sure it does not get too hot or too cold. Never leave your insulin in a parked car. Do not store insulin in the trunk, glove compartment or on the dashboard where it could be subject to high temperatures. Pack your insulin between layers of clothing in a bag you will be hand carrying, instead of packing it in luggage that might be subject to temperature extremes. Store your insulin in a refrigerator as soon as possible after arriving at your destination. If refrigeration is not available, keeping your insulin in a wide-mouth insulated Thermos™ bottle can help. Fill the bottle with cold water or ice to cool it, pour the cold water or ice out, then put the insulin vials inside the bottle and tighten the cap. *Insulin should never be frozen.* Allow insulin to warm to room temperature to avoid painful injections.

If you are going to visit a country where English is not spoken, carry an "I Have Diabetes" identification card in the local language and try to learn enough phrases to enable you to order meals, describe emergencies, and get medical care. Keep carbohydrate snacks available for those unforeseen delays in obtaining regular meals.

You will want to continue some form of exercise program while away from home. This may take the form of walking while sightseeing. Alternating your footwear with an extra pair of comfortable walking shoes will help to prevent sore feet and callouses.

Traveling companions and friends should know about your diabetes so that they can be of assistance should the need arise. Be sure to take a glucagon kit with you and instruct one of your travelling companions in its use.

If you are traveling long distances by car, stop every few hours for short walks to improve circulation. Prolonged sitting, particularly for those over the age of forty, interferes with the circulation of the lower extremeties and predisposes to phlebitis, a potentially dangerous condition.

If you are driving yourself, it is important to avoid hypoglycemia by eating regularly, avoiding fatigue and keeping snacks on hand.

Thousands of diabetic patients who have traveled the world over report that they have had exciting times and wonderful experiences without concerns as long as they planned ahead and took the few common sense precautionary steps described in this chapter.

C H A P T E R
• 21 •

Hygiene

Skin Care
Dental Care
Eye Care
Urinary Tract Infections

U ncontrolled elevated blood sugar levels increase the risk of infections, as well as interfering with wound healing. For this reason, it is important that you familiarize yourself with the simple precautions to be taken in the routine of daily life to prevent, whenever possible, future bothersome complications.

Hygiene is the art of the preservation of physical health. Diabetics must take special care of their skin, hair, eyes, teeth and feet. Daily routines should be established to allow adequate time for meals, exercise, recreation, rest and sleep. Emotional stresses such as worry and anxiety have the physiological effect of raising blood sugar, making control more difficult. The following sections outline the steps you must take for satisfactory personal care.

CARE OF THE SKIN

The skin, particularly that of the hands, may harbor bacteria that can cause infections. Bathe at least once daily with mild soap and water. Dry yourself thoroughly after washing. Avoid extremely hot baths or showers because neuropathy can cause a loss of protective pain perception. Protect your skin by avoiding scratches or punctures by wearing gloves when you work at tasks that might injure your hands. Treat all injuries promptly.

Wash cuts with warm, soapy water and hydrogen peroxide, then apply a dry sterile dressing. Do not apply iodine, merchurochrome, alcohol or other strong antiseptic to wounds. Although these substances kill bacteria, they also destroy healthy body tissues. Notify your doctor if cuts or scrapes show any signs of infection (redness, heat, swelling, tenderness, throbbing, or pus formation). If an infection does occur, use an antiseptic soap like Betadine that kills skin bacteria and may prevent the spread of infection.

Wear only all-cotton underwear, which allows air to circulate freely. The use of baby powder, particularly in areas where the skin rubs together, helps to prevent irritation. After a shower or swimming, drying the ear canals may help avert bacterial or fungal infection. If you develop a fungal infection—jock itch, athlete's foot, ringworm, vulvar or vaginal infections—notify your doctor.

Avoid sunburn by using sunscreen and common sense. Prevent frostbite by dressing wisely and avoiding excessive exposure during the cold weather. On cold, windy days, use a moisturizing cream. Select hypoallergenic deodorants and cosmetics. At the first sign of increased sensitivity, change to another brand. Women should not shave their legs with a safety razor; an electric razor is preferable. Chapping of hands can be prevented by thorough drying and the use of a bland cream. Fingernails should be kept the proper length. The cuticle may be gently pushed back with an orangewood stick, never with a pointed instrument.

CARE OF THE HAIR

Hair should be shampooed at least once or twice weekly with a hypoallergenic commercial preparation. Hair cuts, shaves and removal of hair should be done with scrupulously clean instruments.

CARE OF THE TEETH AND GUMS

Proper care of the teeth and gums are excellent examples of how simple daily prophylactic measures can prevent long-term problems.

Elevated blood sugar levels can affect all the tissues of the body, including the gums and teeth. There is a higher incidence of plaque and bacteria in the mouth and gums in uncontrolled diabetes. In addition, the inclination of capillary blood vessels to narrow and deliver less oxygen and nourishment to gum tissues leads to delay in healing of tiny cuts or bruises made by too vigorous brushing of the teeth or other trauma inflicted by such objects as hard candies, fish bones or leathery and fibrous foods. Use only soft bristle tooth brushes. Hard bristles are prone to cause minor gum irritations which can lead to periodontal disease.

While diabetes probably does not initiate periodontal or gum disease, it does delay the healing process and makes good dental care critical.

A dental abscess or severe periodontal disease can exacerbate the underlying diabetic condition by contributing to infection, interfering with proper eating, and causing stress, all tending to raise blood sugar levels.

Patients should make sure their dentist is aware of their diabetic status. The dentist or the dental hygienist can then give proper instructions regarding dental care: brushing, using floss, and massaging the gums periodically. The diabetic patient should visit his dentist at least every six months to have his teeth cleaned and checked. When sores or painful, reddened gums occur, the dentist should be promptly notified.

Brush and floss every day after meals. Use a soft, nylon brush with rounded ends on its bristles. Brush gently with a scrubbing motion while holding the bristles at approximately a 45 degree angle to the gum line. Brush the front, back and chewing surfaces. Some dentists recommend the "Water-Pic" to reduce the formation of plaque while others instruct the patient in the use of electrically-operated toothbrushes. This will also aid in keeping the teeth and gums and the bone structure underneath the gums healthy. Use dental floss at least once a day to remove food that may have become lodged between teeth, promoting bacterial growth, and to curtail plaque formation. Special floss holders and devices to facilitate cleaning between teeth are available at most pharmacies. Dentists recommend strict control of blood sugars before rendering any dental treatment — including even such minor procedures as dental cleaning or minor fillings. Before beginning intensive dental or gum treatment, antibiotics may be prescribed to prevent infection as well as the possibility of bacteremia — release of bacteria into the blood stream as a result of dental manipulation.

Blood on the toothbrush or noted in expectorated saliva may be the first sign of gingivitis. A special type of gingivitis due to the herpes simplex virus can cause inflammation and bleeding that may be particularly severe in diabetes. Most of these infections are self-limited and require only symptomatic therapy, but antibiotics may be necessary to treat secondary infections.

Infections of the roots of the teeth (endodontal infections) are usually associated with the rarer strains of anaerobic bacteria and are best treated by an endodontist.

Call your dentist promptly if any of the following occurs:

1. Gums bleed easily when you brush your teeth.
2. Gums are red, swollen or tender.
3. Pus is expressed from pockets between teeth when gums are pressed.
4. You develop a persistent bad taste in the mouth.
5. You notice a change in the way your denture or partial plate fits.

REVIEW OF DENTAL CARE AND DIABETES

Although a diabetic may not necessarily be more prone to infection than a non-diabetic, once an infection develops it tends to be more severe and last a longer period of time. Probably one of the most common types of chronic infection is inflammatory periodontal (gum) disease. It is also called pyorrhea, periodontitis or gingivitis. Gingivitis is the beginning stage of gum disease in which the soft tissue surrounding the teeth becomes inflamed. If the inflammation extends to include the supporting bone surrounding the teeth, the condition is then called periodontitis. (See illustration on the following page.)

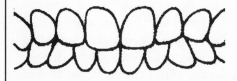

NORMAL HEALTHY GUMS

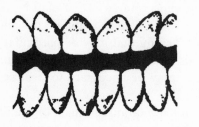

PLAQUE

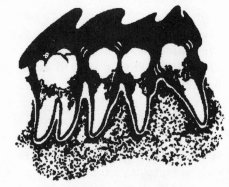

PERIODONTITIS

1. Daily Brushing and

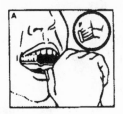 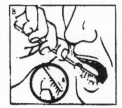 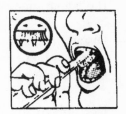

2. Dental Flossing

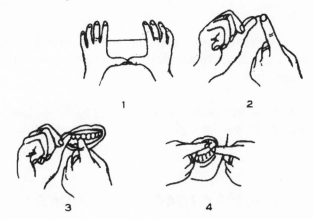

CARE OF THE EYES

The eye damage that diabetes may cause was discussed in Chapter 19, *Long Term Complications of Diabetes.* Take the steps listed below to further reduce the risk and danger of eye problems.

— Have a complete eye exam every year by an ophthalmologist. Remember, eye damage has NO symptoms in the early, most treatable stages.

— Visit an ophthalmologist, a medical doctor who specializes in eye care, at once if you have any of these symptoms:
    1. Blurred or double vision. (In addition to opthalmological conditions, high or low blood pressure can sometimes cause blurring of vision.)
    2. Narrowed field of vision.
    3. Seeing dark spots.
    4. Feeling of pressure or pain in the eyes.
    5. Difficulty seeing in dim light.

— Have your blood pressure checked regularly.

— Discuss exercise activities with your ophthalmologist. Strenuous exercises that raise the pressure within the eye can lead to retinal hemmorrhages.

— Keep blood sugar controlled. This helps to prevent retinal blood vessel disease.

— Do not smoke.

— If you have retinopathy, don't take birth control pills. They can adversely affect the blood clotting mechanism as well as raise the blood pressure.

— Seek medical treatment early for eye problems. Laser treatment for retinopathy can be highly effective when instituted early in the course of the disease.

URINARY TRACT INFECTIONS

Women with diabetes are especially prone to urinary tract infections. The lower urinary tract consists of the bladder, which collects the urine, and the urethra, the canal through which the urine is voided. The most common lower urinary tract infection occurs when bacteria gain entry to the bladder from the outside through the urethra, causing inflammation of the bladder, or cystitis. Common symptoms of cystitis are any or all of the following: urinary frequency; a constant desire to urinate, even within a short time of having done so; straining at the end of urination, feelings that the bladder has not been completely emptied; burning with urination and decreased strength of the urinary stream.

Anatomically, women are susceptible to bladder infections because the female urethra is a rather short channel that is located close to the vagina and rectum. The rectum, because of bowel movements, is a source of bacteria that can contaminate the urethra and enter the bladder. Once bacteria get into the vaginal area, entry into the bladder is easy, again because the uretha is an extremely short channel. Bacteria can reproduce every twenty minutes. Prompt and adequate treatment of urinary tract infections is essential to effect a complete cure and prevent recurrence.

C H A P T E R
• 22 •

Care of the Feet

How to Avoid Ulcers and Infections
Importance of Early Diagnosis and Treatment
Routine Foot Care

Many diabetics develop serious foot problems, as a result of poor circulation to the lower extremities (due to hardening of the arteries or atherosclerosis and neuropathy), resulting in chronic skin ulcers, numbness, and burning of the lower legs and feet. These conditions can be painful and in some cases, particularly when untreated, lead to gangrene, requiring amputation.

Any injury of the feet, in those whose circulation is already compromised, may precipitate infection and delayed healing. The best approach to the problems of the diabetic foot is to prevent the development of foot ulcers with knowledge and prophylactic foot care. It is wise to make sure shoes have adequate toe room to prevent rubbing, which can cause ulcerations or blisters. Soft, well-fitting shoes play an important role in preventing serious foot problems. Don't plan on breaking in new shoes; they should feel comfortable when first worn. Diabetics should wear shoes at all times to avoid tiny cuts and splinters that can become infected. Cotton socks are preferable to nylon. Moisturizers may be applied when the feet are dry and talc can be used for excessive perspiration. On the beach, the feet must be covered to avoid sunburn. Swelling, change in color, or texture of the foot's skin are significant symptoms and should be followed up promptly by a visit to the family doctor or diabetes specialist.

Nerve damage may cause your feet to lose feeling. If this happens, a simple cut or sore can go unnoticed and lead to problems. Nerve damage predisposes to blisters, sores, and foot ulcers. Poor blood flow to the feet causes injuries to heal more slowly.

Cramps in the leg while walking, particularly in the calf muscle area, may signal the beginning of circulatory problems. The same is true for redness of the feet or darkening of the skin when the legs are in a dependent position. Circulation may deteriorate rapidly causing night pain, which can be relieved by hanging the legs over the side of the bed.

"Athlete's Foot" must be looked for between the toes and treated with anti-fungal agents. Poor control of blood sugar interferes with the ability of the white blood cells to fight off infection. Frequent glucose monitoring becomes mandatory in order to ascertain the amounts of insulin required to keep sugar levels near normal.

The foot may become infected, but diabetic neuropathy may mask the pain associated with this serious condition, allowing progression of the process before consultation with a physician is sought. Unless treatment is started promptly, the infection may spread rapidly and gangrenous changes could make amputation a necessity. Charcot's joint, a rare condition named after a famous French neurologist of the 19th century, results when neuropathy is severe, causing the ligaments to be damaged and allowing the bones to rub against each other. The bones of the arch of the foot may collapse and result in pressure points and irritation, leading to additional ulcers and infection. When this ominous chain of events occurs, the patient may require prolonged bed rest for two to four months before healing can take place. In spite of the changes in the feet that prevent walking, it is important that the patient continues to use as many muscles as is prudent. This may include arm exercise and upper body movements.

The feet should be inspected before and after any form of exercise, and instructions from the diabetic educator and permission from your physician must be obtained before embarking on an exercise program. (See Chapter 17, *Benefits of Exercise.*)

When circulation is impaired, it takes longer for sores to heal and makes it easier for infection to develop. The vast majority of the 20,000 foot and leg amputations performed in this country each year can be traced to some degree of neglect. Prevention and attention to minor problems before they become major could help the diabetic population avoid as many as 75 percent of these devastating procedures.

People who are markedly overweight are more susceptible to foot problems because they cannot reach down to inspect their feet properly for sores, blisters, and infections. Visual problems may also prevent close inspection of the feet.

Any injury to the skin, particularly when there is a laceration or break in the skin, can become infected and destroy underlying tissues. Instituting prompt medical treatment may prevent progression to the point where surgery becomes necessary.

Factors that contribute to the development of the diabetic foot ulcer are:

1. Microvascular disease (atherosclerosis) of the small arteries and capillaries supplying oxygen and nutrients to the foot.
2. Damage to nerve tissue (neuropathy), denying the patient awareness of traumatic injuries to the foot from such things as heating pads or carpet tacks, etc.
3. Macrovascular Disease (atherosclerosis) of the large vessels causing narrowing and/or blockage of major arteries to the lower legs and feet.
4. Structural deformities such as hammertoe, cocked toes, bunions, and corns predispose to the development of ulceration and infection.
5. Poorly fitting shoes can cause undue pressure on the feet, increasing the risk for callouses or corns. Callous formation is a thickening of the outer layers of the skin (hyperkeratosis) that causes some loss of cushioning of the bottom of the foot.

Risk factors for peripheral vascular disease include smoking, hypertension, and dyslipidemia. When blood sugar cannot be controlled, elevation of cholesterol and triglycerides occurs, emphasizing the need for strict, proper diabetic management.

PREVENTION OF FOOT ULCERS

The physician must use every means possible to stop any diabetic patient from smoking. Smoking is particularly harmful to the vascular tree. Nicotine constricts the blood vessels, further limiting the circulation. Treating a patient with peripheral vascular disease who smokes is like treating a burn patient while his hand is still in the fire.

Serum lipids must be measured and if indicated, a rigid low saturated fat, low cholesterol diet must be adopted. If lipids still remain elevated, cholesterol-lowering medications can be utilized. (See Chapter 18, *Cardiovascular Disease and Diabetes.*)

Patients should be taught to examine their feet and toes on a daily basis, checking the spaces between the toes for moisture, and bacterial or fungus infection. Cuts, scratches, blisters, and bruises present potential danger signs. Patients can be taught to examine themselves for decreased sensation, pallor, dryness, or coolness of their lower extremities — signs of impending poor circulation and neuropathy. Molded shoes may prevent formation of bunions, corns and pressure areas. Infection must be treated promptly.

The feet can be washed gently in lukewarm water, *never hot.* Feet should not be soaked or left in the water, as this softens the skin and makes it more susceptible to maceration and to infection. The feet should be dried gently and thoroughly. Moisture restoring cream should be applied to hold moisture in the skin. Lotions or creams should not be placed between the toes. Talcum powder is used for feet that have a tendency to perspire. (Caution: Do not let the powder cake between the toes.) Toenails should be clipped straight across. Use an emery board to smooth nails. Corns and calluses should never be cut. Ideally, a podiatrist should be consulted for routine foot care, particularly if vision or dexterity is in question. Cotton or wool socks are best for diabetics and should be changed daily. Electric heating pads and hot-water bottles may cause serious burns to the legs and feet that can progress to gangrene and should never be used by diabetics. Debridement of callous formation, trimming, and other forms of foot care should be done by a podiatrist, when feasible, rather than by the patient.

When there is evidence of narrowing or blockage of the blood vessels supplying the lower extremities, consultation with a vascular surgeon is in order. Surgical procedures are available to compensate for blockage of involved blood vessels. Vascular bypass operations that shunt blood around the arteriosclerotic vessels are now done routinely. The bypass procedure consists of dissecting a length of vein from the leg to be used as a shunt around the obstructed artery. An opening is made in the artery below the point of obstruction and the vein is sutured to the artery, end to end. The other end of the vein is re-attached to the artery above the point of obstruction, thus serving as a bridge between the unclogged portions of the artery.

Angioplasty is another procedure employed to improve the blood flow through blocked arteries. This operation consists of threading a narrow catheter (tube) into the diseased artery until it reaches the point of obstruction. A small balloon at the tip of the catheter is then inflated, exerting pressure against the wall of the blood vessel, flattening the fatty deposits. The inflation and compression procedure is repeated as required to achieve an adequate opening of the vessel to allow a satisfactory blood supply, avoiding the more invasive open surgical bypass procedures.

Progression of the ischemia (lack of adequate blood supply), development of infection around the ulcer (cellulitis), and erosion of muscle or bone tissue requires immediate hospitalization. Saving the extremity may then require the expertise of such specialists as vascular and plastic surgeons, and orthopedists.

Treatment of diabetic foot infections can be a therapeutic dilemma due to the difficulties in obtaining accurate bacterial cultures that could serve as a guide for appropriate antibiotic therapy. Infections may spread to bones, causing osteomyelitis, a complication that often proves very difficult to treat.

There are many hospital centers today that specialize in the treatment of diabetic foot ulcers that have achieved marked success in managing infections and saving limbs from amputation. The American Diabetes Association can supply you with the location of nearby centers that can accept referrals from your family doctor or diabetologist. Prompt care can make the difference between saving a limb or disastrous consequences.

REVIEW OF FOOT CARE PROCEDURES

Diabetics should be under the care of a podiatrist for routine foot care. If this is not possible, employ the following daily foot care measures.

Daily Foot Care Measures

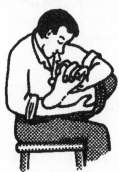

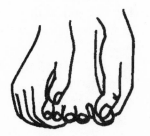

1. Inspect the feet daily —
   Note the presence of:
   a. Cuts, ulcers, scratches, bruises, blisters, corns and callouses.
   b. "Athletes Foot" — especially between the toes.
   c. Lack of feeling — numbness — in the feet or any change in feeling such as tingling or burning.
   d. Changes in color of the feet, e.g., blue or purple may indicate poor circulation.
   e. Change in temperature — e.g., cold feet may indicate poor circulation. Warm areas could mean infection.

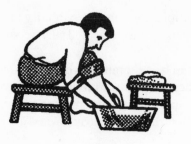

2. Wash feet daily. Bathe, do not soak, feet daily using warm water and mild soap. Test water temperature with elbow.

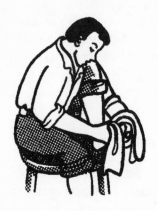

3. Dry feet well, especially between toes. You may use a small hand towel for this purpose.

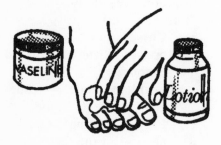

4. For excessively dry feet, apply a good lotion (lanolin, oil, vaseline) to prevent skin from cracking. Do not apply between toes.

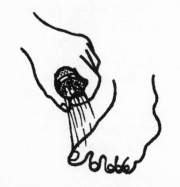

5. When feet sweat, apply a foot powder. If fungus infection develops, use an anti-fungal powder. Consult with your doctor immediately.

Trimming Toenails

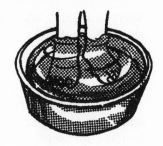

1. Soak feet in basin of warm water for 10-15 minutes. Dry feet well.

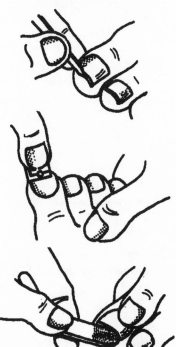

2. Use an orange stick to remove debris from under the nail.

3. Trim nails with toenail clipper or special toenail scissors. Cut nails straight across, clipping small sections of the nail at a time. This helps to avoid ingrown toenails.

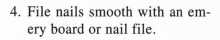

4. File nails smooth with an emery board or nail file.

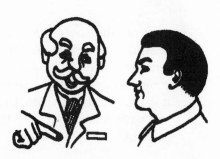

5. Do not trim your own nails if your vision or circulation is poor. Instead, consult with a foot doctor (podiatrist).

Care of Corns and Callouses

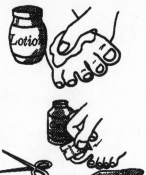

1. Keep corns and callouses soft with a lotion.

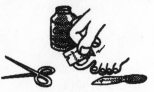

2. Never use: commercial corn removers, razor blades, knives or household scissors

3. Consult with a podiatrist if corns and callouses become a major problem.

Treatment of Foot Injuries

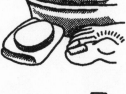

1. Wash affected area with soap and warm water.

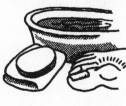

2. Apply a mild antiseptic — hydrogen peroxide (H_2O_2). Do not use Iodine.

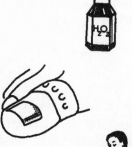

3. If necessary, wrap affected area with sterile gauze or a Band-Aid to keep wound clean.

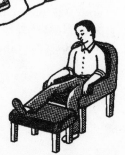

4. Stay off the foot as much as possible to allow it an opportunity to heal. If an area becomes red, painful or swollen, it is likely to be infected. Consult with your physician IMMEDIATELY. Do not wait!

DIABETIC SELF-FOOT CARE CHECK LIST

1. Control your diabetes carefully.

2. Keep feet clean and dry.

3. Always protect feet and legs from injury.
    a. Wear fresh, clean wool or cotton socks or stockings every day.
    b. Wear comfortable, soft, well-fitting leather shoes.
    c. Avoid open-toe shoes.
    d. Don't expect to have to break in new shoes. They should be comfortable when first worn.
    e. If you have neuropathy you might not be able to judge how a shoe feels. Consult a shoewear specialist who is trained to fit people with diabetes.
    f. Avoid use of hot water bottles or heating pads which can burn the skin.
    g. Never walk around barefooted—always wear shoes or slippers.
    h. Never use corn plasters, wart removers or other over-the-counter foot medications.

4. Promote good circulation.
    a. Avoid smoking. Tobacco in any form produces constriction of the blood vessels.
    b. Do not cross legs at the knees or hook legs around a chair.
    c. Avoid use of restrictive garters, socks, girdles.
    d. Exercise feet and legs daily. Walking is excellent.

C H A P T E R
• 23 •

Diabetes and Impotence

Causes
Medical Treatment
Surgical Treatment

W omen with diabetes may experience problems with vaginal lubrication, and during periods of poor glycemic control they are prone to vaginal yeast infections. However, the sexual drive, desire, performance and fulfillment of diabetic women remains relatively unimpaired even among females with evidence of diabetic neuropathy. The same cannot be said of male diabetic patients, of whom at least 25-35 percent will develop problems with erection by middle age. Thereafter an age-related decline in erectile function, unrelated to sexual drive or libido, continues in a steady but often slow fashion.

Libido and potency are the two components of male sexual activity. Libido consists of sexual desire, thoughts, drive and fantasies. Potency is the ability to have and maintain an erection and ejaculate. Erectile dysfunction (ED) or impotence is the consistent inability for a man to have an erection sufficiently firm for penetration and satisfactory sexual performance. Although ED increases with age, it is not an inevitable consequence of the aging process. It is true, however, that as men get older they require a longer time and direct physical stimulation to achieve erection. Additionally, with age erections may become less firm and more time may be required for ejaculation to occur and, following ejaculation, the refractory period—the length of time between erections—increases.

It now appears that strict diabetic control may lessen the incidence of ED. The risk factors for ED are similar to those for coronary heart disease: smoking, high blood pressure, dyslipidemia, and diabetes. Diabetic smokers are seven times as likely to be impotent as non-smokers. Of course, impotence in the younger Type 1 diabetics may have a more devastating impact than when it occurs in older Type 2 patients, although men of all age groups experience severe psychological stress when this "symbol" of manhood is lost. As in the male population at large, diabetics vary widely in their prediabetic libido, due to the same factors that affect everyone: fatigue, performance anxiety*, depression, emotional stress (job related, relationship discord, financial problems, etc.), circulatory problems, low levels of hormones (from liver disease or alcoholism), neuropathy or other serious health problems, including cardiac, pulmonary and liver disease, and as a side effect of medications used to treat these disorders.

The physiology underlying an erection involves complex changes in the penis from a flacid (soft) to a tumescent (swollen) to an erect (rigid) state. With sexual arousal, nerve impulses from the brain travel along nerve fibers to the smooth muscles in the walls of the corpora cavernosa (the spongy vascular chambers of the penis), causing them to relax. This allows more blood to enter the chambers, and like a sponge, they swell as they fill with blood.

Many things can upset the complex physiologic and psychological functions of the body involved in attaining and maintaining an erection. The psychological role is certainly highly significant. The mind has been called the most important sexual organ.

For many years researchers believed that psychological rather than physical (organic) factors were responsible for most cases of ED. However, recent developments in research techniques that enable investigators to apply objective methods for determining organic causes of ED has added to our understanding of this disorder. This increased knowledge has led experts to believe that the vast majority of cases of ED have a physical cause, with only 10-20 percent being attributable to psychological factors. However, we must not forget that there is a very delicate interaction and balance between the physical and the emotional or mental components of sexual arousal which must function in harmony for satisfactory sexual performance.

Evaluation of a diabetic patient who suffers from ED requires a thorough general medical examination and psychological evaluation. As noted,

* Performance anxiety happens occasionally to many men. If it persists it can lead to ED. Fear of failure can start a self-perpetuating cycle.

ED is either predominantly psychological or predominantly organic in nature. Psychological impotence usually begins rather abruptly, whereas impotence caused by physical problems usually has a more gradual onset. A sleep monitoring examination can help to differentiate these two categories of ED.

PHYSICAL CAUSES OF ED

Vascular Causes

The primary physical cause of ED in diabetic men is believed to be atherosclerosis, which leads to plaque deposits in the walls of the blood vessels, causing a reduction of the arterial blood flow to the penis. An ample penile blood supply is a pre-requisite for erection to occur. Penile doppler testing is a simple non-invasive procedure that can help to evaluate blood flow through the penis. A far more sensitive test called penile duplex ultrasonography uses a two-dimensional doppler assessment of the penile arteries. The results of this test can be used to predict a patient's response to the penile injection vasodilator drug treatment. Associated risk factors for ED caused by vascular disease are dyslipidemia, cigarette smoking, high blood pressure, and diabetes. Smoking cessation can sometimes result in a significant improvement in penile blood flow within a relatively short period of time. Venous leak impotence is caused by an inability of the corpora cavernosa—the penile vascular chambers—to occlude the penile veins, a requirement to maintain an erection. Failure of venous closure is responsible for the ED in 90 percent of men who are not responsive to the penile injection of vasodilator drugs.

Endocrine Causes

ED may be associated with disorders of the thyroid gland, pituitary gland, testes and the pancreas. The role of the male sex hormone testosterone in ED is unclear. Although hormone deficiency is associated with decreased libido and frequency and magnitude of nocturnal erections, it is noteworthy that men who have been castrated after reaching puberty can still achieve erection. This would suggest that the male hormone does not play an essential role in the erectile process.

Both an over-active and under-active thyroid can cause ED which is associated with low testosterone levels. Treatment of the thyroid disorder may restore erectile function. However, testosterone treatment alone does not affect ED in these patients.

Pharmacological Causes

Medications are a frequent cause of ED. The most common offenders are high blood pressure medications that affect the central nervous system such as Clonidine, Methyl Dopa, alpha/beta blockers, and diuretics*. Ace inhibitors, calcium channel blockers and peripheral vasodilator drugs are associated with a much lower incidence of ED. *Psychotropic* medications — antidepressants and antianxiety drugs — are frequently associated with ED. Heroin, cocaine, alcohol, digoxin and finasteride (which is used to treat benign prostatic enlargement) may also cause ED.

Neurogenic Causes

Because erection requires the brain to transmit impulses along nerve pathways to the vascular chambers of the penis, any malfunction or disease that affects the brain, spinal cord or the nerves that stimulate the smooth muscles in the walls of the penile vascular chambers to relax, can cause ED. Neuropathy is a frequent cause of diabetic ED. The nerves supplying the penis run close to the prostate gland and are often damaged during radical prostate surgery.

TREATMENT OF IMPOTENCE

A patient with ED whose wife or companion has retained a normal sexual drive should take into consideration his mate's feelings before making a decision regarding therapy for his ED. The type of treatment selected should be a joint decision. Sex therapy can be helpful by opening lines of communication between the partners. Sexual health should be viewed as an intimate relationship of love, trust, sharing and pleasure. We should not forget that it takes more than an erection to have a satisfactory sex life. Erectile functioning is certainly important, but it is only one of many factors that contribute to a rewarding relationship.

ORAL DRUG TREATMENTS

Viagra

Viagra (sidenafil) is the first oral drug available for improving male sexual function that has received FDA approval. Its main attractions are that it is easy to use, relatively inexpensive and is believed to be effective

---

*Examples of possible offending agents in each category: Clonidine (Catapres), Methyl Dopa (Aldomet), Alpha/Beta Blockers (Normodyne, Trandate, Tenormin, Lopressor, Toprol-XL), Diuretics (Dyazide, Maxzide, Hydrochlorothiazide).

about 70 percent of the time. Until the advent of Viagra, the majority of men suffering from impotence did not seek treatment because they were either too embarrassed to seek help, or they found the currently available remedies unacceptable.

Viagra's pharmacological action is unique. It enhances an erection when a man is aroused by amplifying the effects of an erection-promoting chemical normally produced in the penis, which results in a more fully developed and longer-lasting erection.

Unlike the injectable drugs or urethral suppositories which produce an erection regardless of an emotional or mental component of sexual arousal, Viagra requires an erection to be initiated through desire, attraction or physical stimulation. In other words, it is not an aphrodisiac and will not work in the absence of sexual desire.

Under normal conditions of sexual arousal, a man's brain sends nerve signals to his penis which trigger the release of nitric oxide and guanosine monophosphate (GMP), a chemical messenger that causes the spongy vascular chambers within the penis to dilate and fill with blood.

For a full erection to occur, the veins that normally drain the penis must be squeezed closed by the expanded penile vascular chamber. In men suffering from ED, the expansion of the erectile tissue is inadequate to squeeze and collapse the penile veins due to a shortage of cyclic GMP. When blood flow out of the penis is not restricted an erection cannot be achieved. Viagra works by blocking the effects of a naturally occurring enzyme, phosphodiesterase type 5 (PDS5), which causes an erection to subside by breaking down cyclic GMP, thus prolonging its effects. The number of chemical receptors in the penis for cyclic GMP is limited. These receptors can be acted upon by only a limited number of cyclic GMP molecules. This means a large dose of Viagra will not necessarily have a more profound physiological effect than a smaller one.

Viagra can undoubtedly help many men, but it is not a cure-all. It is, however, an excellent drug that can restore sexual potency.

Viagra produces firm, long-lasting erections. The increased sexual response lasts for about four to six hours. For many men the results have been dramatic, enabling them to enjoy sex for the first time in many years.

One in ten men taking Viagra are unable to tolerate the drug because of side effects—headaches (whose severity appears to be dose related), indigestion, facial flushing and subtle visual disturbances ranging from blurred vision to disturbances in blue-green vision, sometimes manifested as a halo effect. The most significant side effect of Viagra is a sudden drop in blood pressure which can occur when the drug is taken in combination with nitroglycerine or other nitrate containing drug even when they are taken only periodically. *The drug is contraindicated in patients using organic nitrates in any form, at any time.* The danger of severe—*at times fatal*—hypotension (drop in blood pressure) which can occur when Viagra is used by patients who are taking medications containing nitrates is well known to physicians and has been widely publicized in the press. However, patients may fail to disclose to their doctor the use of any illicit drugs. Therefore, physicians may be unaware that their patient is using a street drug that is purported to enhance sexual pleasure; called "Poppers"—so named because they come in a glass ampule which must be popped open. "Poppers" — are ampules of amyl or butyl nitrate which are inhaled, and like any nitrate, their concomitant use with Viagra can have lethal consequences.

Patients with heart disease, particularly those with angina, congestive heart failure with low blood pressure, and those taking multiple drugs for high blood pressure, are at special risk for severe drops in blood pressure when taking Viagra. Angina developing within 24 hours of taking Viagra must not be treated with nitrates. Patients taking Erythromycin, Tagamet or those with kidney or liver disease, have delayed excretion of Viagra and retain the drug in the body longer than usual, making them vulnerable to delayed drug interactions. Therefore, it may be undesirable to use Viagra with these patients.

The long-term effects of Viagra are still unknown. Although it does appear to have a satisfactory safety profile when taken according to the manufacturer's directions. The possibility of psychological dependence on the drug may occur in some patients. The effectiveness of Viagra was the same whether the cause of the impotence was physical or psychological.

Viagra is effective in about 70 percent of men with diabetes who are impotent. It worked 35-40 percent of the time for patients whose ED resulted from nerve damage that occurred during prostate surgery. It also benefited many paraplegic men.

Viagra can be taken anywhere from four hours to one-half hour before sexual activity. For most patients, the recommended dose is 50 mg taken as needed one hour prior to sexual activity. For those over age 65, a starting dose of 25mg is recommended. A lower dose is also indicated when taking the antibiotic Erythromycin, or the antifungal drugs, Ketoconozole or Itraconazole. These drugs (as well as some others) are metabolized in the liver with the same enzyme system (P4503A4) as Viagra. Eating a fatty meal prior to taking Viagra hinders its absorption. A wafer form of Viagra dissolves in the mouth and has a more rapid onset of action than the oral tablets.

NOTE: Fatal heart attacks that are precipitated by shoveling snow or other strenuous physical activity in older persons unaccustomed to such endeavors are not rare occurences and come as no surprise. When millions of senior citizens are given a medication that suddenly restores their virility, they proceed to engage in sexual initimacy, an activity that speeds up the heart and may, at times, qualify physiologically as a strenuous physical activity. Therefore it is to be expected, that occasionally, heart attacks may be precipitated by the use of this drug. All elderly persons taking Viagra should have a cardiac evaluation before initiating therapy.

External Vaccum Devices

This non-surgical treatment consists of a suction chamber operated by a hand or battery pump that creates a vacuum around the penis. These devices are a simple and safe method for generating an erection in those with partial or complete impotence. They may be used regardless of the cause of the ED. An airtight plastic cylinder is fitted over the penis and the air is pumped out of the cylinder, creating a vacuum. Venous drainage is inhibited by the use of a specially designed tension ring placed around the base of the penis. This treatment can produce an erection that will last for about 30 minutes. Newer models utilize a battery operated pump to create the vacuum. A good vacuum system will provide a safety valve to allow the rapid release of the vacuum if the patient feels discomfort during the procedure. Vacuum devices allow successful intercourse in more than 70-80 percent of cases with few side effects. Occasionally, they may cause slight bruising of the penis (echymosis), diminished ejaculation and coolness at the tip of the penis. This therapeutic approach has been met with widespread acceptance by many patients suffering from ED and more than 55,000 of these devices are currently in use.

Penile Self-Injection Therapy

Local injection into the penis of a vasodilator drug (Papaverine or Alprostadil) produces an erection if the penile blood supply is adequate. This procedure helps to differentiate ED due to neuropathy from vascular causes. This form of treatment requires the patient to inject a vasodilator drug directly into his penis. Many patients find the thought of inserting a needle into one of the most sensitive areas of their body repugnant, but the needle employed is quite small and the injection into the side of the penis usually causes little or no pain. However, some lingering discomfort at the site of the injection is not uncommon—response to the medicine rather than from the injection itself. The medication causes the vessels of the penis to dilate, increasing the circulation and reproducing the physiologic changes that normally cause erection.

The urologist instructs the patient (and in some cases the partner) in the proper aseptic techniques for these injections. Side effects such as painful persistent erections (priapism), bleeding or bruising and penile fibrosis (scar tissue) can occur. The main significant complication from this therapy is priapism. Erections that persist for more than four to six hours can cause damage to penile tissue. Patients must seek emergency treatment when erections are prolonged. Treatment consists of withdrawing blood from the corpora cavernosa or injecting a drug such as epinephrine into the penis.

It is very important to individualize the dosage of Alprostadil used for treatment. Patient response varies and excessive dosage can cause serious side effects including permanent damage. Frequent consultations with a urologist are necessary. Alprostadil generally causes an erection that lasts an average of 40 to 60 minutes.

Urethral Suppositories

This relatively new and unique approach to treating ED involves the insertion of a delivery tube into the urethral opening of the penis and the insertion of a small pellet of alprostadil into the urethral channel. The pellets are easy to use and obviate the need for needle injections into the penis. Side effects are penile aching, burning sensation in the urethra, aching around the base of the penis, and rarely a drop in blood pressure.

C H A P T E R
• 24 •

Diabetes in
Black Americans

*Epidemiology of Diabetes
in Black-Americans
Need for Increased Awareness
and Treatment*

Today, diabetes mellitus is one of the most serious health challenges facing the more than 30 million black Americans. The following statistics illustrate the magnitude of this disease among black Americans.

• Approximately 2.3 million or 10.8 percent of all black Americans have diabetes. The actual number of black Americans who have diabetes is probably more than twice the number diagnosed because previous research indicates that for every black American diagnosed with diabetes there is at least one undiagnosed case.

• For every white American who gets diabetes, 1.6 black Americans get diabetes.

• One in four black women, 55 years of age or older, has diabetes. (Among blacks, women are more likely to have diabetes than men.)

• Twenty-five percent of blacks between the ages of 65 and 74 have diabetes.

• Black Americans with diabetes are more likely to develop diabetes complications and experience greater disability from the complications than white Americans with diabetes.

WHAT RISK FACTORS INCREASE THE CHANCE OF DEVELOPING TYPE 2 DIABETES?

The frequency of diabetes in black adults is influenced by the same risk factors that are associated with Type 2 diabetes in other populations. Three categories of risk factors increase the chance of developing Type 2 diabetes in African Americans. The first is genetics, which includes inherited traits and group ancestry. The second is medical risk factors, including impaired glucose tolerance, hyperinsulinemia and insulin resistance, and obesity. The third is lifestyle risk factors, including sedentary living with a lack of physical activity.

FIGURE 1.— *Prevalence of Diagnosed Diabetes Among Blacks and Whites, US, 1991–92.*

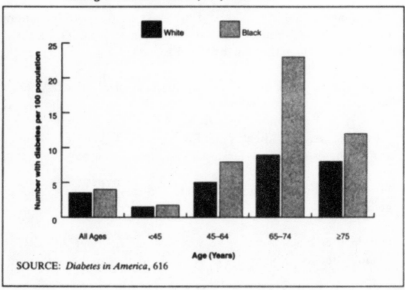

SOURCE: *Diabetes in America,* 616

GENETIC RISK FACTORS

Inherited Traits

Researchers suggest that black Americans—and recent African immigrants to America—have inherited a "thrifty gene" from their ancestors. Years ago, this gene enabled blacks, during "feast and famine" cycles, to use food energy more efficiently when food was scarce. Today, with fewer "feast and famine" cycles, the thrifty gene that developed for survival may instead make weight control more difficult. This genetic predisposition, along with impaired glucose tolerance (IGT), often occurs together with the genetic tendency toward high blood pressure.

Group Ancestry

Black-American ancestry is also an important predictor of the development of diabetes. To understand how rates of diabetes vary among black Americans, it is important to look at the historical origins of black populations in America. Genetic predisposition to diabetes is based, in part, on a person's lineage. The black American population formed from a genetic admixture across black ethnic groups with other racial groups, primarily European and North American Caucasian.

MEDICAL RISK FACTORS

Impaired Glucose Tolerance (IGT)

People with IGT have higher-than-normal blood glucose levels—but not high enough to be diagnosed as diabetes. Some argue that IGT is actually an early stage of diabetes. Black American men and women differ in their development of IGT. As black men grow older, they develop IGT at about the same rates as white American men and women. Black women, who have higher rates of diabetes risk factors, convert more rapidly from IGT to overt diabetes than black men and white women and men.

Hyperinsulinemia and Insulin Resistance

Higher-than-normal levels of fasting insulin or hyperinsulinemia, are associated with an increased risk of developing Type 2 diabetes. Hyperinsulinemia often predates diabetes by several years. One study showed a higher rate of hyperinsulinemia in black American adolescents in comparison to white American adolescents. To date, insufficient information is available on the relationship between insulin resistance or hyperinsulinemia and the development of Type 2 diabetes in black Americans.

Obesity

Obesity is a major medical risk factor for diabetes in black Americans. The National Health and Nutrition Survey (NHANESII), conducted between 1976 and 1980, showed substantially higher rates of obesity in black Americans aged 20 to 74 years of age who had diabetes, compared to those who did not have diabetes. NHANESII also showed higher rates of obesity among black American women and men than white Americans without diabetes.

As noted in Chapter 16, *Obesity and Diabetes*, the degree to which obesity is a risk factor for diabetes may depend on the location of the excess weight. Upper body obesity is a greater risk factor for Type 2 diabetes, compared to excess weight carried below the waist. One study showed that black Americans have a greater tendency to develop upper-body obesity, which increased their risk of Type 2.

Although black Americans have higher rates of obesity, some researchers do not believe obesity alone accounts for their higher prevalence of diabetes. Even when compared to white Americans with the same levels of obesity, age, and socioeconomic status, blacks still have higher rates of diabetes. Other factors yet to be understood appear to be at work.

LIFESTYLE RISK FACTORS

Physical Activity

Physical activity is a strong protective factor against Type 2 diabetes. Researchers suspect that a lack of exercise is one factor contributing to the unusually high rates of diabetes in older black women.

HOW DOES DIABETES AFFECT BLACK AMERICAN YOUNG PEOPLE?

Black American children have lower rates of Type 1 diabetes than white American children. The prevalence of Type 1 diabetes in white American children aged 15 and younger is nearly twice as high as in black American children of the same age.

Researchers tend to agree that genetics probably makes Type 1 diabetes more common among children with European ancestry. In fact, black children with some European ancestry have slightly higher prevalence of Type 1 diabetes. This incidence is also influenced by environmental and lifestyle factors.

HOW DOES DIABETES AFFECT BLACK AMERICAN WOMEN DURING PREGNANCY?

Gestational diabetes, which develops in about two to five percent of all pregnant women, usually resolves after childbirth. Several studies have shown that black American women have a higher rate of gestational diabetes. An Illinois study showed an 80 percent higher incidence of gestational diabetes in black women compared with white women. Once a woman has had gestational diabetes, she has an increased risk of developing gestational diabetes in future pregnancies. In addition, experts estimate that about half of women with gestational diabetes—regardless of race—develop Type 2 diabetes within 20 years of the pregnancy.

HOW DO DIABETES COMPLICATIONS AFFECT BLACK AMERICANS?

Compared to white Americans, black Americans experience higher rates of three diabetes complications—blindness, kidney failure, and amputations. They also experience greater disability from these complications. Some factors that influence the frequency of these complications, such as delay in diagnosis and treatment of diabetes, denial of diabetes, abnormal blood lipids, high blood pressure, and cigarette smoking, can be influenced by proper diabetes management.

KIDNEY FAILURE

Black Americans experience kidney failure, also called end-stage renal disease (ESRD), from 2.5 to 5.5 times more often than white Americans. Interestingly though, hypertension, not diabetes, is the leading cause of kidney failure in black Americans. Hypertension accounts for almost 38 percent of ESRD cases in blacks, whereas diabetes causes 32.5 percent. In spite of their high rates of the disease, black Americans have better survival rates from kidney failure than white Americans.

VISUAL IMPAIRMENT

The frequency of severe visual impairment is 40 percent higher in black Americans with diabetes than in white Americans. Blindness caused by diabetic retinopathy is twice as common in blacks as in whites. Compared to white women, black women are three times more likely to become blind from diabetes. Black American men have a 30 percent higher rate of blindness from diabetes than white American men. Diabetic retinopathy may occur more frequently in black Americans than whites because of their higher rate of hypertension.

AMPUTATIONS

Black Americans undergo more diabetes-related lower-extremity amputations than white or Hispanic Americans. One study of 1990 U.S. hospital discharge figures showed amputation rates for black Americans with diabetes were 19 percent higher than for white Americans. In a 1991 California study, however, black Americans were 72 percent more likely to have diabetes-related amputations than white Americans.

DOES DIABETES CAUSE EXCESS DEATHS IN BLACK AMERICANS?

Diabetes was an uncommon cause of death among black Americans at the turn of the century. By 1993, however, according to the Center for Disease Control and Prevention's National Center for Health Statistics, death certificates listed diabetes as the fifth leading cause of death for blacks aged 45 to 64, and third leading cause of death for those 65 and older. Diabetes is more dangerous for black American women, for whom it was the third leading cause of death.

Diabetes death rates may actually be higher than these studies show for two reasons. First, diabetes might not have been diagnosed. Second, many doctors do not list diabetes as a cause of death, even when the person was known to have diabetes.

The National Diabetes Information Clearinghouse has compiled a directory of programs and other resources to help health educators, public health officials, community leaders, and others, in developing educational programs to foster awareness of diabetes and its management among black Americans. The directory, *Diabetes-Related Programs for Black Americans: A Resource Guide,* includes descriptions of diabetes-related programs that are targeted to black people or that serve communities with substantial black populations.

Single copies of the directory are available free from:

National Diabetes Information Clearinghouse
Box NDIC, 9000 Rockville Pike
Bethesda, MD 20892
(301) 468-2162

C H A P T E R
• 25 •

Straight Talk to Teenagers and Young Adults With Diabetes

What to Tell Friends and Teachers
How to Live a "Normal Life"
Answers to Frequently Asked Questions

"**O**h, you're a diabetic? Don't worry about it. You can live a normal life." I'll bet you've heard that before. You know better. People mean well when they say, "You can lead a normal life." Maybe they don't realize that you have to take "shots" of insulin every day. And stick your finger for blood sugar two or three times a day, and say "no thanks" when someone offers you a piece of cake or candy.

The truth is that through no fault of your own, you've got diabetes. The truth also is that you can live out a full, productive, and meaningful life.

You're still the same person, the same personality, with the same hopes and ambitions for the future that you have always had. Diabetes can never change that.

Your aim, then, is to manage the diabetes and not let it manage you. There are some questions that will need answers. In this chapter, we answer questions that are frequently asked by friends and family. They mean well, but frankly, most people are misinformed about diabetes and maybe, just maybe, you can enlighten them and make *them* feel more comfortable.

Question 1: What should I tell my friends?

Answer:

Explain that when a person eats, the food is digested and then is broken down and passes into the body's cells to supply energy. This requires a hormone called insulin. Since you don't have enough insulin, you take insulin injections.

It's a good idea to let them know that sometimes your sugar may get too low, causing you to act "shaky and confused." They can help by getting you some sweets or a Coca-Cola, fast.

Question 2: What should I tell my teachers at school?

Answer:

You can tell them the same information you gave your friends. It's a good idea to let them know you may be late on occasion in order to test your blood glucose and to take the proper dose of insulin. It is wise to acquaint the teacher with the symptoms of "low blood sugar" so that she/he can help in an emergency situation. Teachers should be informed about the need for glucose tablets or carbohydrates for treatment of hypoglycemic reactions. Show your teachers and school nurse how to do a blood glucose test and inform them of your target range. There are brochures giving excellent information for teachers that are available through the American Diabetes Association and the Juvenile Diabetes Foundation.

Question 3: Will having diabetes have any effect on my dating?

Answer:

No. Hopefully, you will be with someone who knows your needs and understands the possibility of hypoglycemia or the rare occasion of "running to the bathroom." Your date should be aware of your diabetes and not be surprised by your selection of a proper diabetic diet in a restaurant.

Question 4: Can I participate in sports?

Answer:

As long as you control your blood sugar and monitor it regularly, you can participate in most sports. In fact there are only a few that should be avoided, including skydiving, scuba diving, or auto racing. An episode at the wrong time in these sports could cause dangerous problems.

But look what's left: tennis, team sports, biking, swimming, hiking, skiing, and hundreds of other games and activities.

I'm sure you know there have been outstanding stars in major league football, tennis, and baseball, who have had diabetes since childhood. Of course, they are sure to adjust food requirements and insulin dosage before, during, and after strenuous activity. Remember, when you increase physical activity, your insulin and food requirements change. So, plan for this in advance. Contact the International Diabetic Athletes Association for membership and a newsletter.

Question 5: Can I participate at parties?

Answer:
Of course. You can even be the "life of the party."
You are the one who knows what you can eat and how much insulin you must take before going out for the evening. And always have a hard candy or piece of sugar handy, just in case you feel symptoms of low blood sugar. Make sure to check your blood sugar regularly.

Question 6: Will diabetes affect my physical appearance?

Answer:
No. With good diabetic control, your physical development will be right on track. Continue to pay attention to good dental, foot, and skin hygiene, especially around the areas where you give your insulin injections.

Question 7: Will I have difficulty getting a driver's license?

Answer:
No. Usually a doctor's note indicating your diabetes is under good control is sufficient for the license bureau or State Police.

Question 8: Will I be limited in my choice of a career?

Answer:
There are only a few types of work that a person with diabetes would be wise to avoid. These include jobs that carry a great responsibility for the lives and safety of others, such as a commercial airline pilot, bus driver, or an operator of trains or other public vehicles. I can't think of any other fields that would bar a well-controlled diabetic from participation.

Question 9: What about marriage?

Answer:
There is no reason whatsoever that a diabetic cannot have a long and happy married life. A thorough discussion with your future marital partner should convince you that you have found someone who loves you and can be trusted to aid you in case some unforeseen diabetic emergency arises. You should be ready to do the same for your future spouse.

Question 10: Will I be able to have children?

Answer:
Modern management has taken away the fear and consternation that existed years ago in regard to pregnancy and fatherhood. With skilled and careful attention to glucose control, there is no contraindication to pregnancy. Remember that it is especially important for the diabetic woman to be well managed *before*, during, and after pregnancy.

Question 11: What about smoking?

Answer:
In this day and age, the general public is well aware of the terrible health consequences of smoking. For the diabetic, it is an absolute no-no. The effect on the lungs, heart, and blood vessels is magnified even more in diabetics. The combination of diabetes and smoking will almost certainly lead to heart and circulatory problems.

Question 12: What about "recreational" drugs?

Answer:
So-called "recreational drugs" such as marijuana, anti-depressants, amphetamines, and cocaine are not only dangerous to your health, but could mask an insulin reaction with all its harmful consequences. All of these drugs have adverse affects on the diabetic in particular by, in some cases, raising the blood sugar, increasing appetite, raising blood pressure, and causing abuse and dependence.

Question 13: What is the effect of alcohol?

Answer:

Alcohol is by far the most addictive drug in general use today in America. While alcohol in small amounts may have a favorable effect on lipids, in larger amounts it can contribute to cardiovascular disease, head and neck cancer, and cirrhosis.

Question 14: How does diabetes effect sexual activity?

Answer:

In women, there is little if any effect. In men, good control of blood sugars should allow full sexual activity and enjoyment. Some men who have had diabetes for many years will develop sexual problems. Talk to your parents and your doctor or nurse if you have any problems or questions. Sex counts as a physical activity, so you may need an extra snack.

Question 15: What effect do the oral contraceptive drugs have on diabetics?

Answer:

It is probably best to avoid the "pill" since it will affect blood sugar, interfere with insulin action, and cause some retention of fluids. Other side effects include high blood pressure and a tendency to form thromboses (blood clots) in the lower extremities. It is best to seek advice from your physician regarding the best method of birth control for you.

Question 16: Must I continue to test my blood sugar for the rest of my life?

Answer:

The answer to this question is "yes," until a practical cure for diabetes becomes available. In order to avoid acute and chronic complications of diabetes, the blood glucose must be kept within a certain prescribed range. The only way you can do this at the present time is by finger-stick blood sugar determinations. Technical advances to obtain the blood sugar without the necessity of a finger-stick will become available soon.

Question 17: How do I explain to my friends my special needs for injections, glucose monitoring, and meal planning?

Answer:

In a matter-of-fact manner. You will find that people aren't really all that interested and take you as a person, soon forgetting your special needs. You will still be judged on your merit, conversation and personality, just as before.

Question 18: Can I look forward to a cure for diabetes?

Answer:

Definitely. Scientists are at work in major medical centers throughout the world. The outlook for a practical cure has never been brighter. There is, at last, a light at the end of the tunnel.

Question 19: What can I do to maintain a good management program?

Answer:

Knowledge is power! Learn as much as you can. Put your knowledge about diabetes to use— test your blood glucose regularly, stick to your meal plan, take your medication, and exercise regularly. Enroll in a formal course on diabetes if available. Make sure that you see your doctor for an HbA1c assessment *at least every four months.*

Question 20: Will my insulin requirements change?

Answer:

Probably. Growth, hormone changes with puberty, emotional stress, illness or infection, and changes in exercise and lifestyle may all affect your insulin dose. Write down your blood glucose results so that your doctor can review them and look for "patterns." Changes in the "patterns" of your test results are a signal that adjustments may be needed in your meal plan, insulin dose, or exercise program. See Chapter 13, *Patterns of Control & Sick Day Care.*

C H A P T E R
• 26 •

Alternative Therapies for Diabetes

The Role of Alternative Treatments
Natural Treatments for Type 2 Diabetes
Botanical Hypoglycemics
Chromium and Other Minerals
Vitamins

CAUTION: Always consult your doctor before using any alternative therapy. Never substitute an alternative treatment program for standard therapy. Alternative treatments should be used only as an adjunct to conventional therapy, not in place of mainline medical treatment. No reputable health practitioner would ever advise you to stop taking your oral agents or insulin without the approval of your doctor. Herbal remedies can interact with prescription or over-the-counter medications. Under the guidance and supervision of your physician, it may be possible to try alternative treatments and even gradually decrease medication doses if there is sufficient improvement in blood sugar control. However, these decisions can be made only by your personal physician.

I n recent years, alternative therapies for many disorders have become increasingly popular among an American public that has eagerly rushed to embrace non-conventional medical treatments. Some patients seek to replace orthodox treatments that have not worked. Others are concerned about adverse effects that may be associated with some standard medical treatments. The vast majority of people, however, use these therapies to supplement, not replace, conventional treatment.

Modern medicine's reliance on expensive laboratory tests, drugs and space age diagnostic and therapeutic technologies has not only contributed to the sky-rocketing cost of medical care, but has also left many patients feeling isolated as they are referred from one specialist to another for evaluation and treatment. Aside from the perceived coldness of conventional medical treatment, many patients are caught up in the red-tape of managed care.

In brief, the major draws of many alternative medicine treatments (sometimes called complimentary medicine) is the belief that they offer a more holistic approach, treating the whole person—mind and body—in an affordable and sympathetic setting which encourages patients to participate in their own care.

Alternative therapies that supposedly help people gain optimum health by utilizing the body's own healing powers include an extremely varied group of practice disciplines as disparate as nutritional therapy, physical medicine including massage, oriental medicine and acupuncture, manipulation, herbal therapy, ayurveda, chiropractic, homeopathy, and many, many more, including a wide range of cultural practices and disciplines.

In addition to extolling the benefits of their individual therapeutic approach with its emphasis on holistic treatment, many also stress prevention of disease through diet, supplements, anxiety reduction and the elimination of unhealthy lifestyle habits such as smoking, excessive alcohol intake and lack of exercise—sage advise also shared by standard medical practitioners.

Some alternative therapies are based on treatments whose benefits rely on anecdotal patient reports of benefit which have not been substantiated by controlled research studies. Nevertheless, they enjoy widespread popularity and some do seem to be effective. *Others have no valid rationale and are completely worthless or even worse, harmful or potentially fatal.*

Medical doctors are trained to examine facts and evaluate controlled research studies, not anecdotal patient reports. No medical condition exists that can not be resolved by the observation, "I once saw a case.....". Hippocrates advised physicians that the first rule of medicine was, "Above all else....do no harm." This basic tenet remains as valid today as it was in ancient Greece. Medical doctors generally shun unproven treatments, particularly when their safety has not been established. Dr. York Coble of the American Medical Association said, "In God we trust . . . all others must have (research) data." The fact that a treatment is based on a naturally occurring substance does not always mean that it is safe. "Natural" does not necessarily equate with safety.

When dealing with herbal remedies or other substances of purported medicinal value, only scientific research can determine if they are truly safe and effective.

We now know that the mind plays an important role in maintaining the health of the immune system. Emotional health is important for physical well being. The human body is an amazing self-regulating bio-chemical machine with the mind (the software) directing the brain (the hardware) to orchestrate the many bio-chemical and physiologic processes necessary to maintain health.

The apparent benefit of certain alternative treatments that have no basis in fact, and which have not been able to withstand the close scrutiny of scientific study, is due to the "Placebo Effect." A placebo is an inert substance that serves as a control during a drug evaluation study. Research participants are not told whether they are taking the drug under investigation or the inert look-alike. The belief by the recipient of the placebo that he is taking the "real thing" is often sufficient to induce physiologic responses similar to those seen when taking the genuine medication. This process may be thought of as a sort of waking hypnosis. When the subconscious mind believes that something is true, it will often cause the body to respond in a manner that substantiates that belief, in the same way that a hypnotized subject acts out the suggestions of the hypnotist. Much of the whoop-la and testimonials that attest to the benefits of worthless medical treatments can be ascribed to the placebo effect. It is the placebo effect and lack of scientific studies that have made testimonials for some unorthodox alternative treatments highly suspect. Despite this caveat, some unproven alternative therapies based on anecdotal claims do appear to work, even though we may not understand their mechanism of action, and research studies to substantiate their benefits are lacking.

Conventional medicine, too, reports anecdotal type case reports which are published in highly respected medical journals. However, these peer reviewed cases differ substantially from the typical anecdotal reports of many alternative treatments. Standard medicine's case reports are well documented in clinical terms and their publication is motivated by a desire to contribute to our understanding of an illness which might lead to a theory of its etiology that warrants further investigation. In other words, isolated cases are not necessarily used to claim a general remedy for the malady under consideration.

Many alternative treatments not only lack scientific studies, but their proponents often deny the need for such evaluations. Admittedly, many standard medical treatments also have not undergone rigorous scientific testing and scrutiny, a deficit that mainstream medicine acknowledges needs to be rectified. Some alternative therapies not only ignore biological rationales, but often disparage modern scientific methods as unnecessary when dealing with ancient or "natural" folk remedies. Today medical doctors expect statistically significant clinical evidence that validates a treatment regimen before incorporating it into their practice. Recent studies of many widely practiced alternative disciplines have failed to demonstrate any scientific evidence for the therapeutic benefits ascribed to them. Some, however, have been shown to be efficacious.

Patients often fail to disclose to their physician the fact that they may be incorporating alternative treatments along with their standard medical care because they fear rejection and scorn by their doctor. The physician's role, however, is to simply protect patients from harmful treatments and to permit those that are safe, effective and not unreasonably expensive.

So called "natural" treatment techniques are not the sole domain of alternative practitioners. Dietary advice, counselling on lifestyle modifications and preventive health measures are all part of the standard advice conventional doctors give to their patients. For example, for the Type 2 diabetic, modifications in diet, weight control, lifestyle and emotional health are all recognized to play key roles in controlling blood sugar levels and at times reducing the dose or eliminating the need for oral agents or insulin. More than 80 percent of Type 2 diabetics are significantly overweight when first diagnosed with their disease. Many live a sedentary lifestyle and do not follow a healthy diet. Doctors are concerned with not only how much fat a person has but where the fat is distributed on the body. Women typically collect fat in their hips and buttocks, resulting in a "pear" shape. Men, on the other hand, usually build up fat around their bellies, giving them more of an "apple" shape. This is not a hard and fast rule though. Some men are pear shaped and some women are "apples," especially after menopause. People whose fat is concentrated mostly in the abdomen are more likely to develop many of the health problem—including diabetes—associated with obesity. The distribution of body fat may be as important a factor in predisposition to Type 2 diabetes as the Body Mass Index. See Chapter 15, *Obesity and Diabetes.*

HERBAL THERAPY FOR DIABETES

Of all the forms of alternative treatments, the most common is herbal therapy. Until the 20th Century, the vast majority of all medical remedies were herbal in origin. Herbal medicine is based on the fact that many plant leaves, stems, seeds or roots possess medicinal qualities. The scientific study of traditional herbal medicine is called "ethnopharmacology." Through the ages more than 1200 different plants have been said to possess health benefits. Scientific research has verified the effectiveness and safety of many of these substances which have long played an important role in folk medicine. Indeed, many traditional medicines got their start as folk remedies. The foxglove plant, for example, was first used in China over three hundred years ago, to treat edema. This treatment was effective when the swelling was a result of congestive heart failure because the leaves of the foxglove plant contain digitalis, a botanical now known to strengthen heart action and improve vascular hemodynamics.

Ephedra, the main ingredient of some over-the-counter asthma medications, has been used in China to relieve breathing problems for more than 5000 years.

Morphine and codeine were originally derived from the poppy plant. Poppy extract was used to quiet colicky infants in the time of the pharoahs. Penicillin was first discovered when penicillium mold contaminated a laboratory bacterial culture dish. In the seventeenth century a Jesuit priest brought back to Europe a Peruvian native treatment for fever, derived from the bark of the cinchona tree, which proved to be very effective in controlling malaria. We now know that the active ingredient is quinine, an antimalarial suppressive drug that was widely employed during World War II. The willow tree was the source of a widely used folk remedy for arthritic pain and fever which now enjoys worldwide popularity and is known as aspirin. These are but a few examples of the many drugs which were first introduced to civilization by shamans and medicine men. It has been estimated that 25 percent of all modern pharmaceuticals were originally derived from herbs.

The World Health Organization, recognizing that primitive cultures often employ herbal remedies with apparently satisfactory results have urged pharmaceutical companies and researchers to investigate this vast untapped source of potential new drugs throughout the world. The tropical rainforests of the world are a virtual treasure chest of plants with potential medicinal compounds. Notwithstanding, a certain amount of caution is in order. Congress has passed the Dietary Supplement Health and Education Act which exempts supplements from federal regulation as long as the manufacturer makes no therapeutic claims. Accordingly, they are now sold under the euphemistic umbrella of "dietary supplements." There are no safeguards in place to protect the public against impurities or dangers in any of these substances. The fact that they are natural and sold in health food stores does not necessarily mean they are harmless. Ma Huang, for example, is marketed under many brand names as an energy booster and weight control substance. The active pharmacological ingredient is ephedrine. This substance is known to raise blood pressure, as well as cause disturbances in heart rhythm, which on occasion has caused fatalities. Beigel, et al, recently published a report of a patient who developed lead poisoning after taking an Indian herbal remedy for diabetes. Never assume because a supplement is a natural herbal substance that it must be safe.

Because of the lack of governmental controls, herbs have been sold that were contaminated with heavy metals or other harmful substances. Some have been fortified with tranquilizers or non-steroidal anti-inflammatory drugs to enhance their effects. Additionally, many herbal preparations may have ingredients that could interact adversely with standard medications. Despite the fact that some herbal preparations are worthless or downright dangerous, many others appear to be safe and effective against a variety of conditions, including diabetes. To insure product quality, purchase only those that are produced by the larger reputable manufacturers and then ***ONLY WITH THE APPROVAL OF YOUR PERSONAL PHYSICIAN.***

BOTANICAL HYPOGLYCEMICS

Many plants are known to have blood sugar lowering properties in people with diabetes. Although scientific studies are lacking for most of the hypoglycemic botanicals, they have enjoyed widespread popularity in folk medicine and many primitive cultures. Controlled studies are currently underway to verify the therapeutic benefits of many of these herbs. Although botanical hypoglycemics may help to control diabetes, don't expect them to replace an unhealthy lifestyle. *No herb can replace a healthy diet and exercise regimen.*

Bitter Gourd—The most widely employed anti-diabetic herb is bitter gourd (momordica charantia) known as balsam pear. This tropical vegetable is widely cultivated in Asia, Africa and South America. One quarter of a cup of bitter gourd extract daily is purported to lower blood sugar up to twenty percent. A study of Type 2 diabetics showed an improvement in glucose tolerance in three quarters of the subjects tested. The blood sugar lowering ability of the fresh juice or of extracts of the unripe fruit is also reputed to be beneficial. Charantia is made up of several sterols that have a hypoglycemic affect similar to the sulfonylurea drugs. The drug, as its name implies, is quite bitter and unpalatable.

Fenagreed Seed—Fenagreed seed is another herb that is believed to affect glucose metabolism favorably. The chopped seeds (which taste like maple syrup with a bitter twang) are generally regarded in the United States as an exotic kitchen spice. Fenagreed seeds have enjoyed considerable popularity in India and the Middle East as a diabetes treatment. The seeds are usually soaked overnight and then eaten or used as a condiment. Some studies have demonstrated that when ground up seeds were fed to diabetics, there was an improvement in glucose tolerance with a fall in fasting blood sugar levels. Because the seeds are high in a gel-like soluble fiber that binds to bile acids they also help to lower cholesterol. To show beneficial results, it requires about 3-1/2 ounces to be consumed daily. Asians accustomed to consuming large herbal doses are more likely to commit to the large intake required.

Gymnema Sylvestre—This plant, native to the forests of India has long enjoyed a key place in an alternative medical practice popular in India called ayurveda. The theory of ayurveda medicine is based on the theoretical existence of various centers within the body that control all functions. Regardless of the validity of the theories of ayurvedic medicine, this herbal treatment for Type 1 and Type 2 diabetes is said by its proponents to offer benefit. The mechanism of action is claimed to be mediated by a direct effect on the pancreas to enhance insulin production by stimulating regeneration or revitalization of the insulin producing beta cells. One limited study reported a decrease in insulin requirements of Type 1 diabetics. Another supposedly showed an improvement of blood sugar control in Type 1 diabetes. The drug is also said to be effective in Type 2 diabetes, causing a decrease in the dosage of oral agents and sometimes even an improvement in blood sugar control sufficient to permit oral agents to be discontinued completely. Its blood sugar lowering potential is said to work only in the presence of abnormal blood sugar levels. Gymnema Sylvestre has not been subjected to controlled studies to evaluate its purported benefits.

Blueberry Leaf Tea—Blueberry leaves (vaccinium myrtillus) are said to have blood sugar lowering qualities. Several cups a day prepared as a decoction (the leaves are soaked in cold water and then brought to a boil for five to ten minutes) is said to lower blood sugar. Three months are said to be required before benefits become apparent. The blueberry leaves contain anthcyanic acid which is believed to be the active ingredient responsible for improvement in carbohydrate metabolism. Anthcyanic acid is also available in capsule form in many health food stores.

Prickly Pear Cactus—Prickly pear cactus is used as a food in Mexico where it is called nopal. It is believed to have hypoglycemic effects. The prickly pear pads are diced and prepared as a salad or used when preparing tacos. A recent study by Mexican researchers reported that the boiled cactus stem was capable of causing a significant drop in blood sugar within one hour, with glucose levels continuing to decline for two hours. It is believed that the nopal cactus decreases insulin resistance.

Broccoli — Broccoli is an excellent source of fiber, anti-oxidants, vitamins and other nutrients. It is particularly beneficial for diabetics because it is such a rich source of the essential trace mineral, chromium, which plays an important role in glucose metabolism and is believed to enhance insulin efficiency. Broccoli contains about 10mcg (one millionth of a gram) of chromium per cup. Therapeutic benefits for diabetics are said to require between 200-400mcg per day. If adequate amounts are not obtained from dietary sources, supplements may be required to reach a therapeutic dose. More about this in the next section when minerals that play an important role in glucose metabolism are discussed.

Onions and Garlic — The common bulbs, onions and garlic have long been believed to possess sugar-lowering qualities and have played an important role as an adjunct in the treatment of diabetes in folk medicine. Scientific evidence now points to their content of disulfides (sulfur containing compounds) such as allyl propyl and diallyl disulfide as the pharmacologically active ingredients. These chemicals are closely related to the first generation sulfonylurea drug Tolbutamide (Orinase). Like the sulfonylureas, onions and garlic work by stimulating insulin production in the pancreas and therefore offer benefit only for Type 2 diabetics. The larger the quantity of these bulbs eaten, the greater their anti-diabetic effect. The oral ingestion of 50ml of their juice daily has been shown to improve glucose control. The blood sugar lowering propensity of onions is unaffected by cooking. Aside from its favorable effects on carbohydrate metabolism, some studies suggest that garlic can lower cholesterol levels, boost the immune system and decrease the risks for some cancers.

Bitter Herbs and Spices — Bitter herbs have been widely employed by herbalists from Europe to Asia for the treatment of diabetes. Some commonly used spices have been subjected to study which suggest that they may stimulate insulin secretion in response to dietary demand. Ginger, cinnamon, clover, bay leaf, tumeric, nutmeg and coriander seed are but a few of many that are believed to have a favorable affect on carbohydrate metabolism. One study showed cinnamon to have a beneficial hypoglycemic effect, with only a relatively small amount of the condiment being needed to achieve a significant response.

Dandelion Greens — Dandelions have long enjoyed a reputation as a botanical hypoglycemic. Dandelion greens may be used in a salad or the freshly squeezed juice may be included in the diet.

PREVENTING TYPE 2 DIABETES

Fish — Retrospective studies of subjects who had neither diabetes nor impaired glucose tolerance, indicated that those who regularly included fish that were high in omega-3 fatty acids in their diet had a lower incidence of Type 2 diabetes, heart disease, and colo-rectal cancer. It is believed that the Omega-3's contribute to preventing the development of insulin resistance, which in turn, plays a major role in developing obesity and Type 2 diabetes. The preventive protective benefit of including fish in the diet has been known for many years. However, only in recent times has it been determined that the ingredient responsible for the protective benefits are a pair of polyunsaturated fats—the omega-3 fatty acids, eicosapentaenoic acid (EPA) and decosahexaenoic acid (DHA). Only a relatively small amount of fish is necessary to obtain sufficient EPA and DHA to offer benefit. It was long thought that eating a small amount of fish once per week sufficed. Recent evidence points to the necessity of eating fish two or three times per week to reduce or prevent insulin resistance. Those fish that come from cold, deep water have the highest levels of the omega-3 acids. Poaching, baking or broiling are the preferred way to prepare fish to preserve their omega-3 content. Corn oil as well as some other cooking oils are rich in omega-6 fatty acids which have a propensity to neutralize omega-3 fatty acids. Therefore, fish should not be prepared by frying or sauteing. Omega-3 fatty acids are available in capsule form. However, diabetics should never consume more than 3 grams a day because high doses can adversely affect blood sugar. For vegetarians or those who do not eat fish, flaxseed oil contains alpha-linoleic acid, an omega-3 oil, that is found in plants. Flax seeds contain about 3 grams of linoleic acid per tablespoon.

Fish oils slow the blood clotting time, but this is generally not of great enough magnitude to cause significant bleeding. Nevertheless, if you are taking an anti-coagulant medication such as coumadin, or if you suffer from attacks of bronchial asthma which sometimes occur more frequently among people taking fish oil capsules, caution is in order. Because omega-3 supplements may be contraindicated, discuss their use with your doctor.

VITAMIN AND MINERAL SUPPLEMENTS

Although not a panacea, certain vitamins and minerals have been shown to play key roles in glucose metabolism and should be included in every diabetic diet. Less than one percent of the American population eats a balanced diet that adequately meets all of their vitamin and mineral needs. Furthermore, even if you are getting the recommended daily allowance (RDA) for all the nutrients, you may still not be getting enough for maximum well-being. Higher amounts than the RDA of certain vitamin and minerals have been found to be protective against many degenerative diseases, including cardiovascular disease. If adequate amounts cannot be obtained from dietary sources, the use of a supplement may be indicated.

Chromium—Chromium has been purported to lower fasting blood sugar levels in many Type 2 diabetics as well as to lessen the insulin requirements of Type 2's who take insulin by improving carbohydrate metabolism. Chromium is an essential nutrient that is required for normal carbohydrate metabolism. It plays a key role in processing sugar. The amount of chromium a person needs varies considerably, increasing with glucose intolerance and diabetes. Because chromium works by enhancing the action of insulin, for chromium to be of benefit, an individual must be capable of producing insulin. Therefore, it is of no benefit in Type 1 diabetes. A recent study of 180 Type 2 diabetics by the United States Department of Agriculture (USDA) scientists evaluated patients taking 1000 micrograms of chromium picolinate daily. "Nearly all of them no longer had signs or symptoms of diabetes," said chief researcher, Richard Anderson. *Other studies with chromium suggest that adequate chromium intake may sometimes help to prevent the onset of Type 2 diabetes as well as gestational diabetes.* **It is important to note that this study was conducted in China on a population group that was chromium deficient. The dramatic results noted have not been duplicated in the United States in a population group that is not normally markedly chromium deficient.**

The USDA analysis of the typical American well-balanced diet yielded only 24 micrograms of chromium per 1000 calories of food ingested. For many years, the accepted daily requirement for chromium was set at 50mcg/day. The National Research Council now recommends 50-200 mcg/day. The element chromium is difficult to scrutinize in laboratory studies because of the tiny amount involved. Future studies will undoubtedly clarify more precisely human needs.

Although the USDA study used 1000 micrograms of chromium, 200-400mcg/day would have been adequate according to researcher Anderson.

He suggests that biologically active chromium binds to insulin making the hormone more efficient in carrying out its many physiologic functions.

Throughout the evolutionary process adequate chromium was present in nature and gained entry into the body. However, in modern times few foods contain a significant amount of chromium according to recent USDA analysis. Best sources are brewer's yeast, whole grains and whole grain cereals—particularly bran cereals, cocoa, tea, black pepper, corn chips, bacon, and canned products such as pineapple or tomatoes that get chromium leached during the canning process, shell fish, apples, vegetables—especially potato skins (which should never be eaten raw because the potato eyes contain toxins that are detoxified only by heat during the cooking process), prunes and American cheese.

If you have Type 2 diabetes and wish to try chromium supplements, be sure to check with your physician and get his or her approval.

WARNING: Two recent studies have found that when hamster ovary cells were exposed to high doses of chromium picolinate, the cells suffered DNA damage. The researchers believe that high doses (15 times the normal dose) might cause damage to human chromosomes as well. Additional studies will need to be done to evaluate any potential toxicity of high doses of chromium on human DNA. There are no studies that have evaluted the long-term safety of chromium supplementation at high doses in humans. Additionally, excessive chromium intake inhibits zinc and iron absorption which can lead to a deficiency of these two elements.

Manganese—Manganese plays an important role in assisting enzymes that have key roles in glucose metabolism. Manganese deficiency in diabetic laboratory animals resulted in birth defects including offspring with pancreatic abnormalities or congenital absence of the pancreas. Diabetics have a higher need for manganese than non-diabetics. A daily supplement of 30 milligrams will prevent the signs or symptoms associated with deficiencies of this mineral. Manganese is abundant in whole grains, nuts, legumes and fruits.

Magnesium—Magnesium plays an important role in glucose metabolism. Diabetics often have significantly low levels of magnesium and should be sure magnesium is included in their vitamin and mineral supplement. The RDA for magnesium is 350mg per day for men and 300mg per day for women. Diabetics probably require one and a half to two times the RDA which explains why deficiency is common in diabetics. The average adult intake in the United States ranges from 150 - 250mg daily. Food processing destroys much of this mineral. The best dietary sources are whole grains, nuts, seeds, legumes and green leafy vegetables. Because the typical American diet is high in refined foods, meat and dairy products, it is often magnesium deficient.

Pyradoxine (vitamin B-6)—Peripheral neuropathies are known to be associated with pyradoxine deficiency. It is now believed that B-6 may also play a role in diabetic retinopathy with some studies suggesting an improvement in retinopathy with B-6 supplements.

Vitamin C—Insulin plays a role in facilitating the entry of vitamin C into the cells. Vitamin C requirements in diabetes may be increased because of a relative vitamin C deficiency. Vitamin C is a potent anti-oxidant that scavenges free radicals.

Zinc—Excessive zinc excretion in the urine is often seen with diabetes. It is believed that zinc may play a role in maintaining beta cell integrity. Some studies point to improved glucose tolerance when zinc deficiencies are corrected. Too much zinc, however, can cause a copper deficiency. A satisfactory zinc/copper ratio of 10:1 is contained in many multi-vitamin/mineral supplements.

Biotin—This B vitamin increases the activity of glucokinase, an enzyme that plays an important role in the metabolism of glucose by the liver. Blood glucose control is purported to improve when biotin supplements are taken.

C H A P T E R
• 27 •

Diabetes: The Cure

Regeneration of insulin producing beta cells
Pancreatic and Islet Cell Transplants
Overcoming Host vs. Graft Disease
Gene Therapy
Islet Cell Neogenesis
Co-Transplantation of Islet & Sertoli Cells
The Closed Loop
Prevention of Diabetes

Note: Research into the causes, prevention and cure for diabetes is constantly adding to our knowledge and understanding of this complex metabolic disorder.

In this chapter, we shall explore some of the more promising credible research that is going forward in laboratories all over the world, by scientists seeking a practical, lasting diabetes cure.

Some of the experimental protocols which have been effective in laboratory animals have progressed to successful outcomes in humans. Phase III human trials, the final phase before FDA approval, is currently underway for the promising islet regeneration protocol.

INGAP AND PANCREATIC ISLET REGENERATION

Dr. Aaron Vinik of the Eastern Virginia Medical School(EVMS), Norfolk, Virginia and Dr. Lawrence Rosenberg from McGill University in Montreal have collaborated since the 1980's on research with the ultimate goal of regenerating insulin producing pancreatic islet tissue. Rather than seeking a treatment for the metabolic consequences of diabetes —the most notable of which is the derangement in glucose metabolism— their efforts were directed toward a permanent physiological cure for diabetes. The initial discovery that started them on their quest for a cure was their demonstration that they could induce new islet cell growth when they wrapped hamster pancreases in saran wrap. This serendipitous discovery that cell proliferation induced by the saran wrapping technique produced a neogenesis of islet tissue with functioning beta cells was an epiphany. The cellophane wrapping technique became known as "Sarandipity." This discovery was followed by a twenty year journey that would culminate in the discovery of INGAP (Islet Neogenesis Associated Protein). This protein was shown to be the substance that stimulated regeneration of a patient's own islet cells which functioned without requiring immunosuppressive drugs to prevent rejection. Theoretically the regenerated pancreatic beta cells would function normally producing both insulin and glucogon, thus raising or lowering the blood sugar as is normally done by a healthy functioning pancreas. TOO GOOD TO BE TRUE? Only a relatively short time ago this would have appeared to be a distant science fiction vision of the future. However, the future is here now. The INGAP protein has been synthesized in the laboratory.

Laboratory studies on diabetic animals showed that INGAP could reverse their diabetes. Preliminary safety studies on human subjects have been successfully completed and stage III human trials are currently underway.

This therapeutic approach has an excellent rationale and thus far in animal and limited human trials has lived up to expectations. Let's take a closer look at the road traveled by Drs. Vinik and Rosenberg that has brought their protocol to its present state of refinement. In Dr. Vinik's own words, "In the 80's, our scientific team started out on a heretical journey by asking what would be the perfect world to create new islets? We proposed to regenerate islets from endogenous adult stem cells in one's own pancreas. These islets could express the full complement of the hormones that were needed —insulin and glucagon— so that in a person's system, blood sugar would be lowered as well as raised when needed to prevent hypoglycemia. There would be no need for immunotherapy, and we could use benign drugs. This approach could treat both Type 1 and Type 2 diabetes. There would be sufficient insulin production to combat the diabetes as well as the resistance to insulin. Insulin secretion would be regulated. The effect would persist beyond the treatment periods. The treatment would not be associated with any toxicity whatsoever. And we would target only the adult pancreatic stem cells. That was a very tall order. This mythical approach to the treatment of diabetes —recapitulating the normal development of the pancreas in the fetus— has actually now become a reality.

In the 80's our journey began with what we call "Sarandipity." Dr. Lawrence Rosenberg and I were conducting experiments to induce pancreatitis. During these tests, we wrapped hamster pancreases with saran. This process led to a completely unexpected discovery —instead of damaging a pancreas, it produced new islet generation. We continued to follow this new line of research and demonstrated that the saran wrapping reversed streptozotocin-induced diabetes in hamsters. At that point, we realized that we had discovered an active principle that we called "ilotropin." We spent years working on that protein, trying to isolate it to its pure form so that we could administer it to animals made diabetic and later to people with diabetes. The nature of ilotropin eluded us. We had to change the process around. We had to look within the pancreas that was growing again for a protein that was capable of stimulating new growth. A new technology became available that enabled us "shake the genetic haystack" and watch the needles, or proteins, drop out. We found the genetic message and then went after the gene itself. And in doing that, we discovered INGAP (Islet Neogenesis Associated Protein). Dr. Ronit Rafaeloff showed that the protein product was capable of simulating islet neogenesis and lower blood glucose levels. This finding was published in 1997 in the Journal of Clinical Investigation. We found that INGAP has 766 bases. The path that we've become interested in is a mature protein. We created the protein by recombinant (molecular biologic) techniques, and then we investigated if this new construct could treat and reverse diabetes in animals. We gave this recombinant form of INGAP to animals made diabetic with streptozotocin. Several things happened. It stimulated pancreatic duct proliferation; it turned out to be the major component of ilotropin; and, antibodies to INGAP could neutralize the effect. Then we asked if INGAP caused the formation of new islets. Low and behold, it did. We could have been on a wild goose chase. We'd been investigating a product called ilotropin for fifteen years, and we couldn't find its active ingredient. Now, after pursuing a gene that's expressed, it turns out that that gene encodes a protein that is buried in the protein mixture that is doing what we want it to do. We got lucky! From our work with hamsters made diabetic, we found that for every log dose increase of INGAP, there was a progressive reduction in blood glucose concentration. Each dose we gave dropped the blood glucose 35 mg per deciliter translating into about a 1% drop in blood hemoglobin A1c. It was then just a question of how the process worked, what was the biologic effect, and how often we could repeat the outcome. By repeating the process, we were able to reverse diabetes 30 - 40% of the time. Next, we began investigating if a protein fragment could successfully duplicate the action of the whole INGAP protein. We cut up the protein into little pieces to find a smaller protein, a string of 15 amino acids that could do the same work. We synthesized this new INGAP Peptide in vitro and began further testing to see if the INGAP Peptide would reach its target and stimulate islets in the normal hamster.

In an attempt to simplify the problem, Drs. Gary Pittenger and Dr. David Taylor-Fishwick, directors of the Strelitz Diabetes Institute (SDI) laboratories, produced a synthetic peptide fragment of the material and gave it intraperitoneally with a fluorescent tag. They watched where it went in the body. The results were incredible. The injected material went straight to the pancreas and the ducts, and it didn't go anywhere else. Nature has made us very lucky —it has given us a lock that is present in this pancreatic cell. No matter where you put in the INGAP Peptide, the "key" will find the lock and hone in on it. Subsequently, we found that once the Peptide got to the pancreas' ductal cells, it stimulated them to make new islets. We then knew that the biological activity of INGAP was capable of stimulating new islets. We had the answer —INGAP Peptide goes where it is supposed to go and reverses diabetes like the whole INGAP protein. We moved on to investigate if this Peptide could reverse streptozotocin-induced diabetes in another species. We used the C57BL/bt black mouse that when made diabetic gets inflammation of the pancreas, and the cells look exactly like a person with Type 1 diabetes. We began to investigate if increasing the dose could attain a greater effect. The answer was, yes, in a small study with eight animals. With the animals that received salt water nothing happened, the diabetes remained. With all the animals that received INGAP Peptide, the diabetes was reversed.

Our next step was to ascertain how the INGAP Peptide reversed diabetes. With the animals that received saline treatment, the blood glucose remained elevated. With those that were treated with INGAP Peptide, the blood sugars started coming down. Stop giving INGAP Peptide, and the blood sugar stayed down. That means it's not insulin that was producing the effect because insulin only works while it's around in the body. INGAP Peptide had a biological effect to create new cells in the body that make insulin -new cells that the body recognized as its own.

The INGAP Peptide represents a potentially novel anti-diabetic therapy directed at the basis of the disease because it stimulates the growth of insulin-producing cells in the pancreas, rather that treating the metabolic consequences of diabetes such as high blood sugar. It is very encouraging that INGAP in humans appears to be remarkably like that in hamsters, and the antibodies that we have made to different portions of the hamster INGAP molecule cross-react very well with INGAP in the human and other species. We have been able to synthesize the gene down to a small peptide made up of a string of 15 amino acids that is responsible for inducing new islet production in the pancreas. The simpler the compound when administered for treatment, the less likely complications will occur in other areas. In our research with small animals, we experienced no complications, and we saw a reversal of diabetes when INGAP was administered at an adequate dose and for a sufficient period of time. There are only a limited number of pancreases that become available for islet transplants, and even if all were harvested for the purposes of islet transplantation, then only a few thousand people with diabetes would benefit. In contrast, every person with diabetes, even if they have had diabetes for a long time, may have precursor cells in their pancreases that can be trans-differentiated into islets, and there appears to be no limit in the capacity."

Researchers believe that islet cell regeneration has the potential for treating Type 1 and Type 2 diabetes. People with Type 1 diabetes have had their beta cells destroyed by an autoimmune assault in which the body's immune protective system attacks its own pancreatic beta cells as though they were a foreign substance. Although the beta cells are destroyed, other cells within the islets that produce hormones that are precursor cells appear to survive the assault. In Type 2 diabetes the beta cells don't produce enough insulin to overcome the body's insulin resistance. In both cases the pancreas may harbor enough precursor cells that can be turned on to become beta cells with the administration of INGAP.

Dr. Vinik says, "For people with Type 1 diabetes, the good news is that after a person has had diabetes for many years, the autoimmune process tends to die down. It seems that the body has to see foreign material to keep the autoimmune flames alive. When there is sufficient destruction of islets that have been damaged by the process, then the body no longer recognizes these as foreign and loses interest in further destruction. In people with Type 2 diabetes, the beta cells do not function effectively. It was once thought that people with Type 2 diabetes are merely resistant to the insulin their bodies produce. It is now known that people with Type 2 diabetes do not produce the number of beta cells that they need. SDI researchers anticipate that if they can over come the deficit in pancreatic insulin secretion, then islet cell regeneration will treat people with Type 2 as well.

Dr. Vinik compares the replacing of beta cells faster than they are destroyed to filling a bucket that has a hole in the bottom. He says, Even if there is a hole, as long as one pours faster than the bucket leaks, the bucket will fill. I believe that the same is true for producing insulin through islet cell regeneration —if islets are regenerated faster than they may be lost, sufficient islets can still be made to reverse diabetes. The interesting thing is that one needs only about 2% of the total islet mass to be free of diabetes. Say we were to stimulate the formation of a reserve mass, then that would be equivalent to plugging the hole part. We could always go back to the well if necessary."

Dr. David Taylor-Fishwick, Director of the Cell Molecular Biology Laboratory at the SDI, says, "Understanding the process of how INGAP works to regenerate islet cells is extremely important. It can open up new possibilities for treatment —possibly without even using the INGAP Peptide. We may find an alternate way of going into the beta cell and turning on insulin production. The more we know about how INGAP works, the greater our ability to treat diabetes and to identify risk factors for developing the disease."

Looking to the future, SDI researchers believe that someday basic islet cell regeneration research may allow scientists to be able to predict and identify susceptible individuals, and then prevent diabetes from ever occurring.

Dr. Leon-Paul Georges, Director of SDI and Chairman of EVMS's Department of Internal Medicine, explains, "Much research lies ahead, but the most exciting thing is that we are now working with humans; a goal that Dr. Vinik has been working toward since 1983 when he first discovered that the pancreas could grow new islets."

So where are we now? We think that it is not beyond the realms of reason to anticipate that INGAP alone or in combination with other factors, or small molecules that activate the receptor, or gene manipulation will provide a cure

There are currently many research approaches to replicate the worn-out or destroyed insulin producing beta cells of the pancreas. In this chapter we shall focus on those approaches which hold the most promise to do away with the need for insulin shots in Type 1 and Type 2 diabetes and the measures Type 2 diabetics can take to prevent, ameliorate or cure their diabetes.

CURES FOR DIABETES

Pancreatic and Islet Cell Transplantation

Even with the improved outlook of present day knowledge, including diet, exercise, weight control, insulin pumps, and rigid monitoring of glucose, diabetologists have not been able to completely eliminate the formidable long term complications of diabetes. However, for autoimmune (Type 1) diabetes, the successful transplantation of the pancreas or pancreatic islet cells *is* associated with freedom from depending on insulin injections and a dramatic improvement of the patient's quality of life as well as a marked reduction or elimination of long-term complications of diabetes.

The ultimate goal is to have long lasting "normal" glucose-insulin synchronization without reliance on potentially harmful immunosuppressive agents to prevent rejection.

Transplantation of islet cells isolated from the human pancreas was first performed in 1974. The initial exciting results of islet cell transplantation, first observed nearly 30 years ago, suggested that a permanent cure for Type 1 diabetes was at hand. This early optimism was dampened by the many technical problems facing islet cell replacement which became apparent and had to be overcome if long term successful outcomes were to be routinely achieved.* The main obstacles are the limited sources of available islet cells and poor graft survival due to susceptibility of transplanted tissue to immune system attack. *However, recent advances in genetic engineering technology now offer great promise for overcoming the problems which have frustrated researchers in the past.*

Overcoming Host vs. Graft Disease (HVGD)

The major problem confronting successful transplantation of insulin-producing pancreatic tissue from donor organs has been the rejection of these "foreign cells" by the recipient over time. It is the rejection process, refered to in medical terminology as Host vs. Graft Disease (HVGD) that has frustrated researchers in their search for a permanent transplant cure for diabetes. Organ rejection occurs because no two individuals, with the exception of identical twins, have the same DNA and protein components in their cells. When cells from one individual are transplanted to another, the recipient's body responds as though a hostile invader has entered its domain. It does not differentiate between an invading bacterium and a transplanted cell. The immune system response includes the manufacturing of antibodies and mobilization of macrophage and T-cells to seek out and destroy the intruder.

As noted, the problem of HVGD has been the chief stumbling block to the long-term survival of transplanted islet tissue. Were it not for HVGD, this relatively simple, noninvasive procedure of islet cell transplantation would have long ago become routine, and many diabetics could forego their need for insulin and live lives free from the scourge of diabetes.

THE EDMONTON PROTOCOL

Dr. James Shapiro is a Canadian surgeon who has performed many kidney-pancreas transplants. This major surgery, with its risks as well as practical availability for most diabetic patients motivated Dr. Shapiro to form a group with the goal of developing an islet cell transplant protocol that would be safe and have a high rate of success. Since the mid 1980's research focused on islet cell transplantation showed only a temporary success rate of 8%. Additionally, the anti-rejection drugs employed were quite toxic. In April 2000, Dr. Shapiro and his associates at the University of Alberta, Edmonton, Canada released the results of their islet cell transplantation study following their newly devised protocol which represented a major breakthrough. They developed a new technique for isolating and preserving islet cells as well as a safer anti-rejection cocktail. Fifteen patients with unstable diabetes underwent the Edmonton protocol. All of them became insulin-independent after the procedure and twelve have remained so. The "Edmonton Protocol" appears to be so successful that it has been adopted by diabetic research centers around the world.

The drugs employed by the Edmonton group represented a significant improvement in the anti-rejection drug cocktail. The Edmonton protocol drugs were well tolerated with a reduced incidence of side effects. However, one of the drugs used to prevent rejection, Tacrolimus, did provoke some renal side effects in those with pre-existing kidney disease. At the present time the Edmonton protocol is reserved for relatively severe unstable diabetics. Although it is true that the islet transplant procedure is not complex and is sometimes referred to as the "drive through" transplant, it is not without risks. Technically the procedure consists of inserting a catheter (a hollow tube) into the portal vein (the main blood vessel leading to the liver). A solution containing the islet cells is then injected into the catheter and carried by the bloodstream to the liver where they spread out and implant themselves. Possible side effects include bleeding, rarely clotting of the portal vein and on very rare occasions liver failure requiring a liver transplant. As with all anti-rejection drugs, the Edmonton protocol suppressive drugs interfere with the normal functioning of the body's immune protective system although admittedly to a lesser degree than those previously employed. Also, steroids which can raise blood sugar are no longer used. Suppressing the body's immune protective system increases the risks for infections as well as certain cancers.

The main source of human pancreases are those from auto accident victims. The average pancreas has about 1 million islet cells, half of which are lost in the islet cell extraction process. It therefore takes 2 pancreases to supply enough islet cells for an average size person for one transplant. New isolation techniques have now preserved the majority of islet cells. In the United States the six or seven thousand accident donor pancreases available yearly as islet cell sources are sufficient for only a small fraction of those required if the procedure is to become widespread. Islet cells have a short shelf life. In the past the transplant team had only six hours from the removal of the donor organ to transplantation. The Edmonton team has devised methods to hold them for several days.

The Technique of Transplantation
of Islet "Beta Cells"

Islet cell transplantation involves a relatively simple, non-invasive, out-patient procedure. The donor islet cells are suspended in a plastic bag which is connected by a plastic tube to a small catheter which is inserted into a vein that leads to the liver. The transplanted donor islet cell suspension drains by gravity into the catheter and is carried by the bloodstream to the liver where they seed themselves.

The Surgical Technique of Whole Pancreatic Transplant

The technique employed for transplanting the whole pancreas allows the surgeon to place the "new" organ in the right side of the patient's pelvis and attach it to the major vessels that traverse the pelvis. A drainage mechanism is provided by a graft to the bladder for excretion of the digestive enzymes that continue to be secreted by the pancreas.

In the past, because the immunosuppressive drugs are potentially toxic, most recipients of whole pancreatic transplants were chosen from those persons who also required kidney transplants. With the introduction of safer and more effective immunosuppressive drugs, side effects have decreased and the graft survival rate has markedly improved.*

Work done by Drs. Camillo Ricordi and Rodolfo Alejandro at the DRI, has shown that these drugs can be used to decrease the incidence of rejection and reduce some of the short term and long term side effects.

Nevertheless, patients must remain alert and report to their physician on a regular basis, to avoid complications and reduce some of the short term and long term toxic side effects of the drugs currently approved by the FDA for human use.

In one study from Giessen, Germany, islet transplants using various combinations of these anti-rejection drugs, 70 percent had normal glucose metabolism and 33 percent were insulin independent one year after the islet cell transplant.

Candidates for Islet Cell Transplantation

Type 1 diabetics are the most obvious candidates for islet cell transplantation because their disease is caused by the autoimmune destruction of their insulin-producing beta cells. The sub-group of diabetes known as Latent Autoimmune Diabetes of Adults (LADA) would also qualify for islet cell transplantation. This group accounts for 10 percent of all cases of diabetes.

Insulin resistance is the main defect in Type 2 diabetes. However, over time, many of the Type 2 diabetics' overworked, worn-out pancreases begin to fail and their output of insulin declines. Approximately 40 percent of Type 2 patients eventually require insulin to achieve satisfactory blood sugar control. These patients have defects in both insulin production and insulin resistance. Without aggressive treatment, their chronically elevated blood sugar levels increase their risk of developing the long-term complications of diabetes. Elevated blood sugar levels have an adverse affect on the pancreas and further suppress pancreatic insulin output. This phenomenon, called glucose toxicity, is discussed in Chapter 2, *Type 1 & Type 2 Diabetes: Two Different Disorders*. Controlling blood sugar helps to overcome glucose toxicity. These patients, too, might possibly be candidates for islet cell transplantation. The role of islet cell transplantation in Type 2 diabetes, however, is still a clouded issue.

Overcoming the Difficulty of Harvesting an Adequate Supply of Islets

Islets form only approximately 2 percent of the entire pancreas, and isolating them from the rest of the pancreas that does not produce insulin has long been a very time-consuming procedure. The invention of an automated method of islet isolation by Camillo Ricordi, M.D., at the DRI, has made it possible for scientists to obtain larger numbers of islets from a human pancreas.

The Ricordi method has enabled researchers to isolate enough islets from one donor pancreas to transplant one patient. Until this breakthrough, as many as five to six organs were needed to gather enough islet cells for a single transplant.

Recent progress has also improved the purity, as well as the quality, of the islet cells isolated. Freezing techniques that preserve the donor cells for later use have also been developed.

INGAP AND ISLET CELL TRANSPLANTATION

Experimental test tube studies have shown that INGAP has the potential to expand the quantity of islets cells available for transplantation. The INGAP protein stimulates donor islet cell to proliferate without the limitation of apoptosis (the cell death that normally follows a cells inborn gene programmed limited number of cell divisions). In short, when INGAP is added to islet tissue cultures, the cells divide producing pancreatic cells that produce insulin. This test tube success is important because it suggests that research may soon be able to supply a greatly expanded , indeed a limitless quantity of islet cells for transplantation. Researchers now have the ability to synthesize as much of the INGAP Peptide as they need for therapeutic treatment. Humans will be receiving the same Peptide that was administered to the experimental animals. The ability to create the necessary quantities of INGAP Peptide for therapeutic treatment gives scientists a wide potential for therapeutic applications.

GENE (DNA) THERAPY

The genes (DNA) are the cellular machinery that direct all cellular functions. Gene therapy to cure disease is a relatively new therapeutic approach.

Rather than directing treatment at the signs and symptoms a disease produces gene therapy is aimed directly at the genetic code responsible for the disorder. To access the cell's molecular machinery—the DNA—it is necessary to gain passage to the cell nucleus in the interior of the cell where the DNA is located. Therefore, one of the main obstacles that had to be overcome, if gene therapy were to become a practical reality, was the development of a gene delivery system. Viral infections occur because viruses, which are single strands of DNA, enter body cells and duplicate themselves by taking over the cellular DNA reproductive machinery. Space-age bioengineering has enabled scientists to modify harmless viruses to serve as transmission vectors for designer genes that direct the cell to perform new functions. When selected segments of human DNA are transferred into targeted cells, they can improve or restore the defective cellular functioning associated with many diseases—including diabetes.

Developing Surrogate (Copycat) Beta Cells

Type 1 diabetes is caused by the selective destruction of the beta cells by the diabetic's own immune system. This so-called autoimmune attack also limits the survival of transplanted islet cells. To circumvent this attack against beta cells, researchers have engineered non-beta cells to provide insulin. These altered cells *simulate* the ability of beta cells to recognize the blood glucose levels and then secrete the appropriate amount of insulin to maintain equilibrium with blood glucose levels—a balance that physiologists call homeostastis. In short, researchers have already succeeded in manipulating the DNA of non-islet cells to function as though they were insulin-producing beta cells of the pancreas. The altered cells, with their newly incorporated DNA, are not subject to attack by the body's immune defense system because, although they produce insulin, they are not beta cells—the target cells of the autoimmune attack in Type 1 diabetes.

This development of a new source of insulin from non-pancreatic tissues offers the potential for a limitless supply of low-cost islets.

Dr. Christopher Newgard, a pioneer in this cutting edge research, has already developed a procedure for large-scale production of engineered islet cells and their preservation. They have demonstrated that cryo (freezing) preservation does not adversely affect their insulin-producing ability.

The practical application of these techniques not only offers an abundant supply of "islet-like" tissue, but greatly reduces the cost involved. Although technical problems remain and this source of islet tissue is not yet available to patients, it holds great potential to meet the need for insulin-producing tissue in the near future.

Dr. Raquel Faradji and her group have bio-engineered pituitary cells to produce insulin by utilizing recombinant adenoviruses to interpose into pituitary cells, two molecules which are indispensable for glucose metabolism, specifically the glucose transporter (GLUT2) and glucokinase (GK). They have succeeded in inducing the pituitary cells to produce insulin but, not as yet, to secrete it in a glucose-regulated manner. Although further cell engineering refinement to overcome this problem is required, these promising results show the potential of utilizing pituitary cells for beta cell replacement.

Employing cells from the liver (hepatocytes), and also using experimental procedures involving bio-engineering, Dr. Peter Thule also used an adenoviral vector to induce insulin production. Using a similar adenoviral insulin-transgene containing vector in diabetic rats, he demonstrated normal glucose-responsive human insulin expression. This study clearly showed the successful use of engineered hepatic (liver) insulin production.

The Gene Gun

A dramatic experimental gene delivery system being developed at the DRI, which seems to be straight out of science fiction, involves a biolistic particle accelerator or "gene gun" that functions as a gene delivery system. When islet DNA-coated gold particles are fired, they retain their normal appearance and continue to produce insulin, even after transplantation. DRI scientists are currently refining techniques that deliver genes (DNA) that would confer immune acceptance around donor islet cells and thus exempt them from immune attack. The successful application of this therapeutic approach would eliminate the need for chronic suppression of the recipient's immune system with immunosuppressant drugs following tissue transplantation.

Preventing the Autoimmune Reaction

Dr. Zandong Yang and co-workers have used adenoviral vectors to introduce the *uteroglobulin* gene into islets transplanted into laboratory animals. Uteroglobulin, a protein which normally is expressed during pregnancy, confers immunologic tolerance and protection from autoimmune attack.

Increased transplant survival was demonstrated in laboratory animals when uteroglobulin was utilized. This research clearly showed the feasability of blocking the autoimmune attack with uteroglobulin.

Gene Manipulation to Expand the
The Available Supply of Beta Cells

Improving the technique of in vitro (in the laboratory) culture of beta cells to meet the demands of researchers and patients worldwide has been the focus of considerable research. To go forth with a transplant cure for the loss of these vital cells, a huge supply of cultured cells that can replicate their function is needed.

Initially, both primary human cells and bio-engineered transformed cell lines did not function for long enough periods of time to be practical. Beta cell enriched primary cell cultures from the human fetal and adult pancreas can be stimulated with the substance known as *hepatocyte growth-factor*. The proliferative response is strong at first but limited over time by aging of the cells. Pancreatic cells transformed by bio-engineering techniques employing the introduction of antigen (SVLT) and reconstituted oncogenes* have helped in increasing the life of the cultured cells. In a complicated research protocol involving knowledge of DNA replication, telomerase* activity has been checked in the oncogene-transformed human pancreatic cell lines, enabling them to escape a premature demise.

Xenotransplantation

The problem of obtaining donor organs or islet tissue in quantity has not yet been solved completely. In the United States today, far too few organs are donated annually for organ transplantation to meet the needs of America's diabetics. The global shortage of organ donors could be counteracted if a way could be found to utilize organs from animals. Transplantation of organs between species, called xenotransplantation, has not been successful in the past because the recipient's immune system immediately recognizes the transplanted tissue as non-human—foreign—and rejection rapidly ensues. To neutralize this defensive reaction, researchers are testing strategies to "trick" the immune system into failing to recognize the foreign nature of the transplanted tissue. At the forefront of this research is a novel type of gene therapy.

Because of their physiological and anatomical similarities to men, pigs have been the focus of study as a potential source of donor organs. DNA in pigs has been genetically engineered to include a segment of human DNA in the chromosome chain to make it more closely resemble human genes. This procedure also alters the surface of the donor cells. These changes make it difficult for the recipient's immune system to differentiate the transplanted tissues from its own.

In New Zealand, Dr. Robert Elliot, of the Aukland School of Medicine, has gone one step further toward making the transplantation of gene altered tissues a practical reality when he successfully transplanted altered animal pancreatic tissues into two human subjects. One of the recipients showed no signs of rejection even though he was not given immunosuppressive drugs at the time of the transplant. The other subject had previously had a kidney transplant and was already taking immunosuppressive drugs at the time of the xenotransplant.

ALGINATE PROTECTED CELLS

Alginate is a highly refined component of naturally occurring sea weed.

For some unknown reason the body's immune protective system does not regard alginate as a substance foreign to the body when it is implanted. One research approach utilizing this unique property of alginate has been to create an artificial pancreas about the size and thickness of an ordinary business card containing islet cells embedded within the alginate material. The card size alginate plaque is then surgically fastened to the liver with sutures on each cover to hold it in place. The body's immune system would destroy the islets if any were not covered with alginate. Even if only a few were exposed, the immune system would destroy all the other transplanted islet cells.

This research is currently being refined and human trials are eventually planned.

In Auckland, New Zealand, Prof. Bob Elliott sought a better way to replace human islets with a form that was more readily available. For many years, following the discovery of insulin in 1921, humans were treated with insulin derived from pigs. Pigs have similar carbohydrate metabolism to humans and their normal blood sugar levels are similar. Until recent years pigs remained the main source of insulin. Prof. Elliott reasoned that pigs offered a limitless source of islet cells. He coated his pig islet cells with alginate and injected them directly into the peritoneal (abdominal) cavity. This protocol reversed diabetes in the treated animals. In 1966, a human transplant was performed utilizing a relatively small dose of alginate coated islets. The subject's insulin dosage was cut in half following transplant. Fearing transmission of a pig virus to humans, the New Zealand government ordered the research to cease. Prof. Elliott has now moved his base of operations to Mexico City. He has treated twelve adolescents, only one of whom was made completely insulin free. His research is ongoing.

Although some researchers have expressed fears that xenotransplantation carries the risk of animal to human transmission of heretofore unknown diseases. Most scientists believe, that theoretically, this certainly could happen, but it is not very likely. Today, there are many successful applications of this type of transplant, e.g. porcine heart valves. The Food and Drug Administration has agreed with those experts who believe that the dangers can be limited and has approved xenotransplantation in humans provided strict safeguard guidelines are followed to monitor recipients as well as the tissues or organs involved.

Thymus Protocols To Induce Tolerance to Transplanted Tissue

A unique project that has thus far been carried out only in rodents, that shows promise in achieving the goal of permanent tolerance to transplanted islet tissue in human subjects, utilizes the thymus gland. The thymus is a glan-

*The factor within the cell that limits the number of times a cell can reproduce without becoming extinct.

dular structure of largely lymphoid tissue, located in the upper anterior chest behind the breast bone. Investigators have shown that by injecting an antigen (a protein or carbohydrate substance that when introduced into the body, stimulates the production of antibodies) into the thymus gland, a tolerance to the protein develops, and it no longer stimulates antibody production. Dr. Rodolfo Alejandro of the DRI has injected transplantation antigens from multiple donors into the thymus gland of rodents. These islet cells functioned normally and subsequently have been able to reverse diabetes following their injection into the kidneys of diabetic rodents without the use of immunosuppressive drugs. This transplant procedure induced tolerance that allowed insulin-producing islet cells to be successfully transplanted without the accompanying use of immuno-suppressive drugs to prevent rejection.

Another thymus research protocol to induce tolerance being carried out at the DRI that has produced encouraging results is the concurrent transplantation of donor bone marrow cells along with organ transplantation including islet tissue. The immune system originates in the bone marrow. Clinical studies indicate that high-dose donor bone marrow infusions greatly enhance graft acceptance in organ transplant patients. In one trial, immunosuppressive drugs will be discontinued and the patients will be followed carefully to determine if the bone marrow cells prevent or forestall rejection. In brief, transplant survival is significantly improved by the addition of donor bone marrow infusions. Randomized studies are currently being performed. Every time an organ is transplanted, there is a two-way traffic of cells. In this experimental protocol, lymphoid cells go from the recipient into the transplanted islet tissue. From the other direction, transplanted bone marrow cells migrate to other locations in the recipients body. This phenomenon—a state of coexistence—is called "chimerism."

Microencapsulation

The ideal transplant goal is to render the transplanted tissue non-immuno-genic—incapable of causing an immune system rejection response by the recipient. A novel experimental procedure that shows much promise to achieve this goal is the introduction of a semi-permeable membrane or microencapsulation coating which covers and isolates transplanted cells from the recipient's immune system. The protective layer over the transplanted cells has pores that are large enough to permit glucose and insulin to pass freely, but small enough to block antibodies and other immune system elements that seek to identify and destroy the transplanted tissue. DRI researchers are currently testing new bio-compatible polymers derived from human tissues, which can serve as chemical shields to protect donor cells from immune attack. This unique material, developed at the DRI, is bio-compatible because of its human origin. These immuno-protective polymers are currently undergoing laboratory animal evaluation studies.

Stem Cell Research

Stem cells are primordial all-purpose cells from which all tissues of the body are derived. Research aimed at producing stem cells that will mimic the insulin-producing B-cells of the pancreas is being actively pursued.

Research institutes working in this field include the Whittier Institute for Diabetes in La Jolla, California. This laboratory uses human fetal pancreatic cells in its effort to develop a cell line that is glucose-responsive. Thus far, they have achieved success in rodents.

The Scripps Research Institute is in the process of identifying and isolating pancreatic stem progenitor cells, and Ixion Biotechnology Inc. of Alachua, Florida, is attempting to develop islet-progenitor stem cells that allow the growth of substantial numbers of islets derived from adult donors for transplantation therapy.

Research investigators are awaiting approval from the Food and Drug Administration to perform trials on humans, utilizing stem cells from *bone marrow* instead of cord blood from embryos or fetal tissues. Also, experiments are now being carried out on the *placenta* (that is usually discarded after all births), again eliminating the major controversies regarding ethical implications.

THE CLOSED LOOP

The ultimate artificial device to control blood sugar is the closed loop, an "artificial pancreas" that incorporates a glucose sensor permanently implanted in the patient's body. New research to improve insulin pumps has been responsible for the development of sophisticated glucose sensors that permit the blood sugar to be monitored continuously with the information transmitted to a tiny computerized insulin reservoir that metes out insulin as needed. The implanted sensor has a flexible cable that connects the sensing unit to a small monitor that is about the size of a business card.

Although the sensor is located in the subcutaneous tissue and not directly in the blood vessels, it still accurately measures the glucose content of the interstitial fluid correlating with the blood glucose levels. Clinical trials with these devices containing reliable fail-safe mechanisms to avoid run-away high or low blood sugar levels, are now under way.

PREVENTION OF TYPE 1 DIABETES

Type 1 diabetes represents approximately 8 to 12 percent of all cases of diabetes and that accounts for more than one million Type 1 diabetes in the U.S. Unfortunately, the amount of diabetic complications is high in this group of young people who face a difficult time in terms of insulin injections, strict dietary habit and frequent fingerstick blood determinations.

The Diabetes Prevention Trial (DPT-1) uses antigen-based (insulin) treatment of nondiabetic relatives in order to prevent or delay the onset of clinical diabetes. Accurate risk in relatives of diabetics is 15-20 fold higher than in the general population. These youngsters are screened for ICA (islet cell antibodies) to rule out the possibility of already having diabetes.

The rationale for this approach is based upon limited studies in humans as well as rodents that seemed to indicate prevention or decreased severity of diabetes. Various theories have been offered to explain the drug's mechanism of action in protecting against the development of diabetes.

Coming as a great disappointment, the five year study showed no impact of insulin therapy on delaying or preventing the onset of Type 1 diabetes. And, C-peptide levels showed no difference with or without treatment.

REDUCTION OF THE INCIDENCE OF TYPE 2 DIABETES WITH LIFESTYLE MODIFICATION INTERVENTION OR METFORMIN VS PLACEBO

A large study based on the hypothesis that some risk factors for developing diabetes —elevated fasting blood sugar, elevated post-prandial glucose levels, obesity and a sedentary lifestyle are all factors which predispose an individual to developing diabetes. These risk factors are *all potentially reversible*. Over three thousand persons with elevated fasting and post-glucose load elevations beyond the normal range were divided into three groups: placebo, Metformin (850mg twice daily) and a lifestyle modification program. The lifestyle modification group had as its goal at least a seven percent weight loss and at least two and one-half hours of exercise per week. The mean age of the participants was 51 years. After approximately a three year follow up lifestyle modification and treatment with Metformin significantly reduced the incidence of diabetes, with lifestyle changes being more effective than Metformin.

The hypothesis that Type 2 diabetes is preventable has been supported by multiple prior studies that have demonstrated the benefits of diet and exercise. The Metformin - Lifestyle study clearly demonstrated that Type 2 diabetes can be prevented or delayed in individuals at high risk for the disease. The incidence of diabetes was reduced by 58 percent with lifestyle modification and by 31 percent with Metformin, as compared with placebo. The results of the study did not vary with racial, ethnic or gender groups. The intensive lifestyle modification worked equally well in young and older individuals. However, the study design did not assess the relative contributions of dietary change, weight loss and increased physical activity. Metformin was effective in this study, but less so in persons with a lower base-line, body-mass index or lower fasting plasma glucose than in those with higher values of these factors at the start of the study. The reduction in fasting plasma glucose was similar in lifestyle modification and the Metformin group. However, a larger proportion of those in the lifestyle modification group had normal post-prandial glucose levels and they also exhibited a greater beneficial effect on their glycosylated hemoglobin (HbA1c).

In summary, this study showed that treatment with Metformin and lifestyle modification were both highly effective means of delaying or preventing Type 2 diabetes. Lifestyle modification showed the most favorable benefit with one case of diabetes prevented per seven persons treated for three years. It would be interesting to see the results of a study that included a lifestyle modification group that also took Metformin 850mg twice daily.

Thiazolidinedione and a-Glucosidase oral agents as preventative drugs for type2 diabetes

Two studies using oral glucose-lowering agents of classes other than biguanides have also shown a decrease in progression to diabetes in high risk groups. Troglitazone (which has been withdrawn from the U.S. market because of liver toxicity) is a member of the chemical group called thiazolidinediones which also includes Rosiglitazone and Pioglitazone, two widely prescribed oral agents. The Troglitazone study showed a 56% reduction in the progression of diabetes. Eight months after the completion of the study, the protective benefit of the drug was still present. This finding indicated that drugs of the thiazolidinedione class may alter the natural course of the disease and actually prevent diabetes in some subjects rather than just delaying its onset.

In a study that lasted approximately three and a half years,, drugs of the a-glucosidase class were studied as a diabetes preventative. The treated group showed a 36% reduction in progression to diabetes.

To evaluate the risk of developing diabetes in an individual patient such factors as age, family history of diabetes, waist-to-hip ratio, lipid levels, blood pressure and obesity must be considered in conjunction with evidence of impaired fasting glucose and impaired glucose tolerance.

In brief, recognition of the early stages of elevated blood sugar that portends the development of diabetes and the success of multiple protocols shows that progression to diabetes can be delayed and sometimes even prevented. Individuals at high risk for developing diabetes must be identified and afforded preventative treatment to delay or prevent the disease from manifesting itself.

Insulin Production in the Thymus Gland and Prevention of Type 1 Diabetes

Researchers at the DRI have identified the thymus gland as a source of insulin. This discovery of insulin production by non-pancreatic tissue has been the subject of extensive investigation by the Institute's scientists who have learned that lymphocytes—a type of white blood cell that performs important immune defense functions—migrate from the bone marrow, where they are formed, to the thymus, where they undergo maturation. During their stay in the thymus, they are exposed to body elements, including insulin. Lymphocytes that recognize and attack insulin molecules or insulin producing cells are destroyed. Only lymphocytes that do not respond to "self" tissue or body components are allowed to survive and complete their maturation training. Normally this system works efficiently and one's own lymphocytes ordinarily do not attack one's own body. When the protective monitoring of lymphocyte maturation does not work efficiently, defectively programmed lymphocytes that cause auto-immune destruction of pancreatic beta cells escape detection and are released into the bloodstream. These defective lymphocytes seek out normal pancreatic tissue, which they erroneously identify as foreign or "non-self" tissue.

Lymphocyte schooling in the thymus is dependent on adequate thymic insulin production. DRI scientists have learned that insulin production by the thymus is genetically controlled, and low insulin output is associated with a high risk for developing Type 1 diabetes. Current research is directed toward developing a protective version of the genetic factors that increase thymic insulin production. This exciting research is pointing the way to regulating a naturally occurring mechanism for the prevention of Type 1 diabetes.

Following the DRI discovery that insulin found in the thymus plays a key role in teaching our immune system to tell the difference between "self" and "non-self or foreign" tissue, Alberto Pugliese, M.D., summarized the findings as follows: "These studies provide evidence to explain how a genetic factor might protect against Type 1 diabetes. If we could learn more about this naturally occurring mechanism, we might be able to reproduce it and prevent Type 1 diabetes altogether."

HOW TO PREVENT, AMELIORATE OR CURE TYPE 2 DIABETES NATURALLY

Type 2 diabetes can in fact be prevented or cured, particularly if those predisposed to the disease who take corrective measures in the early years of onset. Unfortunately, the early stages of Type 2 diabetes are often asymptomatic for years despite the fact that impaired glucose tolerance with elevation of the blood sugar and damage to body organs is progressing. However, physicians can predict years in advance those at risk for developing Type 2 diabetes by monitoring the close relatives of diabetics.

The epidemic of Type 2 diabetes in America today clearly correlates with the typical Western lifestyle and diet. This diet is high in refined sugars, saturated fats and is low in fiber content. The evidence of the association of diabetes with diet and lifestyle is overwhelming. In so-called "primitive" cultures, even today, whose members eat a plant-based diet, high in fiber and complex carbohydrates, and whose lifestyle demands hard physical exercise, diabetes is rare. This is true even among populations that are genetically predisposed to developing the disease.

The glycemic index is the propensity of a food to raise the level of the blood sugar. In other words, some types of foods may raise the blood glucose levels more quickly than other foods that contain the same amount of calories. High glycemic index foods which are most likely to cause the blood sugar levels to rise quickly include potatoes, white bread, white rice, and sugared soft drinks. Those which have a low glycemic index are whole grain foods high in fiber such as whole wheat bread (not wheat bread) and unprocessed grain cereals, brown rice, legumes and other vegetables and fruits. The process of refining strips cereal of fiber and nutrients.

The benefits of the high fiber, low glycemic index diet was recently verified in a Harvard University study involving 65,000 subjects. The results, published in the *Journal of the American Medical Association*, clearly demonstrated that a high fiber diet with a low glycemic index substantially decreased the risk for developing diabetes. An added bonus of this type of diet is its favorable effect on blood lipids. The Pritikin Diet, discussed in Chapter 18, *Cardiovascular Disease and Dibetes*, qualifies as a low glycemic diet high in fiber and complex carbohydrates.

Exercise is the equally important other half of the diabetes control equation. Physical activity burns sugar and reduces insulin needs. A more important benefit is its favorable effect on insulin resistance, the main physiologic defect of Type 2 diabetes. The many benefits of exercise were examined in Chapter 17, *The Benefits of Exercise*.

The dramatic benefits of diet and exercise in preventing, controlling and curing diabetes can be seen in the plight of the Pima American Indians of Arizona. Seventy-five years ago, diabetes was almost unknown among the Pimas. The dramatic rise in the incidence of this metabolic disorder that has taken place during the past three-quarters of a century can be attributed almost exclusively to changes in diet and physical activity. A diet based on fresh fruits and vegetables produced by hard labor in the field was replaced with a high-fat, low-fiber, Western-style diet.

Although the Pimas were born with the genes that predisposed them to developing diabetes, their former lifestyle was sufficient to prevent the disease from manifesting itself. With the loss of their healthy protective diet and physical activities, obesity has become rampant and diabetes so prevalent that it threatens the very survival of this genetically susceptible population. The Pimas' plight clearly demonstrates that a propensity to develop diabetes is not a significant problem until a diet of fatty, high calorie foods and the development of obesity in association with a sedentary lifestyle are introduced into the equation. Interestingly, a sub-group of Pimas who mi grated to Mexico many years ago have retained their healthy lifestyle, and have not suffered the same fate as their North American relatives. Their rate of incidence of diabetes remains low.

In spite of the familial predisposition to diabetes, one can "prevent" its development or reduce the severe complications of diabetes by adhering to an intelligent way of life—eating the right foods and keeping weight within the normal range.

Achieving normal body weight is often associated with an improvement in glycemic control and sometimes even a restoration of normal glucose metabolism. *In other words, many people with Type 2 diabetes who lose weight, watch their diet and increase their level of physical activity do extremely well.* Their bodies regain some of the lost sensitivity to insulin, and the quantity of insulin produced by the pancreas may once again suffice to meet their needs. If these individuals go off their diet, gain weight, and once again live a sedentary lifestyle, insulin resistance increases, their blood sugar levels rise, and diabetes manifests itself once again.

In brief, by following these few "rules to remain healthy," many diabetics achieve a lowering of insulin resistance, improve their glucose metabolism and sometimes even achieve normal blood sugar level, which helps to avoid the complex of abnormal lipids, hypertension, and many of the chronic complications of diabetes. These "rules" are beneficial for everyone, not just those susceptible to the development of diabetes.

Advance Glycosylation End Products

When sugar (glucose) attaches itself to proteins without the aid of enzymes, a series of chemical reactions results in the formation and eventual accumulation of irreversible bonds, or "cross-links" between proteins. This "molecular glue," known as Advanced Glycosylation End-Products, or AGEs, causes proteins that are normally flexible and separate to become rigid and attached, making cells, tissues and organs stiff and increasingly less functional. This physiologic event is responsible for many of the changes of the aging process and is considered "normal" as we age.

In diabetes, unfortunately, this aging process may be accelerated. Many researchers attribute this to the elevated blood sugar levels and increased AGEs formation which may be the link between diabetes and long-term complications such as retinopathy, nephropathy, neuropathy and cardiovascular disease.

The effect of diabetes has been described by some as an accelerated aging. Indeed, increased AGEs formation may play an important role in the development of cardiovascular disease because of its effect on collagen in blood vessel walls. The non-enzymatic glycosylation of the eye's proteins may contribute to the formation of cataracts.

Current research is focused in two directions: preventing or slowing of AGEs formation and the breaking of AGEs cross-links between proteins.

The DCCT (Diabetes Control and Complications Trial) clearly demonstrated that blood sugar levels as reflected by HbA1c correlated directly with increased risks, incidence and severity of organ damage from diabetes. *As the blood sugar is controlled, the rate of formation of AGEs is reduced.*

Anti-oxidants such as Vitamin E and C, and Selenium are also being evaluated for their ability to prevent non-enzymic glycosylation. Also of importance is the fact that *smoking increases AGEs formations, thus making the nicotine habit particularly deadly for diabetics.*

NEW MODES OF INSULIN DELIVERY

New modes of insulin delivery have simplified the administration of insulin particularly among the elderly or anyone who has difficulty in handling a syringe and insulin. The novolin innolet is a variation of the insulin pen that offers patients with diminished vision and limited dexterity the ability to self administer insulin.

Newer insulin pumps have the potential for communicating with a glucometer and automatically administering appropriate mealtime dosages of insulin eliminating the need to calculate the insulin dose. Additional information about these devices is available on the Internet at www.diabetesinterview.com.

Until recently the scientific quest for an easier way to deliver insulin into the body by injection had eluded scientists. Attempts to design oral forms of insulin that would not be destroyed by digestive enzymes, or nasal spray of insulin particles that could be absorbed through the nasal mucosa had significant drawbacks. A new treatment technique that is now in clinical trials involves the ability to administer insulin in a dry powder that can be stored at room temperature and inhaled directly into the lungs, thus eliminating the need for painful and inconvenient injections.

The insulin inhaler device consists of a two-chamber system. Blister packs of powdered insulin are inserted into the lower chamber. When the device is activated, the packs shatter and the powdered insulin is propelled through the upper chamber, into the patient's mouth and on to the lungs, in a manner similar to the delivery of inhaler asthma medications and simply involves taking a deep, steady breath. With each single use, these devices can deliver either 1 mg. or 3 mg. of powdered insulin, the equivalent of 3 or 8 units of regular insulin. Inhaled insulin is currently being developed by major pharmaceutical companies including Aventis, Pfizer and Lilly for use in both Type 1 and Type 2 diabetes. Their use is similar to the inhalers that deliver asthma medication to patients through the airways of the lungs to the small blood vessels in the alveoli (air sacs) of the lungs. Nasal and aerosolized insulins are currently undergoing phase III human trials.

Tablets of insulin coated with a substance that inhibits the action of the digestive enzymes in the intestinal tract which would degrade and destroy the insulin molecules have been developed and currently are undergoing studies. The limited experimental success of oral insulin tabs has not yet been subject to large scale trial studies. The preliminary studies with human volunteers showed the oral insulin to be well tolerated with a dose-related reduction in blood glucose which is well tolerated.

Administration by inhalation may be able to achieve glucose levels similar to that obtained with present day subcutaneous injections. The inhaler, however, does not eliminate all the pain associated with controlling diabetes. Blood sugar analyses must still be performed and many patients would still require a daily injection of long-acting insulin.

BLOODLESS GLUCOSE MONITORING

Pricking fingers to obtain blood sugar levels may become outmoded soon. Researchers are working on methods to measure blood sugar levels without the need for a finger-stick. One device, that is worn like a wristwatch, uses a micro-electrical current to measure glucose levels within the circulating blood. Another approach that offers promise utilizes an infrared light beam to measure the glucose. A third method under study uses a skin patch that is worn for about five minutes before being removed and placed in a meter that measures glucose levels.

•GLOSSARY•

A

ACE INHIBITOR - ANGIOTENSIN CONVERTING ENZYME. A DRUG USED TO LOWER BLOOD PRESSURE THAT MAY HELP PREVENT OR SLOW THE PROGRESSION OF KIDNEY DISEASE IN DIABETES.

ACETONE - A CHEMICAL FORMED IN THE BLOOD WHEN THE BODY USES FAT INSTEAD OF GLUCOSE FOR ENERGY.

ADRENAL GLANDS - ORGANS LOCATED ON TOP OF THE KIDNEYS THAT MAKE AND RELEASE HORMONES SUCH AS ADRENALIN (EPINEPHRINE).

ALBUMINURIA - ABNORMAL AMOUNTS OF A PROTEIN CALLED ALBUMIN IN THE URINE.

ALPHA CELL - A TYPE OF SPECIALIZED CELL IN THE PANCREAS THAT MAKE THE HORMONE GLUCAGON THAT RAISES THE LEVEL OF GLUCOSE (SUGAR) IN THE BLOOD.

AMINO ACIDS - ORGANIC COMPOUNDS THAT LINK TOGETHER TO FORM PROTEIN.

AMYOTROPHY - A TYPE OF DIABETIC NEUROPATHY THAT CAUSES MUSCLE WEAKNESS AND WASTING.

ANGIOPATHY - DISEASE OF THE BLOOD VESSELS (ARTERIES, VEINS, AND CAPILLARIES). THERE ARE TWO TYPES: MACROANGIOPATHY, INVOLVING THE LARGE BLOOD VESSELS, AND MICROANGIOPATHY THAT INVOLVES SMALL BLOOD VESSELS.

ANTAGONIST - AN AGENT THAT OPPOSES OR FIGHTS THE ACTION OF ANOTHER. FOR EXAMPLE, INSULIN LOWERS THE LEVEL OF GLUCOSE, WHEREAS GLUCAGON RAISES IT. THE TWO DRUGS ARE ANTAGONISTIC TO EACH OTHER.

ANTIBODIES - PROTEINS THAT THE BODY MAKES TO PROTECT ITSELF FROM FOREIGN SUBSTANCES. SEE ANTIGENS.

ANTIGENS - SUBSTANCES THAT CAUSE AN IMMUNE RESPONSE IN THE BODY. THE BODY "SEES" THE ANTIGENS AS HARMFUL OR FOREIGN. TO FIGHT THEM, THE BODY PRODUCES ANTIBODIES, WHICH ATTACK AND TRY TO NEUTRALIZE THE ANTIGENS.

ARTERIOSCLEROSIS - NARROWING OF ARTERIES DUE TO DEPOSITS OF CHOLESTEROL AND CALCIUM. ETC., ALSO KNOWN AS ATHEROSCLEROSIS AND HARDENING AF THE ARTERIES

ARTERY - A BLOOD VESSEL THAT CARRIES BLOOD FROM THE HEART TO OTHER PARTS OF THE BODY.

ASPARTAME - SWEETENER THAT IS SOMETIMES USED IN PLACE OF SUGAR.

ATHEROSCLEROSIS - SEE: ARTERIOSCLEROSIS.

AUTOIMMUNE DISEASE - DISORDER OF THE BODY'S IMMUNE SYSTEM IN WHICH THE IMMUNE SYSTEM MISTAKENLY ATTACKS AND DESTROYS BODY TISSUE THAT IT BELIEVES TO BE FOREIGN. TYPE 1 DIABETES IS AN AUTOIMMUNE DISEASE BECAUSE THE IMMUNE SYSTEM PRODUCES ANTIBODIES THAT ATTACK AND DESTROY THE INSULIN-PRODUCING BETA CELLS OF THE PANCREAS.

B

BACKGROUND RETINOPATHY - EARLY STAGE OF DIABETIC RETINOPATHY; USUALLY DOES NOT IMPAIR VISION.

BASAL RATE - THE CONTINUOUS 24 HR. SUPPLY OF LOW LEVELS OF INSULIN BY THE PANCREAS, AS IN INSULIN PUMP THERAPY.

BETA CELL - A TYPE OF CELL IN THE PANCREAS IN AREAS CALLED THE ISLETS OF LANGERHANS THAT MAKE AND RELEASE THE HORMONE INSULIN.

BLOOD GLUCOSE - THE MAIN SUGAR THAT IS THE BODY'S MAJOR SOURCE OF ENERGY. THE CELLS CANNOT USE GLUCOSE WITHOUT THE HELP OF INSULIN.

BLOOD GLUCOSE METER - A MACHINE THAT MEASURES HOW MUCH GLUCOSE IS IN THE BLOOD.

BLOOD PRESSURE - THE LATERAL FORCE THE BLOOD EXERTS ON THE WALLS OF ARTERIES. TWO LEVELS OF BLOOD PRESSURE ARE MEASURED—THE HIGHER, OR SYSTOLIC, PRESSURE, WHICH OCCURS EACH TIME THE HEART PUMPS BLOOD INTO THE VESSELS, AND THE LOWER, OR DIASTOLIC, PRESSURE, WHICH MEASURES THE PRESSURE AGAINST THE WALL OF THE ARTERY WHEN THE HEART RESTS BETWEEN BEATS. THE SYSTOLIC IS THE MOST IMPORTANT.

BOLUS - AN EXTRA BOOST OF INSULIN GIVEN TO COVER AN EXPECTED RISE IN BLOOD GLUCOSE SUCH AS THE RISE THAT OCCURS AFTER EATING.

BORDERLINE DIABETES - A TERM NO LONGER USED. SEE: IMPAIRED GLUCOSE TOLERANCE.

C

C.D.E. (CERTIFIED DIABETES EDUCATOR) - A HEALTH CARE PROFESSIONAL WHO IS QUALIFIED BY THE AMERICAN ASSOCIATION OF DIABETES EDUCATORS TO TEACH PEOPLE WITH DIABETES HOW TO MANAGE THEIR CONDITION.

C-PEPTIDE - A SUBSTANCE THAT THE PANCREAS RELEASES INTO THE BLOODSTREAM IN EQUAL AMOUNTS TO INSULIN. C-PEPTIDE LEVELS SHOW HOW MUCH INSULIN THE BODY IS MAKING.

CALCIUM CHANNEL BLOCKER - A CLASS OF DRUGS USED TO LOWER BLOOD PRESSURE.

CARBOHYDRATE - ONE OF THE THREE MAIN CLASSES OF FOODS AND A SOURCE OF ENERGY. CARBOHYDRATES ARE SUGARS AND STARCHES THAT THE BODY BREAKS DOWN INTO GLUCOSE (A SIMPLE SUGAR THAT THE BODY CAN USE FOR ENERGY).

CATARACT - CLOUDING OF THE LENS OF THE EYE.

CEREBROVASCULAR DISEASE - DAMAGE TO THE BLOOD VESSELS IN THE BRAIN THAT MAY RESULT IN A STROKE. THE BLOOD VESSELS BECOME BLOCKED BECAUSE OF SPASM, OR PLAQUE DEPOSITS. OR THE BLOOD VESSELS MAY BURST, RESULTING IN A HEMORRHAGIC STROKE. STROKES FROM A BLOOD CLOT WITHIN THE ARTERIOSCLEROTIC VESSEL ARE THE MOST COMMON TYPE. PEOPLE WITH DIABETES ARE AT HIGHER RISK FOR CEREBROVASCULAR DISEASE.

CHARCOT FOOT - A FOOT COMPLICATION ASSOCIATED WITH DIABETIC NEUROPATHY THAT RESULTS IN DESTRUCTION OF JOINTS AND SOFT TISSUE. ALSO CALLED "CHARCOT'S JOINT" AND "NEUROPATHIC ARTHROPATHY."

CHOLESTEROL - A FAT-LIKE SUBSTANCE FOUND IN BLOOD AND BODY TISSUES. THE BODY MAKES CHOLESTEROL WHICH IT USES TO SYNTHESIZE CERTAIN HORMONES. TOO MUCH CHOLESTEROL, HOWEVER, MAY CAUSE A BUILD UP IN ARTERY WALLS CAUSING ARTERIOSCLEROSIS.

CIRCULATION - THE FLOW OF BLOOD THROUGH THE HEART AND BLOOD VESSELS OF THE BODY.

COMA - A SLEEP-LIKE STATE; NOT CONSCIOUS. MAY BE DUE TO A HIGH OR LOW LEVEL OF GLUCOSE (SUGAR) IN THE BLOOD. SEE ALSO: DIABETIC COMA.

COMPLEX CARBOHYDRATE - LARGE CARBOHYDRATE MOLECULES MADE UP OF LONG CHAINS OF SUGAR, BROKEN DOWN BY DIGESTION SLOWLY.

COMPLICATIONS OF DIABETES - HARMFUL EFFECTS THAT MAY HAPPEN AS A CONSEQUENCE OF DIABETES. THEY MAY DEVELOP WHEN A PERSON HAS HAD DIABETES FOR A LONG TIME. THESE INCLUDE DAMAGE TO THE RETINA OF THE EYE (RETINOPATHY), THE BLOOD VESSELS (ANGIOPATHY), THE NERVOUS SYSTEM (NEUROPATHY), AND THE KIDNEYS (NEPHROPATHY).

CONGENITAL DEFECTS - PROBLEMS OR CONDITIONS THAT ARE PRESENT AT BIRTH.

CONGESTIVE HEART FAILURE - DECREASED PUMPING EFFICIENCY AND POWER BY THE HEART, RESULTING IN FLUIDS COLLECTING IN THE BODY. CONGESTIVE HEART FAILURE USUALLY DEVELOPS GRADUALLY. GENERALLY, IT CAN BE TREATED WITH DRUGS.

CONTINUOUS SUBCUTANEOUS INSULIN INFUSION - FORM OF INSULIN DELIVERY WHEN USING AN INSULIN PUMP.

CONTRAINDICATION - A SPECIAL CONDITION OR CIRCUMSTANCE THAT MAKES A PARTICULAR TREATMENT INADVISABLE.

CONVENTIONAL THERAPY - A SYSTEM OF DIABETES MANAGEMENT PRACTICED BY MOST PEOPLE WITH DIABETES; WITH TYPE 1 DIABETES, THE SYSTEM CONSISTS OF INSULIN INJECTIONS EACH DAY, DAILY SELF-MONITORING OF BLOOD GLUCOSE, AND A STANDARD PROGRAM OF NUTRITION AND EXERCISE. THE MAIN OBJECTIVE IN THIS FORM OF TREATMENT IS TO AVOID VERY HIGH AND VERY LOW BLOOD GLUCOSE. ALSO CALLED: "STANDARD THERAPY."

C-REACTIVE PROTEIN- PROTEIN BLOOD ASSOCIATED WITH INFLAMMATION. IF NO FOCUS OF INFLAMMATION IS OBVIOUS THEN THIS SERVES AS A CARDIOVASCULAR DISEASE RISK INDICATOR

D

DEHYDRATION - EXCESSIVE LOSS OF BODY FLUIDS. A HIGH LEVEL OF GLUCOSE IN THE URINE CAUSES LOSS OF WATER BY EXERTING AN OSMOTIC EXCRETORY EFFECT.

DEXTROSE - THE BODY'S MAIN SOURCE OF ENERGY. ALSO CALL GLUCOSE. SEE ALSO: BLOOD GLUCOSE.

DIABETES CONTROL AND COMPLICATIONS TRIAL (DCCT) - A 10-YEAR STUDY TO ASSESS THE EFFECTS OF INTENSIVE THERAPY ON THE LONG-TERM COMPLICATIONS OF DIABETES. THE STUDY PROVED THAT INTENSIVE MANAGEMENT OF TYPE 1 DIABETES PREVENTS OR SLOWS THE DEVELOPMENT OF EYE, KIDNEY, AND NERVE DAMAGE CAUSED BY DIABETES. RECENT STUDIES HAVE VERIFIED THE BENEFITS OF INTENSIVE MANAGEMENT FOR TYPE 2 DIABETES.

DIABETIC COMA - A MAJOR MEDICAL EMERGENCY IN WHICH A PERSON IS UNCONSCIOUS BECAUSE THE BLOOD GLUCOSE   IS TOO LOW OR TOO HIGH. WHEN THE GLUCOSE LEVEL IS TOO HIGH, KETOACIDOSIS MAY BE PRESENT. SEE ALSO: HYPERGLYCEMIA; HYPOGLYCEMIA; DIABETIC KETOACIDOSIS.

DIABETIC KETOACIDOSIS (DKA) - SEVERE, OUT-OF-CONTROL DIABETES WITH ABNORMAL FAT METABOLISM THAT REQUIRES EMERGENCY TREATMENT. DKA OCCURS WHEN BLOOD SUGAR LEVELS ARE ELEVATED. THIS MAY HAPPEN BECAUSE OF ILLNESS, TAKING TOO LITTLE INSULIN, OR GETTING TOO LITTLE EXERCISE. THE BODY STARTS USING STORED FAT FOR ENERGY, AND KETONE BODIES BUILD UP IN THE BLOOD. THE SYMPTOMS INCLUDE NAUSEA, VOMITING AND EXCESSIVE URINATION WITH LOSS OF WATER, WHICH CAN LEAD TO DEHYDRATION, ABDOMINAL PAIN, AND DEEP AND RAPID BREATHING. SEE CHAPTER 5, *DIABETIC KETOACIDOSIS.*

DIABETIC RETINOPATHY - A DISEASE OF THE SMALL BLOOD VESSELS OF THE RETINA OF THE EYE. WHEN RETINOPATHY FIRST STARTS, THE TINY BLOOD VESSELS IN THE RETINA BECOME SWOLLEN AND LEAK FLUID INTO THE RETINA WHICH MAY CAUSE VISION TO BE BLURRED. THIS CONDITION IS CALLED BACKGROUND RETINOPATHY. IF RETINOPATHY PROGRESSES, THE HARM TO SIGHT CAN BE MORE SERIOUS. MANY NEW, TINY BLOOD VESSELS GROW OUT AND ACROSS THE EYE. THIS IS CALLED NEOVASCULARIZATION. THE VESSELS MAY BREAK AND BLEED INTO THE CLEAR GEL THAT FILLS THE CENTER OF THE EYE, BLOCKING VISION. SCAR TISSUE MAY ALSO FORM NEAR THE RETINA, PULLING IT AWAY — DETACHING IT — FROM THE BACK OF THE EYE. THIS STAGE, CALLED PROLIFERATIVE RETINOPATHY, CAN LEAD TO IMPAIRED VISION AND EVEN BLINDNESS WHEN UNTREATED.

DIABETOLOGIST - A DOCTOR WHO SPECIALIZES IN TREATING PEOPLE WITH DIABETES MELLITUS.

DIAGNOSIS - THE ACT OF IDENTIFYING A DISEASE FROM ITS SIGNS AND SYMPTOMS.

DIALYSIS - MACHINE CLEANING OF THE BLOOD WHEN THE KIDNEYS FAIL.

DIETITIAN - NUTRITIONIST WHO HELPS PEOPLE WITH SPECIAL HEALTH NEEDS PLAN THE KINDS AND AMOUNTS OF FOODS TO EAT. A REGISTERED DIETITIAN (R.D.) HAS SPECIAL QUALIFICATIONS. THE HEALTH CARE TEAM FOR DIABETES SHOULD INCLUDE A DIETITIAN.

DIURETIC - A DRUG THAT INCREASES THE EXCRETION OF FLUID FROM THE BODY. THE FLOW OF URINE INCREASES AS THE BODY RIDS ITSELF OF EXTRA FLUID.

DNA (DEOXYRIBONUCLEIC ACID) - THE CHEMICAL SUBSTANCE IN PLANT AND ANIMAL CELLS THAT CONTAINS THE GENETIC FORMULA AND TELLS THE CELLS WHAT TO DO AND WHEN TO DO IT. DNA IS THE GENETIC INFORMATION THAT EACH PERSON INHERITS FROM HIS OR HER PARENTS. SEE ALSO: GENE.

DUPUYTREN'S CONTRACTURE - A CONDITION OF THE TENDONS THAT CAUSES THE FINGERS TO CURVE INWARD;CONTRACTION OF THE PALMAR TISSUE CAUSING PERMANENT FLEXION OF ONE OR MORE FINGERS. THE CONDITION IS MORE COMMON IN PEOPLE WITH DIABETES AND MAY PRECEDE DIABETES.

DYSLIPIDEMIA - ABNORMAL LEVELS OF LIPIDS IN THE BLOOD. SEE CHAPTER 18, *CARDIOVASCULAR DISEASE AND DIABETES.*

E

EDEMA - A SWELLING OR PUFFINESS OF SOME PART OF THE BODY SUCH AS THE ANKLES, CAUSED BY A COLLECTION OF FLUID IN THE TISSUES.

ELECTROLYTES - CHARGED MINERALS OR SALT COMPOUNDS WHICH PLAY A VITAL ROLE IN BODY CHEMISTRY.

EMBOLUS - PORTION OF A BLOOD CLOT OR OTHER SUBSTANCE THAT BECOMES DETACHED AND TRAVELS THROUGH THE BLOODSTREAM UNTIL IT BECOMES LODGED IN A BLOOD VESSEL AT A DISTAL SITE, CAUSING OBSTRUCTION.

ENDOCRINE GLANDS - GLANDS THAT PRODUCE AND RELEASE HORMONES INTO THE BLOODSTREAM. THEY REGULATE MANY BODILY FUNCTIONS. ONE ENDOCRINE GLAND IS THE PANCREAS. IT RELEASES INSULIN WHICH THE BODY REQUIRES TO USE SUGAR FOR ENERGY. SEE ALSO: GLAND.

ENDOCRINOLOGIST - A DOCTOR WHO SPECIALIZES IN THE TREATMENT OF PROBLEMS OF ENDOCRINE GLANDS. DIABETES IS AN ENDOCRINE DISORDER. SEE ALSO: ENDOCRINE GLANDS.

ENDOGENOUS - SYNTHESIZED OR MADE INSIDE THE BODY. THE INSULIN THAT IS MADE BY A PERSON'S OWN PANCREAS IS ENDOGENOUS INSULIN.

END-STAGE RENAL DISEASE (ESRD) - THE FINAL PHASE OF KIDNEY DISEASE, TREATED BY DIALYSIS OR KIDNEY TRANSPLANTATION. SEE ALSO: DIALYSIS; NEPHROPATHY.

ENZYMES - A SPECIAL TYPE OF PROTEIN THAT HELPS THE BODY'S CHEMISTRY WORK BETTER BY FACILITATING CHEMICAL REACTION.

ERECTILE DYSFUNCTION - MALE LOSS OF ABILITY TO FUNCTION SEXUALLY.

ETIOLOGY - THE CAUSE OR CAUSES OF A CERTAIN DISEASE.

EXCHANGE LISTS - A DIETARY PLAN WITH SUBSTITUTION OF FOODS, SIMILAR IN TYPE WITH COMPARABLE CALORIC VOLUME. THESE GROUPS ARE: (1) STARCH/ BREAD, (2) MEAT, (3) VEGETABLES, (4) FRUIT, (5) MILK, AND (6) FATS. WITHIN A FOOD GROUP, EACH SERVING HAS ABOUT THE SAME AMOUNT OF CARBOHYDRATE, PROTEIN, FAT, AND CALORIES.

EXOGENOUS - MADE OUTSIDE OF THE BODY.

F

FASTING BLOOD GLUCOSE TEST - A METHOD FOR DETERMINING HOW MUCH GLUCOSE IS IN THE BLOOD WHEN FASTING. THE TEST IS USUALLY DONE IN THE MORNING AFTER AN OVERNIGHT FAST. THE NORMAL, NONDIABETIC RANGE FOR FASTING BLOOD GLUCOSE IS FROM 70 - 110 MG/DL. IF THE LEVEL IS OVER 126 MG/ DL, (EXCEPT FOR NEWBORNS AND SOME PREGNANT WOMEN), FURTHER EVALUATION IS INDICATED TO MAKE A DIAGNOSIS OF DIABETES.

FATS - ONE OF THE THREE MAIN CLASSES OF FOODS AND A SOURCE OF ENERGY IN THE BODY. FATS ARE THE SOURCE OF VITAMINS A, D, E AND K. THEY MAY ALSO SERVE AS ENERGY STORES FOR THE BODY. IN FOOD, THERE ARE TWO TYPES OF FATS: SATURATED AND UNSATURATED.

FATTY ACIDS - A BASIC UNIT OF FATS. WHEN INSULIN LEVELS ARE TOO LOW OR THERE IS NOT ENOUGH GLUCOSE TO USE FOR ENERGY, THE BODY BURNS FATTY ACIDS FOR ENERGY.

FIBER - A SUBSTANCE FOUND IN FOODS THAT COMES FROM PLANTS. FIBER HELPS INTESTINAL FUNCTION AND IS THOUGHT TO LOWER CHOLESTEROL AND HELP CONTROL BLOOD SUGAR. THE TWO TYPES OF FIBER IN FOOD ARE SOLUBLE AND INSOLUBLE. SOLUBLE FIBER, FOUND IN BEANS, FRUITS, AND OAT PRODUCTS, DISSOLVES IN WATER AND IS THOUGHT TO HELP LOWER BLOOD CHOLESTEROL. INSOLUBLE FIBER, FOUND IN WHOLE-GRAIN PRODUCTS AND VEGETABLES, PASSES DIRECTLY THROUGH THE DIGESTIVE SYSTEM, HELPING TO RID THE BODY OF WASTE PRODUCTS.

FUNDUS OF THE EYE - THE BACK PART OF THE EYE, INCLUDING THE RETINA.

FUNDOSCOPY - THE VISUALIZATION OF THE BACK AREA OF THE EYE TO SEE THE STATUS OF THE BLOOD VESSELS AND OTHER CONDITIONS THAT HAVE OCULAR MANIFESTATIONS. THE DOCTOR USES A DEVICE CALLED AN OPHTHALMOSCOPE TO PERFORM THIS EXAMINATION.

G

GANGRENE - THE DEATH OF BODY TISSUE, MOST OFTEN CAUSED BY A LOSS OF BLOOD FLOW FROM PERIPHERAL VASCULAR DISEASE, ESPECIALLY IN THE FEET AND TOES. (SEE PERIPHERAL VASCULAR DISEASE)

GENE - A BASIC UNIT OF HEREDITY. GENES ARE MADE OF DNA, A SUBSTANCE THAT TELLS CELLS WHAT TO DO AND WHEN TO DO IT. THE INFORMATION IN GENES IS PASSED FROM PARENT TO CHILD.

GESTATIONAL DIABETES MELLITUS - TYPE OF DIABETES MELLITUS THAT CAN OCCUR WHEN A WOMAN IS PREGNANT. HOWEVER, WHEN THE PREGNANCY ENDS, THE BLOOD GLUCOSE LEVELS USUALLY RETURN TO NORMAL.

GINGIVITIS - AN INFLAMMATION OF THE GUMS THAT IF LEFT UNTREATED MAY LEAD TO PERIODONTAL DISEASE, A SERIOUS GUM DISORDER. SIGNS OF GINGIVITIS ARE INFLAMED AND BLEEDING GUMS. SEE ALSO: PERIODONTAL DISEASE.

GLAND - A GROUP OF SPECIAL CELLS THAT MAKE SUBSTANCES THAT HELP BODILY FUNCTIONS. FOR EXAMPLE, THE PANCREAS IS A GLAND THAT MANUFACTURES INSULIN WHICH HELPS OTHER BODY CELLS TO USE GLUCOSE FOR ENERGY.

GLUCAGON - A HORMONE THAT RAISES THE LEVEL OF GLUCOSE IN THE BLOOD. THE ALPHA CELLS OF THE PANCREAS MAKE GLUCAGON WHEN THE BODY NEEDS TO PUT MORE SUGAR INTO THE BLOOD. AN INJECTABLE FORM OF GLUCAGON, WHICH CAN BE BOUGHT IN A DRUG STORE, IS SOMETIMES USED TO TREAT HYPOGLYCEMIA. INJECTED GLUCAGON QUICKLY RAISES BLOOD GLUCOSE LEVELS. SEE ALSO: ALPHA CELL.

GLUCOSE - A SIMPLE SUGAR FOUND IN THE BLOOD. IT IS THE BODY'S MAIN SOURCE OF ENERGY; ALSO KNOWN AS DEXTROSE. SEE ALSO: BLOOD GLUCOSE.

GLUCOSE TOLERANCE TEST - A TEST TO DETERMINE IF A PERSON HAS DIABETES. THE TEST IS GIVEN IN A LAB OR DOCTOR'S OFFICE IN THE MORNING BEFORE THE PERSON HAS EATEN.

GLUCONEOGENESIS - THE SYNTHESIS OF GLUCOSE FROM SUBSTANCES WHICH ARE THEMSELVES NOT CARBOHYDRATES, SUCH AS PROTEIN OR FAT.

GLYCEMIC INDEX - PROPENSITY OF A FOOD SUBSTANCE TO RAISE THE BLOOD SUGAR. SCIENTIFIC MEASUREMENT OF BLOOD GLUCOSE LEVEL RESPONSE TO A FOOD SUBSTANCE.

GLYCEMIC RESPONSE - THE EFFECT OF A FOOD ON BLOOD GLUCOSE (SUGAR) LEVELS OVER A PERIOD OF TIME. SOME TYPES OF FOOD RAISE BLOOD GLUCOSE LEVELS MORE QUICKLY THAN OTHER FOODS CONTAINING THE SAME AMOUNT OF CALORIES.

GLYCOGEN - A SUBSTANCE MADE UP OF SUGARS. A STORAGE FORM OF GLUCOSE IN THE LIVER AND MUSCLES, BREAKS DOWN AND RELEASES GLUCOSE INTO THE BLOOD WHEN NEEDED. GLYCOGEN IS THE CHIEF SOURCE OF STORED CARBOHYDRATE FUEL IN THE BODY.

GLYCOSURIA - HAVING GLUCOSE IN THE URINE.

GLYCOSYLATED HEMOGLOBIN TEST - A BLOOD TEST THAT CORRELATES WITH A PERSON'S AVERAGE BLOOD GLUCOSE LEVEL FOR THE 2- TO 3-MONTH PERIOD BEFORE THE TEST. SEE: HEMOGLOBIN A1c.

H

HEMOGLOBIN A1C (HbA1C) - THE SUBSTANCE FORMED WHEN GLUCOSE BECOMES ATTACHED TO HEMOGLOBIN MOLECULES. THE QUANTITY FORMED SERVES AS AN

INDICATOR OF AVERAGE BLOOD SUGAR LEVELS FOR THE 8-12 WEEK PERIOD PRIOR TO THE TEST. (ALSO KNOW AS GLYCOHEMOGLOBIN AND GLYCOLSYLATED HEMOGLOBIN)

HEPATIC - REFERRING TO THE LIVER.

HIGH DENSITY LIPOPROTEIN (HDL) - "GOOD" CHOLESTEROL.

HIGH BLOOD PRESSURE - BLOOD PRESSURE THAT IS GREATER THAN 120/80.

HLA ANTIGENS - PROTEINS ON THE OUTER PART OF THE CELL THAT HELP THE BODY FIGHT ILLNESS. THESE PROTEINS VARY FROM PERSON TO PERSON. SCIENTISTS THINK THAT PEOPLE WITH CERTAIN TYPES OF HLA ANTIGENS ARE MORE LIKELY TO DEVELOP TYPE 1 DIABETES.

HOME BLOOD GLUCOSE MONITORING - TESTING BY PATIENTS AT HOME TO DETERMINE HOW MUCH GLUCOSE (SUGAR) IS IN THE BLOOD. ALSO CALLED SELF-MONITORING OF BLOOD GLUCOSE. SEE ALSO: SELF-MONITORING OF BLOOD GLUCOSE.

HORMONE - A CHEMICAL PRODUCED BY GLANDULAR CELLS AND SECRETED DIRECTLY INTO THE BLOODSTREAM TO TELL OTHER CELLS WHAT TO DO. FOR EXAMPLE, INSULIN IS A HORMONE MADE BY THE BETA CELLS IN THE PANCREAS. WHEN RELEASED, INSULIN ENABLES OTHER CELLS TO USE GLUCOSE FOR ENERGY.

HUMALOG INSULIN - A SYNTHETICALLY PRODUCED TYPE OF INSULIN WITH MORE RAPID ONSET AND BRIEFER DURATION OF EFFECT THAN REGULAR INSULIN.

HUMAN INSULIN - MAN-MADE INSULINS THAT ARE SIMILAR TO INSULIN PRODUCED BY THE HUMAN BODY. HUMAN INSULIN HAS BEEN AVAILABLE SINCE OCTOBER 1982.

HYPERGLYCEMIA - ELEVATED LEVEL OF SUGAR IN THE BLOOD; A SIGN THAT DIABETES IS OUT OF CONTROL.

HYPERINSULINISM - ELEVATED HIGH LEVELS OF INSULIN IN THE BLOOD AND OFTEN INDICATING INSULIN RESISTANCE. THIS CONDITION IS OFTEN ASSOCIATED WITH TYPE 2 DIABETES.

HYPERLIPIDEMIA - ABNORMALLY HIGH LEVELS OF LIPIDS IN THE BLOOD.

HYPEROSMOLAR COMA - A COMA (LOSS OF CONSCIOUSNESS) RELATED TO HIGH LEVELS OF GLUCOSE IN THE BLOOD REQUIRING EMERGENCY TREATMENT.

HYPERTENSION - BLOOD PRESSURE THAT IS ABOVE THE NORMAL RANGE. SEE ALSO: HIGH BLOOD PRESSURE.

HYPOGLYCEMIA - TOO LOW A LEVEL OF GLUCOSE IN THE BLOOD. THIS OCCURS WHEN A PERSON WITH DIABETES HAS INJECTED TOO MUCH INSULIN OR TAKEN CERTAIN ORAL AGENTS, EATEN TOO LITTLE FOOD, OR HAS EXERCISED WITHOUT EXTRA FOOD INTAKE. SEE INSULIN REACTION.

HYPOTENSION - LOW BLOOD PRESSURE OR SUDDEN DROP IN BLOOD PRESSURE. A PERSON RISING QUICKLY FROM A SITTING OR RECLINING POSITION MAY HAVE A SUDDEN FALL IN BLOOD PRESSURE, CAUSING DIZZINESS OR FAINTING. SOMETIMES SEEN AS A SIDE EFFECT OF CERTAIN MEDICATIONS.

I

IMMUNOSUPPRESSIVE DRUGS - DRUGS THAT BLOCK THE BODY'S ABILITY TO FIGHT INFECTION OR FOREIGN SUBSTANCES THAT ENTER THE BODY. A PERSON RECEIVING A KIDNEY OR PANCREAS TRANSPLANT IS GIVEN THESE DRUGS TO STOP THE BODY FROM REJECTING THE NEW ORGAN OR TISSUE.

IMPAIRED GLUCOSE TOLERANCE (IGT) - BLOOD GLUCOSE LEVELS HIGHER THAN NORMAL, BUT NOT HIGH ENOUGH TO BE CALLED DIABETES. PEOPLE WITH IGT MAY OR MAY NOT DEVELOP DIABETES. OTHER NAMES (NO LONGER USED) FOR IGT ARE "BORDERLINE," "SUBCLINICAL," "CHEMICAL," OR "LATENT" DIABETES.

IMPOTENCE - MALE LOSS OF ABILITY TO FUNCTION SEXUALLY. ALSO KNOWN AS ERECTILE DYSFUNCTION.

INSULIN - A HORMONE THAT HELPS THE BODY USE GLUCOSE (SUGAR) FOR ENERGY. THE BETA CELLS OF THE PANCREAS (IN AREAS CALLED THE ISLETS OF LANGERHANS) MAKE THE INSULIN.

INSULIN ANTAGONIST - A SUBSTANCE THAT OPPOSES OR FIGHTS THE ACTION OF INSULIN. INSULIN LOWERS THE LEVEL OF GLUCOSE IN THE BLOOD, WHEREAS GLUCAGON, AN ANTAGONIST OF INSULIN, RAISES BLOOD SUGAR.

INSULIN BINDING - THE PROCESS BY WHICH INSULIN ATTACHES ITSELF TO SOMETHING ELSE. THIS CAN OCCUR IN TWO WAYS. FIRST, WHEN A CELL NEEDS ENERGY, INSULIN CAN BIND WITH THE OUTER PART OF THE CELL. THE CELL THEN CAN BRING GLUCOSE INSIDE AND USE IT FOR ENERGY. WITH THE HELP OF INSULIN, THE CELL WORKS EFFICIENTLY.

INSULIN-INDUCED ATROPHY - SMALL DENTS THAT FORM ON THE SKIN WHEN A PERSON KEEPS INJECTING INSULIN IN THE SAME SPOT. THEY ARE HARMLESS.

INSULIN-INDUCED HYPERTROPHY - SMALL LUMPS THAT FORM UNDER THE SKIN PRODUCED WHEN A PERSON KEEPS INJECTING INSULIN AT THE SAME SITE.

INSULIN PEN - AN INSULIN INJECTION DEVICE THE SIZE OF A PEN THAT INCLUDES A NEEDLE. IT CAN BE USED INSTEAD OF SYRINGES FOR GIVING INSULIN INJECTIONS.

INSULIN REACTION - TOO LOW A LEVEL OF GLUCOSE IN THE BLOOD; ALSO CALLED HYPOGLYCEMIA. THIS OCCURS WHEN A PERSON WITH DIABETES HAS AN IMBALANCE BETWEEN THE AMOUNT OF INSULIN INJECTED, EATEN TOO LITTLE FOOD, OR EXERCISED WITHOUT EXTRA FOOD. SYMPTOMS ARE HUNGER, NAUSEA, WEAKNESS, NERVOUSNESS, SHAKINESS, CONFUSION, AND SWEATING. TAKING SMALL AMOUNTS OF SUGAR, SWEET JUICE, OR FOOD WITH SUGAR WILL USUALLY HELP THE PERSON FEEL BETTER WITHIN 10 - 15 MINUTES. SEE ALSO: HYPOGLYCEMIA; INSULIN SHOCK.

INSULIN RECEPTORS - AREAS ON THE OUTER PART OF A CELL THAT ALLOW THE

CELL TO JOIN OR BIND WITH INSULIN THAT IS IN THE BLOOD. WHEN THE CELL AND INSULIN BIND TOGETHER, THE CELL CAN TAKE GLUCOSE FROM THE BLOOD AND USE IT FOR ENERGY.

INSULIN RESISTANCE - MANY PEOPLE WITH TYPE 2 DIABETES PRODUCE ENOUGH INSULIN, BUT THEIR BODIES DO NOT RESPOND NORMALLY TO THE ACTION OF INSULIN. THIS DEFECTIVE RESPONSE IS CALLED INSULIN RESISTANCE. ONE OF THE MAJOR CAUSES OF TYPE 2 DIABETES.

INSULIN SHOCK - A SEVERE CONDITION THAT OCCURS WHEN THE LEVEL OF BLOOD GLUCOSE DROPS TOO LOW. THE SIGNS ARE SHAKING, SWEATING, DIZZINESS, DOUBLE VISION, CONVULSIONS, AND COLLAPSE. INSULIN SHOCK MAY OCCUR WHEN AN INSULIN REACTION IS NOT TREATED QUICKLY ENOUGH. SEE ALSO: HYPOGLYCEMIA; INSULIN REACTION.

INTENSIVE MANAGEMENT - A FORM OF TREATMENT FOR TYPE 1 DIABETES IN WHICH THE MAIN OBJECTIVE IS TO KEEP BLOOD SUGAR LEVELS AS CLOSE TO THE NORMAL RANGE AS POSSIBLE. THE TREATMENT CONSISTS OF THREE OR MORE INSULIN INJECTIONS A DAY OR USE OF AN INSULIN PUMP; FOUR OR MORE BLOOD GLUCOSE TESTS A DAY; ADJUSTMENT OF INSULIN, FOOD INTAKE, AND ACTIVITY LEVELS BASED ON BLOOD GLUCOSE TEST RESULTS; DIETARY COUNSELING; AND MANAGEMENT BY A DIABETES TEAM. SEE ALSO: DIABETES CONTROL AND COMPLICATIONS TRIAL; TEAM MANAGEMENT.

ISLETS OF LANGERHANS - SPECIAL GROUPS OF CELLS IN THE PANCREAS THAT MAKE AND SECRETE HORMONES THAT HELP THE BODY BREAK DOWN AND USE FOOD. NAMED AFTER PAUL LANGERHANS, THE GERMAN MEDICAL STUDENT WHO DISCOVERED THEM IN 1869, THESE CELLS SIT IN CLUSTERS SCATTERED WITHIN THE PANCREAS. THERE ARE FIVE TYPES OF CELLS IN AN ISLET: BETA CELLS, WHICH MAKE INSULIN; ALPHA CELLS, WHICH MAKE GLUCAGON; DELTA CELLS, WHICH MAKE SOMATOSTATIN; AND PP CELLS AND D1 CELLS, ABOUT WHICH LITTLE IS KNOWN.

J

JET INJECTOR - A DEVICE THAT USES HIGH PRESSURE TO PROPEL INSULIN THROUGH THE SKIN AND INTO THE BODY WITHOUT A NEEDLE.

JUVENILE ONSET DIABETES - FORMER TERM FOR TYPE I DIABETES. SEE ALSO:INSULIN-DEPENDENT DIABETES MELLITUS.

K

KETOACIDOSIS - SEE: DIABETIC KETOACIDOSIS.

KETONE BODIES - CHEMICALS THAT THE BODY MAKES WHEN THERE IS NOT ENOUGH INSULIN IN THE BLOOD AND FAT MUST BE UTILIZED FOR ENERGY. WHEN THE BODY DOES NOT PRODUCE ENOUGH INSULIN, THE KETONES BUILD UP IN THE BLOOD AND THEN "SPILL" OVER INTO THE URINE AS THE BODY ATTEMPTS TO GET RID OF THEM. THE BODY CAN ALSO RID ITSELF OF ONE TYPE OF KETONE, CALLED ACETONE, THROUGH THE LUNGS. THIS GIVES THE BREATH A FRUITY ODOR. HIGH KETONE LEVELS LEAD TO SERIOUS ILLNESS AND COMA. SEE ALSO: DIABETIC KETOACIDOSIS.

KETONURIA - HAVING KETONE BODIES IN THE URINE; A WARNING SIGN FOR THE DEVELOPMENT OF DIABETIC KETOACIDOSIS (DKA).

KETOSIS - THE CONDITION OF HAVING KETONE BODIES BUILD UP IN BODY TISSUES AND FLUIDS. THE SIGNS OF KETOSIS ARE NAUSEA, VOMITING, AND ABDOMINAL PAIN. KETOSIS CAN LEAD TO KETOACIDOSIS.

KIDNEYS - TWO ORGANS IN THE LOWER BACK THAT CLEAN WASTE AND POISONS FROM THE BLOOD. THE KIDNEYS ARE SHAPED LIKE TWO LARGE BEANS, AND ACT AS THE BODY'S FILTER. THEY ALSO HELP TO CONTROL THE LEVEL OF CHEMICALS IN THE BLOOD SUCH AS SODIUM, POTASSIUM, PHOSPHATE, CHLORIDE, ETC.

KIDNEY THRESHOLD - THE BLOOD LEVEL ABOVE WHICH A SUBSTANCE SUCH AS GLUCOSE "SPILLS" OVER INTO THE URINE.

L

LABILE DIABETES - A TERM USED TO INDICATE THAT A DIABETICS BLOOD GLUCOSE LEVEL OFTEN SWINGS QUICKLY FROM HIGH TO LOW AND FROM LOW TO HIGH. ALSO CALLED BRITTLE DIABETES.

LACTIC ACIDOSIS - THE BUILDUP OF LACTIC ACID IN THE BODY. THE SIGNS OF LACTIC ACIDOSIS ARE DEEP AND RAPID BREATHING, VOMITING, AND ABDOMINAL PAIN. LACTIC ACIDOSIS MAY BE CAUSED BY DIABETIC KETOACIDOSIS, LIVER OR KIDNEY DISEASE. IT IS ALSO SOMETIMES SEEN AS A SIDE EFFECT FROM CERTAIN MEDICATIONS.

LASER TREATMENT - USING A SPECIAL STRONG BEAM OF LIGHT OF ONE COLOR (LASER) TO HEAL A DAMAGED AREA. LASER BEAMS ARE USED TO HEAL BLOOD VESSELS IN THE EYE. SEE ALSO: PHOTOCOAGULATION.

LIPID - A COMPREHENSIVE TERM FOR FATTY ACIDS AND CHOLESTEROL.

LOW DENSITY LIPOPROTEIN (LDL) - "BAD" CHOLESTEROL.

M

MACROVASCULAR DISEASE - A DISEASE OF THE LARGE BLOOD VESSELS THAT SOMETIMES OCCURS WHEN A PERSON HAS HAD DIABETES FOR A LONG TIME. LIPIDS BUILD UP IN THE WALLS OF THE LARGE BLOOD VESSELS. THREE KINDS OF MACROVASCULAR DISEASE ARE CORONARY DISEASE, CEREBROVASCULAR DISEASE, AND PERIPHERAL VASCULAR DISEASE.

MARKERS - GENETIC SIGNPOSTS ON DNA THAT SERVE AS INDICATORS FOR THE DEVELOPMENT, OR PROPENSITY TO DEVELOP, A CONDITION OR DISEASE.

MEAL PLAN - A GUIDE FOR CONTROLLING THE AMOUNT OF CALORIES, CARBOHYDRATES, PROTEINS, AND FATS A PERSON EATS. PEOPLE WITH DIABETES CAN USE EXCHANGE LISTS TO HELP THEM PLAN MEALS THAT CAN KEEP THEIR DIABETES UNDER CONTROL. SEE ALSO: EXCHANGE LISTS.

METABOLISM - THE TERM FOR THE WAY CELLS CHEMICALLY CHANGE FOOD SO THAT IT CAN BE USED TO KEEP THE BODY ALIVE. IT IS A TWO-PART PROCESS. ONE PART IS CALLED CATABOLISM—WHEN THE BODY USES FOOD FOR ENERGY. THE OTHER IS CALLED ANABOLISM—WHEN THE BODY USES FOOD TO BUILD OR MEND CELLS. INSULIN IS NECESSARY FOR THE METABOLISM OF FOOD.

METFORMIN - A MEDICATION USED AS A TREATMENT FOR TYPE 2 DIABETES; BELONGS TO A CLASS OF DRUGS CALLED BIGUANIDES.

MICROALBUMINURIA - SMALL AMOUNTS OF ALBUMIN IN THE URINE AFFORDS A MEASURABLE METHOD TO DETECT EARLY STAGES OF DIABETIC NEPHROPATHY.

MG/DL - MILLIGRAMS PER DECILITER. TERM USED TO DESCRIBE HOW MUCH GLUCOSE IS IN A SPECIFIC AMOUNT OF BLOOD. IN SELF-MONITORING OF BLOOD GLUCOSE, TEST RESULTS ARE GIVEN AS THE AMOUNT OF GLUCOSE IN MILLIGRAMS PER DECILITER OF BLOOD. A FASTING READING OF 70 TO 110 MG/DL IS CONSIDERED IN THE NORMAL (NONDIABETIC) RANGE.

MICROANEURYSM - SWELLING THAT FORMS ON THE SIDE OF TINY BLOOD VESSELS. THESE SMALL SWELLINGS MAY BREAK AND BLEED INTO NEARBY TISSUE. PEOPLE WITH DIABETES SOMETIMES GET MICROANEURYSMS IN THE RETINA OF THE EYE.

MICROVASCULAR DISEASE - DISEASE OF THE SMALL BLOOD VESSELS THAT SOMETIMES OCCURS WHEN A PERSON HAS HAD DIABETES FOR A LONG TIME. THE WALLS OF THE VESSELS BECOME ABNORMALLY THICK, BUT WEAK, AND THEREFORE THEY BLEED, LEAK PROTEIN, AND SLOW THE FLOW OF BLOOD.

MIXED DOSE - COMBINING TWO KINDS OF INSULIN IN ONE INJECTION. A MIXED DOSE COMMONLY COMBINES REGULAR INSULIN, WHICH IS FAST ACTING, WITH A LONGER ACTING INSULIN SUCH AS NPH. A MIXED DOSE INSULIN SCHEDULE MAY BE PRESCRIBED TO PROVIDE BOTH SHORT-TERM AND LONG-TERM COVERAGE.

MONONEUROPATHY - A FORM OF DIABETIC NEUROPATHY AFFECTING A SINGLE NERVE. THE EYE IS A COMMON SITE FOR THIS FORM OF NERVE DAMAGE. SEE ALSO: NEUROPATHY.

MONOSATURATED FATS - FATS THAT ARE LIQUID AT ROOM TEMPERATURE WITH LIMITED SATURATION OF THEIR CHEMICAL CHAIN, BELIEVED TO EXERT BENEFICIAL EFFECT ON LIPID METABOLISM.

MYOCARDIAL INFARCTION - PERMANENT DAMAGE TO AN AREA OF THE HEART MUSCLE FROM A HEART ATTACK. THIS HAPPENS WHEN THE BLOOD SUPPLY TO THE AREA OF HEART MUSCLE IS INTERRUPTED BECAUSE OF NARROWED OR BLOCKED BLOOD VESSELS.

N

NEPHROLOGIST - A DOCTOR WHO SPECIALIZES IN THE TREATMENT OF KIDNEY DISEASES.

NEPHROPATHY - DISEASE OF THE KIDNEYS CAUSED BY DAMAGE TO THE SMALL BLOOD VESSELS OR TO THE GLOMERULI (UNITS IN THE KIDNEYS THAT CLEANSE THE BLOOD).

NEUROPATHY - DAMAGE TO THE NERVOUS SYSTEM ASSOCIATED WITH DIABETES OF LONG-STANDING. THE MOST COMMON FORM IS PERIPHERAL NEUROPATHY, WHICH MAINLY AFFECTS THE URINARY BLADDER, GASTROINTESTINAL TRACT, GALL BLADDER, SWEATING, PARTICULARLY OF THE FEET, AND AND PUPILLARY RESPONSE

TO LIGHT. SEE ALSO: PERIPHERAL NEUROPATHY; **AUTONOMIC NEUROPATHY.**

NPH INSULIN - INTERMEDIATE ACTING INSULIN.

NUTRITION - THE PROCESS BY WHICH THE BODY DRAWS NUTRIENTS FROM FOOD AND USES THEM FOR PHYSIOLOGIC ACTIVITIES.

O

OBESITY - EXCESSIVELY CORPULENT. EXTRA BODY FAT (20 PERCENT OR MORE) FOR AGE, HEIGHT, SEX, AND BONE STRUCTURE. EXTRA BODY FAT IS THOUGHT TO BE A RISK FACTOR FOR TYPE 2 DIABETES.

OPHTHALMOLOGIST - A MEDICAL DOCTOR WHO SPECIALIZES IN THE TREATMENT OF EYE PROBLEMS OR DISEASES.

ORAL HYPOGLYCEMIC AGENTS - MEDICATIONS TAKEN BY MOUTH THAT LOWER THE BLOOD GLUCOSE LEVEL.

P

PANCREAS - AN ABDOMINAL ORGAN BELOW AND BEHIND THE LOWER PART OF THE STOMACH THAT IS ABOUT THE SIZE OF A HAND. IT MANUFACTURES INSULIN. IT ALSO MAKES ENZYMES THAT HELP THE BODY DIGEST FOOD.

PEAK ACTION - THE TIME PERIOD WHEN THE EFFECT OF SOMETHING IS AT ITS STRONGEST; SUCH AS WHEN INJECTED INSULIN HAS THE MOST EFFECT ON LOWERING THE GLUCOSE IN THE BLOOD.

PERIODONTAL DISEASE - GUM DISEASE. PEOPLE WHO HAVE DIABETES ARE MORE PRONE TO PERIODONTAL DISEASE THAN NON-DIABETICS.

PERIPHERAL NEUROPATHY - NERVE DAMAGE, USUALLY AFFECTING THE FEET AND LEGS; CAUSING PAIN, NUMBNESS, OR A TINGLING FEELING. ALSO CALLED "SOMATIC NEUROPATHY" OR "DISTAL SENSORY POLYNEUROPATHY."

PERIPHERAL VASCULAR DISEASE (PVD) - DISEASE OF THE LARGE BLOOD VESSELS OF THE EXTREMITIES (PARTICULARLY LOWER EXTREMITIES). PEOPLE WHO HAVE HAD DIABETES FOR A LONG TIME ARE PRONE TO DEVELOP PVD BECAUSE ARTERIOSCLEROTIC BLOOD VESSELS IN THEIR LIMBS DO NOT SUPPLY ADEQUATE BLOOD. THE SIGNS OF PVD ARE ACHING PAINS IN THE CALF AREA WHEN WALKING, WHICH ARE RELIEVED BY REST, AND FOOT SORES THAT HEAL SLOWLY.

PHOTOCOAGULATION - USING A SPECIAL STRONG BEAM OF LIGHT (LASER) TO SEAL OFF BLEEDING BLOOD VESSELS SUCH AS IN THE EYE. THE LASER CAN ALSO BURN AWAY ABNORMAL BLOOD VESSELS THAT HAVE GROWN IN THE EYE. THE MAIN TREATMENT MODALITY FOR DIABETIC RETINOPATHY.

PLAQUE - ATHEROSCLEROTIC DEPOSITS OF LIPIDS AND FIBROUS TISSUE IN THE WALL OF A BLOOD VESSEL.

PODIATRIST - A DOCTOR OF PODIATRY WHO TREATS AND TAKES CARE OF PEOPLE'S FEET.

PODIATRY - THE CARE AND TREATMENT OF HUMAN FEET IN HEALTH AND DISEASE.